DESIGN and ANALYSIS of QUALITY of LIFE STUDIES in CLINICAL TRIALS

Second Edition

CHAPMAN & HALL/CRC
Interdisciplinary Statistics Series

Series editors: N. Keiding, B.J.T. Morgan, C.K. Wikle, P. van der Heijden

Published titles

Published titles

Chapman & Hall/CRC
Interdisciplinary Statistics Series

DESIGN and ANALYSIS of QUALITY of LIFE STUDIES in CLINICAL TRIALS

Second Edition

Diane L. Fairclough

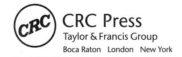

CRC Press
Taylor & Francis Group
Boca Raton   London   New York

CRC Press is an imprint of the
Taylor & Francis Group, an **informa** business

A CHAPMAN & HALL BOOK

Chapman & Hall/CRC
Taylor & Francis Group
6000 Broken Sound Parkway NW, Suite 300
Boca Raton, FL 33487-2742

© 2010 by Taylor and Francis Group, LLC
Chapman & Hall/CRC is an imprint of Taylor & Francis Group, an Informa business

No claim to original U.S. Government works

Printed in the United States of America on acid-free paper
10 9 8 7 6 5 4 3 2 1

International Standard Book Number: 978-1-4200-6117-8 (Hardback)

Library of Congress Cataloging-in-Publication Data

Fairclough, Diane Lynn.
    Design and analysis of quality of life studies in clinical trials / Diane L. Fairclough.
-- 2nd ed.
        p. ; cm. -- (Chapman & Hall/CRC interdisciplinary statistics series)
    Includes bibliographical references and index.
    ISBN 978-1-4200-6117-8 (hardcover : alk. paper)
    1. Clinical trials--Longitudinal studies. 2. Clinical trials--Statistical methods. 3. Quality of life--Research--Methodology. I. Title. II. Series: Interdisciplinary statistics.
    [DNLM: 1. Quality of Life. 2. Statistics as Topic. 3. Clinical Trials as Topic. 4. Longitudinal Studies. 5. Research--methods. WA 950 F165d 2010]

R853.C55 F355 2010
615.5072'4--dc22   2009042418

Visit the Taylor & Francis Web site at
http://www.taylorandfrancis.com

and the CRC Press Web site at
http://www.crcpress.com

Contents

Preface

What's New?

The second edition of *Design and Analysis of QOL Studies in Clinical Trials* incorporates answers to queries by readers, suggestions by reviewers, new methodological advances, and more emphasis on the most practical methods.

Datasets for the Examples

The most frequent request that I had after the publication of my first edition was for the datasets that were used in the examples. This was something I had hoped to provide with the first edition, but time constraints prevented that from happening. I have been able to obtain the necessary permissions (data use agreements)* to be able to do so in this edition. These datasets are available solely for educational purposes to allow the readers to replicate the analyses presented in this edition. In the last few years, more attention has been focused on the protection of patient's health information (PHI). To protect both study participants and sponsors, a number of steps have been taken in the creation of these limited use datasets. First, all dates and other potentially identifying information has been removed from the datasets. Small amounts of random variation have been added to other potential identifiers such as age and time to death; categories with only a few individuals have been combined. Finally, the datasets were constructed using bootstrap techniques (randomly sampling with replacement) and have a different number of participants than the original datasets. Anyone wishing to use the data for any purposes other than learning the techniques described in this book, especially if intended for presentations or publication, MUST obtain separate data use agreements from the sponsors. The datasets and additional documentation can be obtained from *http://home.earthlink.net/~ dianefairclough/ Welcome.html*.

---

*Two of the datasets (Study 2 and 6) were completely simulated.

New Chapters and Sections

There are also several new chapters in this edition as well as new sections in old chapters. I have added a chapter about testing models that involve moderation and mediation (Chapter 5) as I have found myself examining these more often in the analysis of clinical trials. In particular, most trials are based on a conceptual model in which the effects of treatment on health-related quality of life (HRQoL) and other patient reported outcomes are often hypothesized to be mediated by other measurable outcomes. I have revised the discussions of multiple comparisons procedures focusing on the integration of HRQoL outcomes with other study outcomes using Gatekeeper strategies (Chapter 13). There have been numerous methodological developments for the analysis of trials with missing data. I have added a few of these that I have found useful and shortened or dropped discussion of those that have minimal application. A brief discussion of quality adjusted life-years (QALYs) and Q-TWiST specific to clinical trials has also been added (Chapter 15).

Example Programs in SAS, SPSS and R

The first edition almost solely illustrated the implementation of methods using the statistical software package SAS. As I have worked with more international investigators, I have become more aware that many use other packages, often because of cost. In response to this, I have added examples of implementation of the basic models (see Chapters 3 and 4) and other selected applications in R and SPSS. Because of space limitations, I cannot illustrate all the methods with all the software packages, but will continue to add examples, applications and other software (STATA) to the web site (*http://home.earthlink.net/~ dianefairclough/Welcome.html*) as time permits. The interested reader should go to the web site to look for these. If the readers note omissions, it may be that some methods cannot be implemented using a specific software package. But it is also likely I am not fully aware of all the available options in each package. If readers note omissions and are willing to share their programs, please contact me and I would be happy to add them to the web site.

Scope of the Book

For almost 30 years I have been engaged by the challenges of design and analysis of longitudinal assessment of health outcomes in children and adults. Most of my research has been on the psychosocial outcomes for pediatric cancer survivors and health-related quality of life (HRQoL) of adult cancer patients, but has included other diagnoses. As I have designed and analyzed these studies, many of the same themes continued to occur. My intent was to summarize that experience in this book.

There are numerous books that discuss the wide range of topics concerning the evaluation of health-related quality of life. There still seemed to be a need for a book that addresses design and analysis in enough detail to enable readers to apply the methods to their own studies. To achieve that goal, I have limited the focus of the book to the *design* and *analysis* of longitudinal studies of health-related quality of life in clinical trials.

Intended Readers

My primary audience for this book is the researcher who is directly involved in the design and analysis of HRQoL studies. However, the book will also be useful to those who are expected to evaluate the design and interpret the results of HRQoL research. More than any other field that I have been involved with, HRQoL research draws investigators from all fields of study with a wide range of training. This has included epidemiologists, psychologists, sociologists, behavioral and health services researchers, clinicians and nurses from all specialties, as well as statisticians. I expect that most readers will have had some graduate-level training in statistical methods including multivariate regression and analysis of variance. However, that training may have been some time ago and prior to some of the more recent advances in statistical methods. With that in mind, I have organized most chapters so that the concepts are discussed in the beginning of the chapters and sections. When possible, the technical details appear later in the chapter. Examples of SAS, R, and SPSS programs are included to give the readers concrete examples of implementation. Finally, each chapter ends with a summary of the important points.

Self-Study and Discussion Groups

I expect that most readers will use this book for self-study or in discussion groups. Ideally you will have data from an existing trial or will be in the process of designing a new trial. As you read though the book you will be able to contrast your trial with the studies used throughout the book and decide the best approach(es) for your trial. The intent is that readers, by following the examples in the book, will be able to follow the steps outlined with their own studies.

Use in Teaching

This book was not designed as a course textbook and thus does not include features such as problem sets for each chapter. But I have found it to be extremely useful when teaching courses on the analysis of longitudinal data. I can focus my lectures on the concepts and allow the students to learn the details of how to implement methods from the examples.

The Future

One of my future goals is to identify (and obtain permission to use) data from other clinical trials that illustrate designs and analytic challenges not covered by the studies presented in this book. Perhaps the strategies of deidentification and random sampling of subject utilized for the datasets obtained for this second edition can be used to generate more publicly accessible datasets that can be used for educational purposes. If you think that you have data from a trial that could be so used, I would love to hear from you.

Diane L. Fairclough

Acknowledgments

First, I would like to thank the sponsors of the trials who gave permission to use data from their trial to generate the limited use datasets as well as the participants and investigators whose participation was critical to those studies. I would like to thank all my friends and colleagues for their support and help. I would specifically like to thank Patrick Blatchford, Joseph Cappelleri, Luella Engelhart, Shona Fielding, Dennis Gagnon, Sheila Gardner, Cindy Gerhardt, Stephanie Green, Keith Goldfeld, Paul Healey, Mark Jaros, Carol Moinpour, Eva Szigethy and Naitee Ting for their helpful comments on selected chapters.

1

Introduction and Examples

In this initial chapter, I first present a brief introduction to the concept and measurement of Health-Related Quality of Life (HRQoL). I will then introduce the five clinical trials that will be used to illustrate the concepts presented throughout the remainder of this book. The data from each of these trials and all results presented in this book arise from derived datasets from actual trials as described in the Preface. Access is provided to the reader solely for the purpose of learning and understanding the methods of analysis. Please note that the results obtained from these derived datasets will not match published results.

1.1 Health-Related Quality of Life (HRQoL)

Traditionally, clinical trials have focused on endpoints that are physical or laboratory measures of response. For example, therapies for cancer are evaluated on the basis of disease progression and survival. The efficacy of a treatment for anemia is evaluated by hemoglobin levels or number of transfusions required. Although traditional biomedical measures are often the primary endpoints in clinical trials, they do not reflect how the patient feels and functions in daily activities. Yet these perceptions reflect whether or not the patient believes he or she has benefited from the treatment. In certain diseases, the patient's perception of his or her well-being may be the most important health outcome [Staquet et al., 1992]. More recently, clinical trials are including endpoints that reflect the patient's perception of his or her well-being and satisfaction with therapy. Sometimes clinical investigators assume that a change in a biomedical outcome will also improve the patient's quality of life. While in many cases this may be true, sometimes surprising results are obtained when the patient is asked directly. One classic example of this occurred with a study by Sugarbaker et al. [1982] comparing two therapeutic approaches for soft-tissue sarcoma. The first was limb-sparing surgery followed by radiation therapy. The second treatment approach was full amputation of the affected limb. The investigator hypothesized "Sparing a limb, as opposed to amputating it, offers a quality of life advantage." Most would have agreed with this conjecture. But the trial results did not confirm the expectations; subjects receiving the limb sparing procedures reported limitations in mobility and sexual functioning. These observations were confirmed with physical assessments of mobility and endocrine function. As a result of these studies, radiation therapy was modified and physical rehabilitation was added to the limb-sparing therapeutic approach [Hicks et al., 1985].

The World Health Organization (WHO) defined *health* [1948, 1958] as a "state of complete physical, mental and social well-being and not merely the absence of infirmity and disease." This definition reflects the focus on a broader picture of health that includes health-related quality of life (HRQoL). Wilson and Cleary [1995] propose a conceptual modelof the relationships among health outcomes. In their model, there are five levels of outcomes that progress from biomedical outcomes to quality of life (Figure 1.1). The biological and physiological outcomes include the results of laboratory tests, radiological scans and physical examination as well as diagnoses. Symptom status is defined as "a patient's perception of an abnormal physical, emotional or cognitive state." Functional status includes four dimensions: physical, physiological, social and role. General health perceptions include the patients' evaluation of past and current health, their future outlook and concerns about health.

FIGURE **1.1** Five progressive levels of outcomes from Wilson and Cleary's [1995] conceptual model of the relationship among health outcomes.

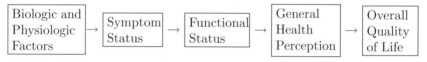

The term *health-related quality of life* has been used in many ways. Although the exact definition varies among authors, there is general agreement that it is a multidimensional concept that focuses on the *impact* of disease and its treatment on the well-being of an individual. In the broadest definition, the quality of our lives is influenced by our physical and social environment as well as our emotional and existential reactions to that environment. Kaplan and Bush [1982] proposed the use of the term to distinguish health effects from other factors influencing the subject's perceptions including job satisfaction and environmental factors. Cella and Bonomi [1995] state

> Health-related quality of life refers to the extent to which one's usual or expected physical, emotional and social well-being are *affected* by a medical condition or its treatment.

In some settings, we may also include other aspects like economic and existential well-being. Patrick and Erickson [1993] propose a more inclusive definition which combines quality and quantity.

the value assigned to duration of life as modified by the impairment, functional states, perceptions and social opportunities that are influenced by disease, injury, treatment or policy.

It is important to note that an individual's well-being or health status cannot be directly measured. We are only able to make inferences from measurable indicators of symptoms and reported perceptions.

Often the term *quality-of-life* is used when any *patient-reported outcome* is measured. This has contributed to criticisms about the measurement of HRQoL. It is recognized that symptoms are not equivalent to quality of life, but they do impact HRQoL and are measurable, thus part of the assessment of HRQoL. As clinicians and researchers, it is important that we are precise in our language, using terms to describe what has been measured. Are we measuring functional status, symptom frequency, general health perceptions, interference with daily activities, etc.? That being said, for the ease of communication, I use the term HRQoL generically throughout this book when describing methods but will attempt to be precise when presenting results of a particular trial.

1.2   Measuring Health-Related Quality of Life

1.2.1   Health Status Measures

There are two general types of HRQoL measures, often referred to as *health status* and *patient preference* [Yabroff et al., 1996]. These two forms of assessment have developed as a result of the differences between the perspectives of two different disciplines: psychometrics and econometrics. In the health status assessment measures, multiple aspects of the patient's perceived well-being are self-assessed and a score is derived from the responses on a series of questions. This score reflects the patient's relative HRQoL as compared to other patients and to the HRQoL of the same patient at other times. The assessments range from a single global question asking patients to rate their current quality of life to a series of questions about specific aspects of their daily life during a recent period of time. These instruments generally take the 5 to 10 minutes to complete. A well-known example of a health status measure is the Medical Outcomes Survey Short-Form or SF-36 [Ware et al., 1993]. Among health status measures, there is considerable variation in the context of the questions with some measures focusing more on the perceived impact of the disease and therapy (How much are you bothered by hair loss?) and other measures focusing on the frequency and severity of symptoms (How often do you experience pain?). These measures are primarily designed to compare groups of patients receiving different treatments or to identify change over time within groups of patients. As a result, health status has most often been used in clinical trials to facilitate the comparisons of therapeutic regimens.

1.2.2   Patient Preference Measures

Measures of patient preference are influenced strongly by the concept of *utility*, borrowed from econometrics, that reflects individual decision-making under uncertainty. These preference assessment measures are primarily used to evaluate the tradeoff between the quality and quantity of life. Values of utilities are generally between 0 and 1 with 0 generally associated with death and 1 with perfect health. These preference measures may be elicited directly from patients or indirectly from the general public depending on the intended use. Utilities have traditionally been used in the calculation of quality-adjusted life years for cost-effectiveness analyses and in analytic approaches such as Q-TWiST [Goldhirsch et al., 1989, Glasziou et al., 1990]. (See Chapter 15).

There are a number of methods to elicit utilities for various health states. Direct measures include *time tradeoff* (TTO) and *standard gamble* (SG). Time tradeoff utilities [McNeil et al., 1981] are derived by asking respondents how much time in their current health state they would give up for a specified period of time in perfect health. If a patient responded that he would give up 1 year of time in his current health for 5 years of perfect health, the resulting utility is 0.8. Standard gamble utilities [Torrance et al., 1971] are measured by asking respondents to identify the point at which they become indifferent to the choices between two hypothetical situations. For example, one option might be a radical surgical procedure with no chance of relapse in the next five years but significant impact on HRQoL and the other option is watchful waiting with a chance of progression and death. The chance of progression and death is raised or lowered until the respondent considers the two options to be equivalent. The direct measures have the advantage that patients identify their own health states and its value [Feeny et al., 2005] and are specific to disease states that are not assessed in the more generic measures. However, these direct assessments are resource intensive and more burdensome to the patients requiring the presence of a trained interviewer or specialized computer program and rarely used in clinical trials.

Multi-attribute measures combine the advantages of self-assessment with the conceptual advantages of utility scores. Patients are assessed using a very brief questionnaire that assess health states in a limited number of domains. Their use is limited by the need to develop and validate the methods by which the multi-attribute assessment scores are converted to utility scores for each of the possible health states defined by the multi-attribute assessments. For example, for 5 domains of HRQoL with three possible levels for each domain, there will be 243 possible health states with a corresponding utility score. For the HUI3 there are 972,000 states. To derive the corresponding utilities, preference scores using direct measures are obtained from random samples of the general population. Examples include the Quality of Well

Being (QWB) [Patrick et al., 1973], Health Utility Index (HUI) [Feeny et al., 1992], the EuroQOL EQ-5D [Brooks, 1996] and the SF-6D [Brazier et al., 2002]. The multi-attribute measures are much less burdensome and have been successfully utilized in clinical trials. However, they may not capture disease specific issues and often have problems with ceiling effects.

1.2.3 Objective versus Subjective Questions

Health status measures differ in the extent to which they assess observable phenomena. Some instruments assess symptoms or functional benchmarks. In these instruments, subjects are asked about the frequency and severity of symptoms or whether they can perform certain tasks such as walking a mile. At the other end of the scale, the impact of symptoms or conditions is assessed. In these instruments, subjects are asked how much symptoms *bother* them or *interfere* with their usual activities. Many instruments provide a combination. The value of each approach will depend on the research objectives: Is the focus to identify the intervention with the least severity of symptoms or to assess the impact of the disease and its treatment?

There may exist a misconception that objective assessments are more valid than subjective assessments. This is generally based on the observation that patient ratings do not agree with ratings of trained professionals. Often we assume that the ratings of these professionals constitute the *gold standard*, when in fact they have more limited information than the patient about unobservable components of health states (e.g. pain), how the patient views his or her health and quality of life. Further, many of the biomedical endpoints that we consider objective include a high degree of measurement error (e.g. blood pressure), misclassification among experts or have poor predictive and prognostic validity (e.g. pulmonary function tests) [Wiklund et al., 1990].

1.2.4 Generic versus Disease-Specific Instruments

There are two basic types of instruments: generic and disease-specific. The generic instrument is designed to assess HRQoL in individuals with and without active disease. The SF-36 is a classic example of a generic instrument. The broad basis of a generic instrument is an advantage when comparing vastly different groups of subjects or following subjects across different phases of their disease or treatment. Disease-specific instruments narrow the scope of assessment and address in a more detailed manner the impact of a particular disease or treatment. As a result, they are more sensitive to smaller, but clinically significant changes induced by treatment, but may have items that are not relevant for patients after therapy or no longer experiencing the disease condition. Examples of disease specific measures include the Functional Assessment of Cancer Therapy (FACT) [Cella et al., 1993b] and the Migraine Specific Quality of Life questionnaire (MSQ) [Jhingran et al., 1998, Martin et al., 2000].

1.2.5   Global Index versus Profile of Domain-Specific Measures

Some HRQoL instruments are designed to provide a single global *index* of HRQoL. Others are designed to provide a *profile* of the dimensions such as the physical, emotional, functional and social well-being of patients. Many instruments attempt to assess both but often in different ways. The index and the profile represent two different approaches to the use of the HRQoL measure. The advantage of a single index is that it provides a straightforward approach to decision making. Indexes that are in the form of utilities are very useful in cost-effectiveness analyses performed in pharmacoeconomic research. Health profiles are useful when the objective is to identify different effects on the multiple dimensions of HRQoL.

A global index measure of HRQoL has the obvious attraction of the simplicity of a single indicator. However, constructing a single score that aggregates the multiple dimensions of HRQoL that is valid in all contexts is challenging. The issues surrounding composite measures are discussed in more detail in Chapter 14. When a construct is quite simple, a single question may be adequate to provide a reliable measure.* As the construct becomes more complex, more aspects of the construct need to be incorporated into the measure, creating a demand for multiple items. At some point the construct becomes so complex that there is no way to identify all the various aspects and a single question is used allowing the subject to integrate the complex aspects into one response.

Two widely used instruments designed for patients with cancer, FACT and EORTC QLQ-30, take very different approaches to obtain global measures. For the FACT measures [Cella et al., 1993b, 1995], the overall score is the summated score from all items in the questionnaire. In Version 4 of the FACT, this consists of 7 questions each measuring physical, functional and social well-being; 6 questions measuring emotional well-being and a variable number addressing disease-specific concerns. In the EORTC QLQ-30, Aaronson et al. [Aaronson et al., 1993] do not propose adding the subscale scores to form an overall score, arguing that a profile of the various domains more accurately reflect the multidimensional character of quality of life. The global score is instead constructed from two questions that are distinct from those used to measure specific domains (Table 1.1).

1.2.6   Response Format

Questionnaires may also differ in their response format. Two of the most widely-used formats are the Likert and visual analog scales (VAS) (Table 1.2). The Likert scale contains a limited number of ordered responses that have a

---

*In general, scales constructed from multiple items have better reliability than single items as the random measurement error tends to cancel.

TABLE 1.1 Questions assessing **Global Quality of Life** in the EORTC QLQ-30.

How would you rate your overall <u>health</u> during the past week?						
1	2	3	4	5	6	7
Very poor						Excellent
How would you rate your overall <u>quality of life</u> during the past week?						
1	2	3	4	5	6	7
Very poor						Excellent

descriptive label associated with each level. Individuals can discriminate at most seven to ten ordered categories [Miller, 1956, Streiner and Norman, 1995, p.35] and reliability and the ability to detect change drops off at five or fewer levels. The number of categories will also vary across different populations. Fewer response categories may be appropriate in very ill patients as well as the very young or elderly.

The VAS consists of a line with descriptive anchors at both ends of the line. The respondent is instructed to place a mark on the line. The length of the line is typically 10 cm. The concept behind the VAS is that the measure is continuous and could potentially discriminate more effectively than a Likert scale. This has not generally been true in most validation studies where both formats have been used. The VAS format has several limitations. First, it requires a level of eye-hand coordination that may be unrealistic for anyone with a neurological condition and for the elderly people. Second, it requires an additional data management step in which the position of the mark is measured. If forms are copied, rather than printed the full length of the line may vary requiring two measurements and additional calculations. Third, VAS precludes telephone and interviewer administered assessments.

1.2.7 Period of Recall

HRQoL scales often request subjects to base their evaluation on the last 7 days or 4 weeks. Symptoms assessment scales often use the last 24 hours or ask about the severity right now. For use in clinical trials, the selection of the appropriate time frame is a balance between being able to detect differences between interventions, detect impact of episodic symptoms and to minimize recall bias and short-term fluctuations (noise) that do not represent real change [Moinpour et al., 1989]. Recall is influenced most strongly by an individual's current status and memorable events, such as the worst intensity of a symptom. Shorter periods of recall are generally more appropriate when assessing severity of symptoms, whereas longer periods are required to assess the impact of those symptoms on activities of daily living. Scales specific to

TABLE 1.2 Example of a Likert and a Visual Analog Scale.

Likert Scale
How bothered were you by fatigue?

Not at all	Slightly	Moderately	Quite a bit	Greatly
0	1	2	3	4

Visual Analog Scale (VAS)
How bothered were you by fatigue?

Not at all   Greatly

diseases or treatments where there can be rapid changes will have a shorter recall duration. HRQoL instruments designed for assessment of general populations will often have a longer recall duration.

1.3 Study 1: Adjuvant Breast Cancer Trial

Increasing dose intensity and scheduling drugs more effectively are two strategies for improving the effectiveness of breast cancer adjuvant chemo-therapy. Although these strategies have advanced the treatment of patients with cancer, the increased toxicity with more aggressive regimens is a concern especially if there are modest improvements in survival. If more aggressive regimens produce comparable disease control and survival benefits, then the selection of optimum therapy should include not only the assessment of toxicity but also the impact of treatment on HRQoL.

In this trial,[†] an experimental 16-week dose-intensive therapy was compared to a conventional 24-week therapy (CAF[‡]) in patients with breast cancer [Fetting et al., 1995]. The primary hypothesis of the study was that disease-free and overall survival would be superior for the experimental regimen. However, the experimental regimen is a more dose-intense therapy than the standard regimen and, in addition to potentially increasing physical symptoms, the inconvenience of the treatment and expected fatigue may also have a greater impact on the psychosocial aspect of patients' lives. Thus, it was hypothesized that HRQoL during the standard therapy is superior to that during the

---

[†]Data presented here are derived (see Preface) from a trial conducted by the Eastern Cooperative Oncology Group funded by the National Cancer Institute Grant CA-23318.
[‡]CAF=cyclophosphamide, doxirubicin and 5-flurouracil.

experimental regimen. This discrepancy in expectations creates a need to reconcile competing outcomes if they indeed occur. Analysis of trials balancing survival and HRQoL is discussed in Chapter 15.

1.3.1 Patient Selection and Treatment

The patients eligible for the treatment trial had hormone receptor negative, node-positive breast cancer. Enrollment in the HRQoL substudy started after the initiation of the treatment trial. Patients registered on the treatment trial who had not yet started therapy on the parent trial were eligible for the quality of life study. Patients were also required to be able to read and understand English to be eligible. Consent was obtained separately for the treatment trial and the HRQoL substudy.

Patients were randomized to receive one of the two regimen [Fetting et al., 1998]. Briefly, the standard therapy consisted of 28-day cycles with 14 days of oral therapy and 2 days of intravenous therapy (days 1 and 8). Thus, patients on this regimen have a 2-week break every 4 weeks. In contrast, the briefer but more intensive experimental regimen consisted of weekly therapy. During odd-numbered weeks patients received 7 days of oral therapy plus 2 days of intravenous therapy. During even-numbered weeks, patients received 2 days of intravenous therapy.

1.3.2 Quality of Life Measure and Scoring

The Breast Chemotherapy Questionnaire (BCQ) was selected among available validated HRQoL instruments that were suitable for cooperative group trials [Moinpour et al., 1989] and also suited to the goals of this study. The BCQ was developed to evaluate treatment-related problems identified by patients and clinicians as most important to HRQoL during breast cancer adjuvant chemotherapy [Levine et al., 1988]. It is a self-administered questionnaire of 30 questions about the past two weeks, answered on a 1 to 7 point scale (Table 1.3). Seven domains were identified: *consequences of hair loss, positive well-being, physical symptoms, trouble and inconvenience, fatigue, emotional dysfunction and nausea.*

The BCQ is scored as follows: The overall raw score (R) is calculated as the mean of answers to the 30 questions; higher scores indicate better HRQoL with a range of possible scores from 1 to 7. The raw score is then rescaled (S=10*(R-1)/6) so that the range of possible BCQ scores (S) is from 0 to 10 points [Levine et al., 1988]. The subscale scores for the seven domains are the mean of the responses to the questions for that domain rescaled in the same manner. If any of the items are skipped, the overall and subscale scores are calculated using the mean of the completed items when at least half of the items were completed.

TABLE 1.3 Study 1: Sample questions from the Breast Chemotherapy Questionnaire (BCQ).

1. How often during the past 2 weeks have you felt worried or upset as a result of thinning or loss of your hair?
   (1)   All of the time
   (2)   Most of the time
   (3)   A good bit of the time
   (4)   Some of the time
   (5)   A little of the time
   (6)   Hardly any of the time
   (7)   None of the time

2. How often during the past 2 weeks have you felt optimistic or positive regarding the future?
   (1)   None of the time
   (2)   A little of the time

   $\vdots$

   (7)   All of the time

3. How often during the past 2 weeks have you felt your fingers were numb or falling asleep?
   (1)   All of the time
   (2)   Most of the time

   $\vdots$

   (7)   None of the time

4. How much trouble or inconvenience have you had during the last 2 weeks as a result of having to come to or stay at the clinic or hospital for medical care?
   (1)   A great deal of trouble or inconvenience
   (2)   A lot of trouble or inconvenience
   (3)   A fair bit of trouble or inconvenience

   $\vdots$

   (7)   No trouble or inconvenience

5. How often during the past 2 weeks have you felt low in energy?
   (1)   All of the time
   (2)   Most of the time

   $\vdots$

   (7)   None of the time

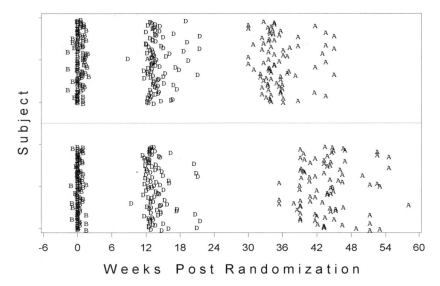

FIGURE 1.2 Study 1: Timing of observations in a study with an event-driven design with assessments before (B), during (D) and 4 months after (A) therapy. Data are from the breast cancer trial. Each row corresponds to a randomized subject. Subjects randomized to the experimental regimen appear in the upper half of the figure and subjects randomized to the standard regimen are in the lower half of the figure.

1.3.3 Timing of HRQoL Assessments

The BCQ assessments were limited to one assessment before, during and after treatment. The assessment prior to therapy was scheduled to be within 14 days of start of chemotherapy. The assessment during treatment was scheduled on day 85 of treatment. This was halfway through the CAF therapy (day 1 of cycle 4) and three quarters of the way through the 16-week regimen (day 1 of week 13). By day 85 it was expected that patients would be experiencing the cumulative effects of both regimens without yet experiencing the psychological lift that occurs at the end of treatment. The third assessment was scheduled 4 months after the completion of therapy. Since the duration of therapy differed between the two treatment regimens (16 vs. 24 weeks), the third assessment occurred at different points in time for patients on the different regimens, but at comparable periods relative to the completion of therapy. Additional variability in the timing of the third assessment was introduced for women who discontinued therapy earlier than planned or for those whose time to complete treatment may have been extended or delayed because of toxicity. The exact timing of the assessments is illustrated in Figure 1.2.

TABLE 1.4 Study 1: Documentation of HRQoL assessments in the adjuvant breast cancer trial.

Status/Reason	Before Therapy N (%)	During Therapy N (%)	After Therapy N (%)
Completed	191 (96)	180 (90)	173 (87)
Too late for baseline*	5 (2)		
No longer receiving therapy**		1 (1)	
Patient refused	1 (1)	2 (1)	3 (2)
Staff oversight	0 (0)	6 (3)	6 (3)
Patient too ill	0 (0)	11 (6)	2 (1)
Other, Early off therapy	0 (0)	0 (0)	11 (6)
Other, Not specified	3 (2)	0 (0)	2 (2)
Not documented	0 (0)	0 (0)	3 (2)
Total expected	200	200	200

* First assessment occurred after therapy began, excluded from analysis
**Second assessment occurred after therapy ended, excluded from analysis

1.3.4   Questionnaire Completion/Missing Data

There were 200 eligible patients registered on the HRQoL study. Assessments were completed by 191 (96%) patients prior to therapy, by 180 (90%) of the patients during therapy and by 173 patients (87%) following therapy (Table 1.4). In an exploratory analysis (Table 1.5), women under 50 years of age were less likely to complete all assessments. Missing assessments during therapy were associated with early discontinuation of therapy (regardless of reason), and concurrent chronic disease. Assessments were more likely to be missing following therapy in women who went off therapy early. The association of missing assessments with factors that are also associated with poorer outcomes suggests that some of these assessments may not be missing by chance. However, the proportion of missing assessments in this trial is small and unlikely to impact the treatment comparisons. (I will develop this argument in Chapter 6.)

1.4   Study 2: Migraine Prevention Trial

Migraine is a common disorder, with a prevalence of approximately 10% of the general population. The impact includes disruption of social life as well as productivity in the work site. Some individuals whose migraines are of sufficient severity or frequency are appropriate candidates for prophylactic therapy. The goal of this randomized, double-blind, placebo-controlled trial is

TABLE 1.5 Study 1: Patient characteristics associated with missing assessments in the adjuvant breast cancer trial (Study 1).

Time of assessment	Characteristic	Odds Ratio (95% CI[3])	
Before therapy	Age(<50 vs. ≥50)	(91 vs. 100%)[1]	
During therapy	Younger Age (<50)	4.9	(1.3, 19.1)
	Concurrent disease	24.1	(2.8, 211)
	Off therapy early	294	(33, 999)
Following Therapy	Younger Age (<50)	3.4	(1.2, 9.9)
	Off therapy early	21.1	(7.0, 63.5)

[1] Proportions in each group. Odds Ratio could not be estimated.

[2] Other potential explanatory variables included minority race, initial performance status, treatment arm, the presence and severity of selected toxicity including vomiting, diarrhea, alopecia and weight loss and discontinuation of therapy.

[3] CI=Confidence Interval

to evaluate the efficacy and safety of the experimental therapy versus placebo in migraine prophylaxis in individuals with an established history consistent with migraine. The primary outcomes of the trial[§] include the frequency and severity of migraines as reported on patient diaries. Secondary objectives include the assessment of the impact of treatment on HRQoL.

1.4.1 Patient Selection and Treatment

Subjects were 18 to 65 years of age with an established history consistent with migraine for at least six months. Subjects who experienced at least three migraine headaches per month during the baseline phase were eligible for randomization to one of the two treatment regimens. Subjects were allowed to continue taking acute migraine medications for the treatment of breakthrough attacks during the trial.

After meeting the criteria previously specified and following a washout period during which any currently used migraine preventive medications were tapered off, patients were randomized to receive either the experimental drug or matching placebo during the 6 month, double-blind phase of the trial. The double-blind phase consisted of a two month titration period and a four month maintenance period. Doses were increased weekly until patients reached their assigned dose or maximum tolerated dose, whichever was lower.

[§]Data presented here are completely simulated (see Preface). The impact of treatment on the measures and the correlations between measures does not correspond to any actual trial data. The correlations of assessments over time within each measure do mimic actual trial data.

TABLE 1.6 Study 2: Sample questions from the Migraine Specific Quality-of-Life questionnaire (MSQ).

1. In the past 4 weeks, how often have migraines **interfered** with how well you dealt with family, friends and others who are close to you? (Select only **one** response.)
    - 1☐ None of the time
    - 2☐ A little bit of the time
    - 3☐ Some of the time
    - 4☐ A good bit of the time
    - 5☐ Most of the time
    - 6☐ All of the time

2. In the past 4 weeks, how often have migraines **interfered** with your leisure time activities, such as reading or exercising? (Select only **one** response.)
    - 1☐ None of the time

      ⋮

    - 6☐ All of the time

3. In the past 4 weeks, how often have you had **difficulty** in performing work or daily activities because of migraine symptoms? (Select only **one** response.)
    - 1☐ None of the time

      ⋮

    - 6☐ All of the time

1.4.2 Quality of Life Measure and Scoring

HRQoL was evaluated using a disease specific measure, the Migraine-Specific Quality of Life questionnaire (MSQ)[Jhingran et al., 1998, Martin et al., 2000] in order to assess the impact of study medication on the activities of daily living of patients with migraine.

The 14-item MSQ is divided into the *role restriction* (RR), *role prevention* (RF), and *emotional function* (EF) domains. Patients were asked to answer to each question in the MSQ using a standard six-point, Likert-type scale with the following choices: none of the time, a little of the time, some of the time, a good bit of the time, most of the time, and all of the time (Table 1.6). Responses to questions are reversed coded, averaged (or summed) and finally rescaled so that scores can range from 0 to 100 with higher scores indicating better functioning.

1.4.3 Timing of HRQoL Assessments

The MSQ data were scheduled to be collected at baseline and 2, 4, and 6 months. If the patient was discontinuing treatment, an assessment was collected if at least 4 weeks had elapsed since the last assessment. Figure 1.3 illustrates the observed timing of assessments. While most assessments occured within the windows specified in the protocol, a substantial number were delayed. Choices among analytic techniques for longitudinal data based on the timing of assessments and inclusion of all available data will be discussed in Chapters 3 and 4.

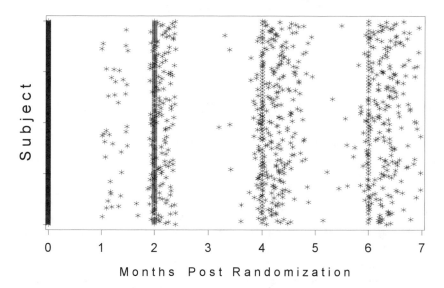

FIGURE 1.3 Study 2: Timing of observations in the migraine prevention trial. Each row represents a subject.

1.4.4 Questionnaire Completion/Missing Data

The number of completed and missing assessments are summarized in Table 1.7. Roughly 70% of the participants completed the final assessments. The most common reason given for dropout was side effects (7% in the placebo arm and 26% in the experimental therapy arm) occuring during the first two months of the study. Lack of efficacy was given as the reason for dropout in 18% of those on the placebo arm and 6% on the experimental therapy arm.

The impact of the differences in the reasons for dropout between the treatment arms on the analysis will be discussed in later chapters. One would expect lack of efficacy to be associated with differences in individual scores of the MSQ subscales. Side effects (typically tingling and fatigue) are less likely to affect the MSQ subscales (as the questions focus on migraine symptoms).

TABLE 1.7 Study 2: Completion of Migraine Symptom Questionnaire (MSQ) in the placebo (Plc) and experimental (Exp) treatment arms.

Status/ Reason Missing	Baseline		2 months		4 months		6 months	
	Plc	Exp	Plc	Exp	Plc	Exp	Plc	Exp
Completed[†]	200	200	192	178	172	145	151	137
Lack of Efficacy	0	0	1	0	14	4	35	12
Side Effects	0	0	7	22	14	51	14	51
Total patients	200	200	200	200	200	200	200	200

1.5   Study 3: Advanced Lung Cancer Trial

To evaluate therapeutic effectiveness of new strategies for non small-cell lung cancer (NSCLC), a multi-center phase III clinical trial[¶] was activated to compare two new Paclitaxel-cisplatin regimens with a traditional etoposide-cisplatin regimen for the treatment of stage IIIB-IV non-small-cell lung cancer (NSCLC) [Bonomi et al., 2000]. In addition to traditional endpoints, such as time to disease progression and survival, HRQoL was included in this trial. The stated objective of the HRQoL component of this study was "to compare quality of life for the three treatment arms and correlate quality of life to toxicity."

1.5.1   Treatment

All three treatment arms included cisplatin at the same dose. The traditional treatment arm contained VP-16 with cisplatin (Control). The other two arms contained low-dose Paclitaxel (Experimental 1) or high-dose Paclitaxel with G-CSF (Experimental 2). The planned length of each cycle was 3 weeks. Treatment was continued until disease progression or excessive toxicity. Of the 525 patients randomized, 308 patients (59%) started four or more cycles of therapy and 198 (38%) started six or more cycles.

[¶]Data presented in this book are derived (see Preface) from a trial conducted Eastern Cooperative Oncology Group funded by the National Cancer Institute Grant CA-23318.

1.5.2 Quality of Life Measure and Scoring

The Functional Assessment of Cancer Therapy-Lung Cancer Version 2 (FACT-L) was used to measure HRQoL in this trial [Bonomi et al., 2000]. It is a self-administered 43-item questionnaire, 33 items of which are general questions relevant to all cancer patients and 10 of which are items relevant to lung cancer. It provides scores for *physical well-being, social/family well-being, emotional well-being, functional well-being and lung cancer symptoms* [Bonomi et al., 2000, Cella et al., 1995]. In addition to the five major subscales, a number of summary scales can be constructed including the FACT-Lung Trial Outcome Index (FACT-Lung TOI) which is the sum of the physical well-being, functional well-being and lung cancer symptom scores. Higher scores imply better quality of life.

Each domain is scored as the sum of the items. If any of the items are skipped and at least half of the items in the subscale are answered, scores are calculated using the mean of the available items times the number of items in the subscale. Examples and details of scoring are presented in Chapter 2. For easier interpretation of the presentations in this book, all scales were rescaled to have a possible range of 0 to 100.

TABLE 1.8 Study 3: Sample questions from the Functional Assessment of Cancer Therapy (FACT)-Lung (Version 2) questionnaire.

Please indicate how true each statement has been for you during the past 7 days					
ADDITIONAL CONCERNS	not at all	a little bit	some-what	quite a bit	very much
34. I have been short of breath	0	1	2	3	4
35. I am losing weight	0	1	2	3	4
36. My thinking is clear	0	1	2	3	4
37. I have been coughing	0	1	2	3	4
38. I have been bothered by hair loss	0	1	2	3	4
39. I have a good appetite	0	1	2	3	4
40. I feel tightness in my chest	0	1	2	3	4
41. Breathing is easy for me	0	1	2	3	4
If you ever smoked, please answer #42.					
42. I regret my smoking	0	1	2	3	4

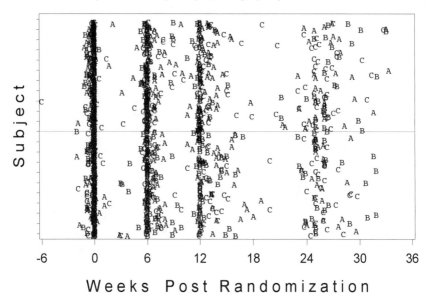

FIGURE 1.4 Study 3: Timing of observations in a time driven design with four planned assessments. Data are from the lung cancer trial (Study 3). Each row corresponds to a randomized patient in this study. Symbols represent the actual timing of the HRQoL assessments relative to the date the patient was randomized. A=Control Group, B=Experimental 1, C=Experimental 2.

1.5.3   Timing of Assessments

Four HRQoL assessments were scheduled for each patient. The assessment times were carefully selected after balancing a number of considerations: 1) concern for excessive burden to this often debilitated group of patients; 2) the relatively short median time to both progressive growth of the tumor and death expected in these patients; and 3) practical matters related to feasibility of the study at multiple clinical treatment sites. These issues contributed to the decision to have relatively few assessments (four) over a fairly brief period of time (6 months from initiation of treatment). Standard community oncology practice for metastatic lung cancer very often involves the administration of two cycles of cytotoxic chemotherapy with re-evaluation at the end of the second cycle (6 weeks) before moving on to further chemotherapy. Because the investigators were particularly interested in obtaining data from this study that would be useful to the community practitioner, they selected the end of the second cycle (3 weeks) as the first clinically relevant assessment after baseline. The third assessment, which occurred at the end of the fourth cycle (12 weeks), was selected because it represents the same interval of time (6 weeks) and we believed it possible that patients' experience with therapy would enable them to tolerate it better over time. The final assessment at 6 months was selected as the best long-term follow up in this population because it was several months before the expected median survival, which ensured that a sufficient number of patients could be studied. Thus, the four assessments were scheduled to be prior to the start of treatment, before the start of the third and fifth courses of chemotherapy and at 6 months (week 26). If patients discontinued the protocol therapy, then the second and third assessments were to be scheduled 6 and 12 weeks after the initiation of therapy.

The actual timing of the HRQoL assessments showed much more variability than the plan would suggest (Figure 1.4). Some of the variation was to be expected. For example, when courses of therapy were delayed as a result of toxicity, then the second and third assessments were delayed. Some variation in the 6-month assessment was also expected as the HRQoL assessment was linked to clinic visits that might be more loosely scheduled at the convenience of the patient and medical staff. There was also an allowed window of 2 weeks prior to the start of therapy for the baseline assessment.

1.5.4 Questionnaire Completion/Missing Data

A total of 1334 HRQoL assessments were obtained in this trial. This represents 98, 75, 63 and 52% of the expected assessments in surviving patients at each of the four planned assessment times (Table 1.9). The most commonly documented reasons for missing assessments are "patient refusal" and "staff oversight". A detailed listing is presented in Table 1.9. A more extensive exploration of the missing data will follow in Chapter 6. Both that exploration and clinical feedback suggest that dropout in this study was likely to be nonrandom [Fairclough et al., 1998b]. Consequently, methods of analysis that address issues of non-ignorable missing data must be considered for this study (see Chapters 9 through 12).

1.6 Study 4: Renal Cell Carcinoma Trial

A multicenter randomized phase III trial was conducted to determine whether combination therapy with 13-*cis*-retinoic acid (13-CRA) plus interferon alfa-2a (IFNα2a) was superior therapy to IFNα2a alone in patients with advanced renal cell carcinoma.[||] The influence of cytokine treatment on quality of life was considered to be an important aspect of the management of advanced renal cell carcinoma. No difference was found for the clinical endpoints [Motzer

---

[||]Data presented in this book are derived (see Preface) from a trial conducted by Memorial Sloan-Kettering Cancer Center and Eastern Cooperative Oncology Group funded by the National Cancer Institute grant CA-05826.

TABLE 1.9 Study 3: Documentation of FACT-Lung assessments.

Status/ Reason Missing	Baseline N (%)	6 weeks N (%)	12 weeks N (%)	6 months N (%)
Completed[†]	513 (98)	362 (75)	276 (63)	183 (52)
Refusal	0 (0)	34 (7)	46 (10)	62 (17)
Patient feels too ill	0 (0)	3 (1)	3 (1)	3 (1)
Staff felt patient too ill	0 (0)	18 (4)	15 (3)	11 (3)
Staff oversight	7 (1)	35 (7)	59 (13)	56 (15)
Other	1 (0)	13 (2)	23 (5)	20 (6)
Unknown	4 (1)	19 (4)	19 (4)	20 (6)
Total expected	525	484	441	355
Patients expired[‡]	0 (0)	41 (8)	84 (16)	170 (32)
Total patients	525	525	525	525

[†] Percent of expected assessments (e.g. patient still alive).

[‡] Percent of all possible assessments.

et al., 2000]. This population experiences considerable morbidity and mortality, with a median survival of approximately 15 months.

1.6.1   Patient Selection and Treatment

Eligibility requirements included histological confirmation of renal cell carcinoma, Karnofsky performance status (KPS) ≥ 70 and estimated life expectancy of more than 3 months.

Patients were randomized to receive either daily treatment with IFNα2a plus 13-CRA (experimental) or IFNα2a alone (control). IFNα2a was given as a single subcutaneous injection and the 13-CRA orally. Doses were adjusted in response to symptoms of toxicity. Treatment was continued until progression of disease, complete response, or development of excessive toxicity.

1.6.2   Quality of Life Measures and Scoring

The trial utilized the Functional Assessment of Cancer Therapy Version 3 (FACT-G) as the tool for HRQoL assessment. Since the effect of biologic response modifiers (BRM) has not been adequately studied, 17 disease-specific questions were appended to the core questionnaire to measure the expected symptoms of 13-CRA and IFNα2a. Validation of the disease-specific questions was undertaken to assess whether these questions are a reliable measure of HRQoL. Using factor analysis and internal consistency coefficients on the 2-week and baseline assessments, the original pool of 17 questions was reduced to a 13-item measure [Bacik et al., 2004]. The factor analysis suggested that two definable dimensions were being measured by this set of questions. Examination of item content of the first dimension or subscale (factor 1) suggests it

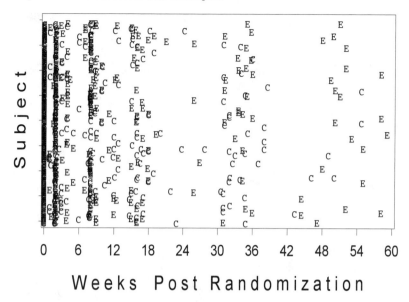

Weeks Post Randomization

FIGURE 1.5 Study 4: Timing of observations in a time driven design with increasing numbers of mistimed observations. Data are from the renal cell carcinoma study [Motzer et al., 2000]. Each row represents a subject.

could be labeled as a *BRM-Physical* component. The second factor included items related to mental or emotional symptoms/side effects (*BRM-Mental*). The initial BRM-Physical subscale included 3 items that were specific to dryness (skin, mouth, eyes) which were specific to the effects of CRA. This subscale was subsequently modified to reflect a more generic class of biologic response modifying therapies. Coefficients of reliability (internal consistency) range from 0.61 to 0.92 for the baseline assessments and from 0.64 to 0.94 for the week 2 assessments. The Trial Outcome Index (*FACT-BRM TOI*), calculated by adding the physical and functional well-being scores and the two BRM subscale scores, was used as a summary measure of HRQoL. Details for scoring the FACT scales are presented in Chapter 2. In the examples presented in this book, the original 0-108 point scale was rescaled to have a 0-100 point range.

1.6.3 Timing of HRQoL Assessments

At the time the study was designed, knowledge about the impact of therapy on the HRQoL of patients with renal cell carcinoma was extremely limited. Six assessments were scheduled. The first was to be obtained in a 2-week period prior to initiating therapy. The second was scheduled 2 weeks after initiation of therapy to assess acute toxicity. The remaining assessments were

TABLE 1.10 Study 4: Sample questions from the Functional Assessment of Cancer Therapy-Biologic Response Modifiers including CRA (FACT-BRM/CRA Version 3) questionnaire.

Please indicate how true each statement has been for you during the past 7 days					
ADDITIONAL CONCERNS	not at all	a little bit	some-what	quite a bit	very much
35.I get tired easily	0	1	2	3	4
36.I feel weak all over	0	1	2	3	4
37.I have trouble concentrating	0	1	2	3	4
38.I have trouble remembering things	0	1	2	3	4
39.My thinking is clear	0	1	2	3	4
40.I have a good appetite	0	1	2	3	4
41.I have pain in my joints	0	1	2	3	4
42.I am bothered by the chills	0	1	2	3	4
43.I am bothered by fevers	0	1	2	3	4
44.I am bothered by dry skin	0	1	2	3	4
45.I am bothered by dry mouth	0	1	2	3	4
46.I am bothered by dry eyes	0	1	2	3	4
47.I get depressed easily	0	1	2	3	4
48.I get annoyed easily	0	1	2	3	4
49.I have emotional ups and downs	0	1	2	3	4
50.I feel motivated to do things	0	1	2	3	4
51.I am bothered by sweating	0	1	2	3	4

to occur at 2, 4, 8 and 12 months (8, 17, 34 and 52 weeks) to assess chronic toxicity. This schedule was to be continued for patients who discontinued the protocol therapy as a result of toxicity or disease progression to assess the continued impact of the disease and toxicity. The exact timing of the assessments became more variable with time (Figure 1.5).

1.6.4 Questionnaire Completion/Missing Data

At least one questionnaire was received from 213 patients with a total of 735 questionnaires. The compliance rates among the 213 patients for the six assessments were 89, 77, 61, 43, 39 and 23% respectively (Table 1.11) Early dropout from the HRQoL study was characterized by poorer prognosis (Kendall's $\tau_b = -0.25$), lower initial FACT-BRM TOI scores ($\tau_b = 0.27$), lower final FACT-BRM TOI score ($\tau_b = 0.22$) and early death ($\tau_b = 0.48$) but not with treatment ($\tau_b = -0.01$). A more extensive exploration of the missing

TABLE 1.11 Study 4: Summary of missing HRQoL assessments over time among 213 renal-cell carcinoma patients with at least one HRQoL assessment (17 patients did not complete any assessments).

Schedule (weeks)	0	2	8	17	34	52
Surviving patients	200	199	191	168	135	112
TOI completed	192	171	140	83	41	14
% of surviving patients	96%	86%	73%	49%	30%	12%
% of total patients	96%	86%	70%	42%	20%	7%

Windows defined as <7 days, 1-<6 weeks, 6-<15 weeks, 15-<30 weeks, 30-<48 weeks, 48-65 weeks.

data will follow in Chapter 4. As in the lung cancer trial, this suggests that dropout in this study was likely to be non-random. Consequently, methods of analysis described in Chapters 7 through 9 must be considered for this study.

1.7 Study 5: Chemoradiation (CXRT) Trial

A single institution trial was conducted to study cancer-related symptoms in patients with non-small cell lung cancer (NSCLC) undergoing current chemoradiation therapy, a standard regimen for patient with stage III lung cancer (e.g. no metastatic disease) for whom no surgery is planned.** This regimen is frequently associated with acute side effects of the radiation and chemotherapy (pain, weight loss, esophagitis and pneumonitis) as well as non-specific symptoms (fatigue, sadness, distress, sleep disturbance, drowsiness, and poor appetite). The primary goals were to determine the prevalence, severity and longitudinal patterns of change that occured during and after CXRT and to assess how each symptom affected the patient's daily activities.[Wang et al., 2006]

1.7.1 Patient Selection and Treatment

Fifty-eight patients were entered into the trial. Patients had to be scheduled for curative CXRT, and have diagnosis of non small cell lung cancer with unresectable non metastatic (stage III) disease. Radiation (50 to 70 Gy) was delivered daily (5 days/week) over 5 to 7 weeks. The chemotherapy (carboplatin plus paclitaxel) was administered concurrently.

**Data presented in this book are derived (see Preface) from a trial conducted by University of Texas M.D. Anderson Cancer Center funded in part by the National Institutes of Health Grants No. R01 CA026582 and R21 CA109286.

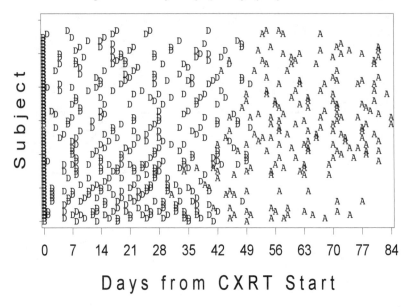

FIGURE 1.6 Study 5: Timing of observations in the chemoradiation trial. Each row represents a subject. Assessments during therapy are indicated by a D and those after therapy by an A.

1.7.2   Patient Reported Outcomes

Symptoms and their impact on activities of daily living were assessed using the M. D. Anderson Symptom Inventory (MDASI)[Cleeland et al., 2000]. The MDASI is a patient-reported outcome tool to assess cancer related symptoms and the impact of those symptoms on activities of daily living. The MDASI includes 13 core symptoms: fatigue, sleep disturbance, pain, drowsiness, poor appetite, nausea, vomiting, shortness of breath, numbness, difficulty remembering, dry mouth, distress and sadness. Two additional symptoms (cough and sore throat) were added in this study. The severity of these symptoms during the previous 24 hours is assessed on a 1 to 10 point numerical scale, with 0 being "not present" and 10 being "as bad as you can imagine." Interference with daily activities was assessed using six questions that describe how much symptoms have interfered with general activity, mood, walking ability, normal work, relations with other people and enjoyment of life. Interference is also assessed on a 0 to 10 point scale, with 0 being "does not interfere" and 10 being "completely interferes." A total score is computed as the mean of the six item scores.

1.7.3 Timing and Frequency of HRQoL Assessments

Symptoms and interference with daily activity were assessed before the start of CXRT, weekly for 12 weeks during and after CXRT. Patient complete therapy between week 5 and 7. The number of assessments varied among patients, mostly due to differences in the length of therapy: 55 patients completed 61 assessments prior to treatment, 58 patients completed 344 assessments (average 5.9) assessments during therapy, and 50 patients completed 181 (average 3.6 assessments). The timing of the assessments is displayed in Figure 1.6. Note that like the breast cancer trial (Study 1), this trial has three distinct phases (before, during and after therapy), but differs as it has multiple assessments of each phase.

1.8 Study 6: Osteoarthritis Trial

A pilot randomized, double blind trial was initiated to assess the efficacy and safety of an experimental drug.[††] The experimental drug is in a class of opioids which may be effective for pain but may also cause side effects (constipation, dizziness, somnolence, etc.) in opioid naive subjects. Lower doses of the drug may not be potent enough for patients with tolerance to opioids. The primary endpoint was pain intensity which was measured on a 0-10 point scale. Higher scores indicate greater pain.

1.8.1 Patient Selection and Treatment

Subjects had moderate to severe chronic pain due to osteoarthritis of the hip or knee. The planned total time on the experimental drug was three weeks. 200 individuals were randomized to one of the two treatment arms.

1.8.2 Timing and Frequency of Assessments

Assessments were scheduled at baseline, 7, 14 and 21 days. The timing of the follow-up assesments varied widely: the median (range) days post randomization was 7 (1-1), 12 (9-18) and 22 (19-28) for the three assessments (Figure 1.7). Of the 200 subjects, 100 (50%) finished the study. The reasons for dropout differed by treatment arm with discontinuation early due to side effects more common in the active treatment arm and to inadequate pain

---

[††]Data presented here are completely simulated. The impact of the hypothetical treatment on the measure does not correspond to any actual trial data. Only the correlations of assessments over time and the trajectories associated with the reason for dropout mimic actual trial data.

relief with the need for rescue medication more common in the placebo arm (Table 1.8.2). The missing data pattern was monotone with one exception of a patient missing the baseline assessment.

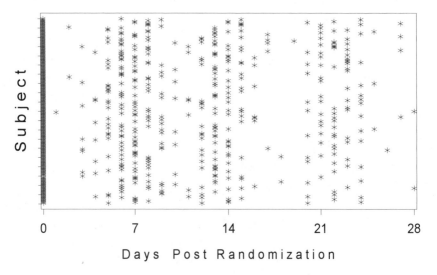

FIGURE 1.7 Study 6: Timing of observations in the osteoarthritis trial. Each row represents a subject.

TABLE 1.12 Study 6: Study completion status/reason for dropout and days to last assessment.

Status	N	Placebo Arm Median	(Range)	N	Experimental Arm Median	(Range)
Completed Study	50	23	(20-28)	50	23	(19-28)
Inadequate Relief	40	10	(3-19)	10	10	(5-16)
Side-effects	10	9	(4-11)	40	9	(2-17)

1.9 Summary

- Health-Related Quality-of-Life (HRQoL)

  1. HRQoL represents the impact of disease and treatment on a patient's perception of their well-being.

  2. HRQoL is multidimensional including physical, emotional, functional and social components.

  3. HRQoL is subjective representing the patient's perspective.

- Measurement

  1. There are numerous measures of health status and patient preferences that are generically referred to as HRQoL measures.

  2. The utility of the various types of measures (health status, preference, disease-specific, general, etc.) will depend on the intended use of the measure.

- Study 1: Breast Cancer Trial

  1. Two-arm study designed to compare a standard and experimental adjuvant therapy.

  2. Simple design with one assessment before, during and after therapy.

  3. Minimal ($< 5\%$) missing data.

  4. Used to demonstrate classical repeated measures model.

- Study 2: Migraine Prevention Trial

  1. Two-arm double-blinded study designed to compare placebo to an experimental therapy.

  2. Four planned assessments: one assessment before therapy and three during or after therapy

  3. Moderate rate of dropout possibly related to HRQoL.

  4. Used to demonstrate that symptom severity/frequency mediates relationship between treatment and HRQoL outcomes.

- Study 3: Lung Cancer Trial

  1. Three-arm trial designed to compare a standard and two experimental therapies

  2. Four planned assessments: one assessment before therapy and three during or after therapy

3. Extensive missing data as a result of death and other reasons probably related to HRQoL. More than 50% missing at time of last assessment.

4. Used primarily to demonstrate methods of analysis when dropout is assumed to be informative (i.e. related to individual trajectories).

- Study 4: Renal-Cell Carcinoma Trial

    1. Two-arm trial designed to compare a standard and experimental therapy

    2. Six planned assessments: one assessment before therapy and five during or after therapy

    3. Extensive missing data as a result of death and other reasons probably related to HRQoL. More than 50% missing at time of last assessment.

    4. Timing of assessments became more variable as the study progressed.

    5. Used to demonstrate mixed-effects growth curve models with non-linear trajectories.

- Study 5: Chemoradiation (CXRT) Trial

    1. Single-arm trial designed to assess symptoms and their impact on activities of daily living

    2. Multiple weekly assessments before, during and after therapy over a 12 week period.

    3. Timing of assessments is variable throughout the trial.

    4. Used to demonstrate mediation in a longitudinal study.

- Study 6: Osteoarthritis Trial

    1. Two-arm trial designed to assess pain intensity in patients with osteoarthritis.

    2. Four weekly assessments planned.

    3. Dropout occurs due to side effects and lack of efficacy and differed substantially across treatment arm.

    4. Used to demonstrate the use of a joint model with two disparate reasons for dropout.

2

Study Design and Protocol Development

2.1 Introduction

> Implicit in the use of measures of HRQoL, in clinical trials and in effectiveness research, is the concept that clinical interventions such as pharmacologic therapies, can affect parameters such as physical function, social function, or mental health.(Wilson and Cleary [1995])

Identification of the components of HRQoL that are relevant to the disease and its treatment, development of specific priori objectives and an analytic plan are essential to both good trial design and subsequent scientific review. This chapter will focus on design and protocol development. Later chapters will deal with strategies for analysis of longitudinal studies (Chapters 3 and 4), definition of endpoints that summarize information over time or domains (Chapter 13), handling multiple endpoints (Chapter 14), development of a statistical analysis plan (Chapter 16), and sample size calculations for studies with dropout (Chapter 16). Figure 2.1 is a checklist for protocol development. All principles of good clinical trial methodology are applicable [Friedman et al, 1985, Meinert, 1986, Fleiss, 1986, Spilker, 1991, Piantadosi, 1997], but there are additional requirements specific to HRQoL. These include clear identification of the construct(s) that are relevant for the disease and treatment, selection of an appropriate measure of that construct and the conduct of the assessment to minimize any bias. The historical tendency to add a HRQoL assessment to a trial often at the last minute without careful thought about all the components of its necessity, implementation and analysis should be just that ... historical! The HRQoL outcomes (using the broad definition) should be a well integrated component of the protocol design.

2.1.1 Purpose of the Protocol

A protocol for a clinical trial has several roles. The primary role is as a *recipe* for the conduct of the study. Thus, the protocol is a public document used by the investigators to conduct the trial and reviewed by IRBs and ethics boards recording the structure of the scientific experiment as based upon a set of

FIGURE 2.1 Checklist for protocol development.

√ Rationale for studying HRQoL and for the specific aspect of HRQoL to be measured

√ Explicit research objectives and endpoints (also see Chapters 13 and 14)

√ Strategies for minimizing the exclusion of subjects from the trial

√ Rationale for timing of assessments and off study rules

√ Rationale for instrument selection

√ Details for administration of HRQoL assessments to minimize bias and missing data

√ Analytic plan (see Chapter 16)

---

hypotheses to be confirmed. It also provides the scientific rationale, study design, and planned analyses so third parties, including regulatory bodies and journal editors, can interpret and weigh the study results. Other important roles include the justification and motivation for the study as well as preliminary evidence that supports the decisions for the intervention and constructs (and measures) assessing the efficacy and safety of the intervention. Thus the protocol is the document that provides the evidence and justification for the *design* and conduct of the trial.

The protocol should include the critical elements of the *analysis* plan. This plan needs to consider the standards that journals may require for publication. The guidelines of the International Committee of Medical Journal Editors (ICMJE) state that in publication the methods section should include only information that was available at the time the plan or protocol for the study was being written; all information obtained during the study belongs in the results section. New standards require that the protocols for clinical trials be placed in the public domain registering with entities such as *ClinicalTrials.gov*. There are multiple motivations for these registries including awareness of other research, but one relevant application is the use by reviewers to assess the reported methods and results against those initially intended as stated in the protocol. In trials that are intended for the approval of new drugs or expanded claims for existing drugs that will be reviewed by regulatory bodies such as the FDA or EMEA, the protocol is often supplemented with a statistical analysis plan (SAP) that provides additional details of the planned analysis.

2.2 Background and Rationale

Providing sufficient background and rationale to justify the resources required for an investigation of HRQoL, one of its components or any patient reported outcome will contribute to the success of the investigation. The rationale should provide answers to such questions as: How exactly might the results affect the clinical management of patients? and How will the HRQoL results be used when determining the effectiveness of the treatment arms? The justification should include a motivation for the particular aspects of HRQoL that will be measured in the trial as they relate to the disease, treatment and its impact.

The HRQoL component is not a separate class of endpoints, but one of the efficacy or safety endpoints. The same demands for a rationale should be applied to all information collected in any clinical trial. However, investigators already have a habit of collecting laboratory and radiological tests so that minimal motivation is required to implement this data collection. The same is not necessarily true for the collection of data that requires patient self assessment and greater motivation may be necessary. Writing a rationale for HRQoL assessments also facilitates the development of well-defined research objectives.

2.3 Research Objectives and Goals

The most critical component of any clinical trial is explicit research objectives and goals; Figure 2.2 is a checklist of questions that must be addressed. It is only when the goals and research objectives provide sufficient detail to guide the design, conduct and analysis of the study that the success of the trial is ensured. If no further thought is given to the specific research questions, it is likely that there will be neither rhyme nor reason to the design, conduct and analysis of the HRQoL assessments. Then, because of either poor design or the lack of a definite question, the analyst and reviewers will ask questions such as What is the question? Why did you collect the data this way? and Why didn't you collect data at this time? There is a real concern that the lack of meaningful results from poorly focused and thus potentially poorly designed and analyzed trials will create the impression that HRQoL research is not worthwhile.

General objectives state the obvious but are insufficient. Regardless of whether HRQoL is considered to be a secondary or primary outcome, a stated HRQoL objective such as *To compare the quality of life between treatment A*

FIGURE 2.2 Checklist for developing well-defined goals and objectives.

√ What are the specific constructs that will be used to evaluate the intervention?

     - If HRQoL, is it the overall HRQoL or a specific dimension?

     - If a symptom, is it severity, time to relief, impact on daily activities, etc.?

√ What is the goal of inclusion of HRQoL?

     - Claim for a HRQoL benefit?

     - Supportive evidence of superiority of intervention?

     - Exploratory analysis of potential negative impacts?

     - Pharmacoecomonic evaluation?

     - Other?

√ What is the population of interest (inference)?

√ What is the time frame of interest?

√ Is the intent confirmatory or exploratory?

---

and B is too nonspecific. The assessment of HRQoL involves changes over time in the various aspects of HRQoL including physical, functional, emotional and social well-being. The detail of the objectives includes identifying 1) relevant dimensions of HRQoL or other constructs such as fatigue, 2) population of interest and 3) the time frame. The stated objectives should refer to the construct being measured (e.g., fatigue) and not the measurement instrument (e.g. SF-36). Hypotheses should be clear as to whether the intent is to demonstrate superiority or non-inferiority and whether the objective is confirmatory or entirely exploratory.

Consider a hypothetical example in which two analgesics (**Pain Free** and **Relief**) are compared for a painful condition. Both drugs require a period of titration in which the dose is slowly increased to a maintenance level. Assessments are obtained during the titration phase and the maintenance phase of the trial. An objective such as *To compare the quality-of-life in subjects receiving* **Pain-Free** *vs.* **Relief** does not provide any guidance. The first step is to be clear about the construct that is being measured. Is it the severity or duration of pain, impact of pain on daily activities or HRQoL. Note that the regulatory agencies (e.g. FDA and EMEA) have indicated that to get a claim for HRQoL, you need to demonstrate that treatment has a significant effect on all domains (i.e., physical, social and emotional functioning). If the condition is permanent and the drugs are intended for extended use, the objective could be restated as *To compare the impact of pain on daily activities while on a maintenance dose* of Pain-Free vs. Relief. Alternatively, if the pain associated with the condition was brief, the drug which provided earlier relief would be preferable and the objective stated as *To compare the time to 20% improvement in the severity of pain with* Pain-Free vs. Relief. These objectives now provide more guidance for the rest of the protocol development. The construct of interest is explicitly defined and will guide the selection of the measure and the timing of assessment. In the first situation, assessments during maintenance are important and in the second, the earlier assessments are the basis of defining the outcome and should be frequent enough to detect differences between the two regimens.

2.3.1 Role of HRQoL in the Trial

The identifying the role of the HRQoL or other patient reported outcomes (PROs) is an important step in the protocol development. Too often this stops with declaring endpoints as primary, secondary or tertiary. The fundamental issue is what decisions will be made based on the results. Which of the endpoints will be used to demonstrate the efficacy of intervention? If more than one, will it be sufficient to demonstrate superiority of only one or will superiority/non-inferiority of all be required? Which of the endpoints will be used to demonstrate the safety/tolerability of the intervention? Which endpoints are solely supportive or exploratory? Answers to these questions will have particular impact on the procedures proposed to adjust for multiple comparisons or design of gatekeeper strategies that are described in Chapter 13.

2.3.2 Pragmatic versus Explanatory Inference

The objectives should clarify to whom the inferences will apply: all study subjects, subjects who complete treatment, or only subjects alive at end of study? A useful terminology for characterizing the trial objectives is described by Schwartz et al. [Schwartz et al., 1980, Heyting et al., 1992]. They distinguish between *pragmatic* and *explanatory* investigational aims. The investigational aims for HRQoL will typically be pragmatic rather than explanatory. The distinction becomes important when the investigators make decisions about the study design and analysis.

Pragmatic objectives are closely related to the *intent-to-treat* analytic strategies. In these trials, the objective is to compare the relative impact of each intervention on HRQoL under practical and realistic conditions. For example, it may not be desirable for all subjects to complete the entire course of intended therapy exactly as specified because of toxicity or lack of efficacy. Some individuals may need to be given additional therapy. Others may be noncompliant for a variety of reasons. In a study with a pragmatic aim, the intent is to make inferences about all subjects for the entire period of assessment. Thus, assessment of HRQoL should be continued regardless of whether the patient continues to receive the intervention as specified in the protocol. HRQoL assessments should not stop when the patient goes *off study*.

In contrast, with an explanatory aim, we compare the HRQoL impact of treatments given in a manner that is carefully specified in the protocol. This is sometimes described as the analysis of the *per-protocol* subgroup. In this setting, HRQoL assessments may be discontinued when subjects are no longer compliant with the treatment plan. The analyses of these studies appear simple on the surface, but there is a real chance of selection bias. The analyst can no longer rely on the principle of randomization to avoid selection bias since unmeasured patient characteristics that confound the results may be unbalanced across the treatment arms.

2.4   Selection of Subjects

Ideally, the subjects who are involved in the HRQoL assessments are the same subjects who are evaluated for all of the study endpoints. This is recommended for several reasons [Gotay et al., 1992]. The first is practical. It is much easier to implement a study if all patients require the same assessments. The second is scientific. The credibility and interpretation of a study is increased when all subjects are evaluable for all endpoints.

In practice, there may be some limitations. Physical, cognitive or language barriers may make self-assessment infeasible. If the exclusions constitute a small proportion of the subjects it is unlikely to compromise the validity of the results. However, if the investigation involves a substantial proportion of subjects either initially or eventually unable to complete self-assessments, a strategy must be developed to deal with the issue. For example, in a study where progressive cognitive impairment is expected, a design option is to start with concurrent subject and proxy assessments, continuing the proxy assessments when the patient is no longer able to provide assessments. The value of this design will be discussed in later chapters.

In some cases, the number of subjects required to detect a clinically meaningful difference in the HRQoL endpoints is substantially smaller than that required for the other endpoints. If the resource savings are substantial enough to warrant the logistical difficulties of obtaining HRQoL assessment on a subset of patients, the selection must be done in a completely random manner. It is not acceptable to allow selection of the subjects by the researchers or even by the patients themselves as these methods are likely to introduce a selection bias.

Care should be taken when defining which subjects are excluded from an analysis. It is not uncommon to read a protocol where the analyses are limited to subjects with at least two HRQoL assessments (baseline and one follow-up). This criterion may change the population to which the results can be generalized by excluding all patients who drop out of the trial early. If this is a very small proportion of patients it will not matter. But if a substantial number of subjects on one or more arms of the trial drop out before the second HRQoL assessment, this rule could have a substantial impact on the results.

2.5 Longitudinal Designs

Longitudinal data arise in most HRQoL investigations because we are interested in how a disease or an intervention affects an individual's well-being over time. The optimal timing of HRQoL assessments depends on the disease, its treatment and the scientific question. The number and timing of HRQoL assessments is influenced by both the objectives and practical considerations such as when the investigators have access to the subjects. Some studies have event- or condition-driven designs. Other studies have periodic evaluations based on the time elapsed since the beginning of treatment or the onset of the disease. Some studies incorporate a mixture of these two designs. The timing of assessments influence how we approach the analysis of each study (see Chapters 3 and 4).

2.5.1 Event- or Condition-Driven Designs

When the objective of the study is to compare HRQoL in subjects experiencing the same condition, assessments are planned to occur at the time of clinically relevant events or to correspond to specific phases of the intervention. These designs are more common when the intervention or therapy is of limited duration. For example, one might consider a simple design with a pre- and post-intervention assessment when comparing the HRQoL after two surgical procedures. The adjuvant breast cancer trial (Study 1) provides a second example in which therapy is of limited duration. The design includes one assessment to measure HRQoL during each of the three phases: prior to, during, and after therapy. Many variations are possible. For example, there may be reasons to believe that differences in HRQoL may exist during only the early or later periods of therapy. In this case, the design would include a minimum of two assessments during therapy. Studies with a limited number of phases of interest in the scientific investigation, where HRQoL is expected to be constant during those phases, are amenable to an event-driven design. Analysis of this type of trial is described in detail in Chapter 3.

2.5.2   Time-Driven Designs

When the scientific questions involve a more extended period of time or the phases of the disease or its treatment are not distinct, the longitudinal designs are based on time. These designs are appropriate for chronic conditions where therapies are given over extended periods of time. In the migraine prevention (Study 2), lung cancer (Study 3) and renal cell carcinoma (Study 4) trials, therapy is intended to be given until there is evidence that it is ineffective or produced unacceptable toxicity. Thus the duration of therapy was indeterminate at the onset of the study. More obvious examples would include treatment of chronic conditions such as diabetes and arthritis. Timing in these designs is based on regularly spaced intervals (e.g., every three months), sometimes more frequent initially (e.g. every month for three months then every three months). Analysis of this type of trial is described in detail in Chapter 4.

2.5.3   Timing of the Initial HRQoL Assessment

It is critical that the initial assessment occurs prior to randomization. Because the measurement of HRQoL is generally based on self-evaluation, there is a potential that the knowledge of treatment assignment will influence a subject's responses [Brooks et al., 1998]. This is especially true when the patient is aware that one of the interventions is new, possibly more effective than standard therapy and exciting to his or her physician. The possible exception occurs if the intervention is double blinded. In this case, it is allowable to obtain initial assessment prior to the beginning of treatment but after randomization.

2.5.4   Timing of the Follow-Up HRQoL Assessments

Similar attention should be paid to the timing of follow-up assessments. Assessments should be made consistently across treatment arms. Attention should be paid to the timing of diagnostic procedures. Especially with life-threatening diseases, the choices are not particularly easy. Prior to the testing patients are likely to be experiencing stress in anticipation of the yet unknown results. After the procedure, the patients will either be experiencing great relief or anxiety depending on the results.

Individuals have better recall of major events and more recent experiences. The period of accurate recall for some constructs (e.g. physical well-being) is between one and four weeks. Recall of the frequency and severity of symptoms (e.g. pain) is accurate over shorter periods of time. There is an important distinction between questionnaires that are designed to specifically assess a symptom (e.g. pain or fatigue) and questionnaires that include symptoms in order to measure a construct involving the impact of symptoms. Shorter recall periods are appropriate for the former and longer for the later. Schipper [1990]

TABLE 2.1 Timing of HRQoL assessments relative to clinical and laboratory assessments.

Design 1: HRQoL less frequent								
Clinical/Labs	X		X		X		X		X
HRQoL	Q				Q				Q

Design 2: HRQoL linked with clinical								
Clinical	X		X		X		X		X
Labs	L	L	L	L	L	L	L	L	L
HRQoL	Q		Q		Q		Q		Q

Design 3: HRQoL linked with labs								
Clinical	X		X		X		X		X
Labs	L	L	L	L	L	L	L	L	L
HRQoL	Q	Q	Q	Q	Q	Q	Q	Q	Q

Design 4: HRQoL more frequent								
Clinical/Labs	X		X		X		X		X
HRQoL	Q	Q	Q	Q	Q	Q	Q	Q	Q

notes that the side effects of chemotherapy in cancer patients may have a less adverse effect on a patient's HRQoL than similar side effects attributable to the disease. This observation may be true in other disease conditions as well. Testing immediately after toxicity occurs will emphasize that experience and deemphasize the benefits of treatment and disease symptoms. It is important not to pick a particular timing that will automatically bias the results against one treatment arm. In studies where the timing and length of treatment differ across arms this may be challenging, if not impossible.

2.5.5 Frequency of Evaluations

The frequency of the assessments should correspond appropriately to the natural history of the disease and the likelihood of changes in HRQoL within that period. Other considerations are a practical follow-up schedule and the timing of therapeutic and diagnostic interventions. The assessments should be frequent enough to capture meaningful change but not so frequent as to be burdensome to the patient or incongruent with the assessment tool. If rapid change is expected during the early part of the study, more frequent early assessments are needed. In the renal cell carcinoma study (Study 4), assessments were planned more frequently during the early phase of the study than toward the end. However, in retrospect, even more assessments during the early phase of therapy would have been informative as HRQoL changed very rapidly during the early weeks of the treatment. Tang and McCorkle [2002] recommend weekly assessments in terminal cancer patients because of the short duration of survival and the dramatic changes in symptoms that occur in some patients.

Assessments should not be more frequent than the period of recall defined for the instrument. The quality of the patient's life does not generally change on an hourly or daily basis as one would expect for symptoms. HRQoL scales often request the subjects to base their evaluation on the last 7 days or 4 weeks. Thus, if the HRQoL instrument is based on recall over the previous month, assessments should not be weekly or daily. Scales assessing symptoms (Study 5) where there can be more rapid changes generally have a shorter recall duration.

2.5.6   Duration of HRQoL Assessments

First, it is important that the assessments take place over a period of sufficient duration to observe changes in HRQoL. Physiologic responses to a therapy may occur more rapidly than changes in HRQoL, especially social or emotional well-being. This is especially true for chronic diseases that have associated physical or functional disabilities.

For practical reasons it is wise to define a specific limit to the duration of assessment specifically avoiding statements such as "and every 6 months thereafter." This is another situation that illustrates the need to have a well-defined objective. For example, are the investigators interested in the HRQoL of subjects while on a therapy that is of limited duration or is it especially important to understand the long-term impact of the treatment on HRQoL? If the former, the additional information that can be obtained from continued assessments may diminish after some point either because there is little or no change or because the number of subjects with assessments is too small to analyze. If none of the objectives of the study requires continued assessment, then follow-up beyond that point is unwarranted.

2.5.7   Assessment after Discontinuation of Therapy

A very clear policy needs to be developed for following patients who cannot follow the treatment protocol. There are two major considerations when developing this policy. The first aspect is practical; the off-treatment assessments are often difficult to obtain, especially if the patient no longer remains under the care of the same physician.

The second aspect to be considered is scientific and depends on the research question. If the discontinuation of treatment limits any future therapy to more intensive and toxic treatments or eliminates treatment options altogether as the disease progresses, the failure to continue HRQoL assessment can lead to selection bias and over optimistic estimates. A treatment arm with a high rate of dropout may appear artificially beneficial because only the healthiest of the patients remain on the treatment. On the other hand, discontinuation of assessment may make scientific sense in other disease settings. The conservative approach is to continue HRQoL assessment; the off-therapy assessments can always be excluded if later deemed uninformative with respect to the research question. The opposite is not true; one can never retrospectively obtain the off-therapy assessments at a later date if they are determined to be of interest.

2.6   Selection of Measurement Instrument(s)

Guyatt et al. [1991] define an *instrument* to include the questionnaire, the method of administration, instructions for administration, the method of scoring and analysis and interpretation for a health status measure. All these aspects are important when evaluating the suitability of an instrument for a clinical trial (Figure 2.3). Many of the steps in the selection of the HRQoL instrument(s) for a trial can be accomplished by examining the literature and the questions posed in the instrument. However, empirical data are also valuable especially with diseases or treatments that have not been previously studied. Bouchet [2000] describe a pilot study in which they evaluated three possible measures for a primary prevention trial. Included in the evaluation were ceiling effects, convergent validity, known-groups discrimination, reproducibility among individuals reporting no change, responsiveness among individuals reporting change.

Selecting a previously validated instrument is vastly preferable to the use of a new unvalidated instrument [Streiner and Norman, 1995]. Developing a new instrument is expensive, time-consuming and should be undertaken only when existing instruments clearly are unsuitable. Clinical researchers who have never undertaken this task may severely underestimate the time and effort required. Instrument development is not limited to the generation of a list of questions and use in a single clinical trial. Development involves numerous steps of item generation (patient input and expert panels), cognitive interviews evaluating comprehension of questionnaire wording (pilot tests with probing questions), data collection in a wide range of patients receiving the entire range of treatment options, item reduction, validation studies, translation and cultural adaptation. Development of a new instrument can easily require 3 or more years and is often a career consuming endeavor. The final limitation is that unvalidated instruments or questions may not be accepted in trials used for regulatory approval.

FIGURE 2.3 Checklist for the selection of measurement instrument(s) for a clinical trial.

√ Identification of the construct to be measured.

√ Does the instrument measure what it proposes to measure?

√ Is the information relevant to the research question?

  – How well does the instrument cover the important aspects of what is to be measured?

  – Is a generic or disease-specific instrument more appropriate?

  – Heath status (rating scale) vs. patient preference (utility)?

√ Will the instrument discriminate among subjects in the study and will it detect change?

√ How well does the instrument predict related outcomes?

√ Are the questions appropriate for the subjects across time?

√ Are the format and mode of administration appropriate to the subjects and the trial?

√ Has the instrument been previously validated in the target or similar population? If not, what are the plans to do so for current study?

√ If using new instrument or items, the rationale and reasons they are indispensable

---

2.6.1 Trial Objectives

Ware et al. [1981] suggests:

> when searching for measures of health status, one first needs a clear understanding of the reasons for studying health status. A second requirement is a clear statement of the aspect of health being studied.

It is important to be clear on which of the different dimensions (physical, cognitive, emotional and social) are relevant to the specific research questions and verify that all relevant domains are included. If the objective is to provide data for economic evaluations a utility measure will facilitate the calculation of quality-adjusted life years. If the objective is to compare the impact of two therapies for the same condition on specific domains of disease specific HRQoL, a disease-specific instrument is the most suitable.

2.6.2 Validity and Reliability

There are numerous aspects and terms for the various components of reliability and validity of an instrument. For formal presentations of these concepts in greater depth, the reader is referred to one of the numerous textbooks presenting these definitions. A partial list specific to HRQoL includes Streiner and Norman [1995], McDowell and Newell [1996, chapters 1 and 2], Juniper et al. [1996], Naughton et al. [1996], Frank-Stromborg and Olsen [1997], Staquet, Hayes and Fayers [1998, Part IV] and Fayers and Machin [2000, chapters 3-7].

The validity of a measure in a particular setting is the most important and the most difficult aspect to establish. This is primarily because there are no gold standards against which the empirical measures of validity can be compared. In establishing the validity of measures of HRQoL, we compare the measure to other potentially flawed measures of HRQoL. Nonetheless, we can learn a good deal about an instrument by examining the instrument itself and the empirical information that has been collected.

The first questions about the content of an instrument "Does the instrument measure what it proposes to measure?" and "Are the questions comprehensible and without ambiguity?" are referred to as *face validity*. Note that across instruments the same label or descriptor is sometimes given to groups of questions that measure different constructs. The wording of the questions should be examined to establish whether the content of the questions is relevant to the population of subjects and the research question. Although expert opinion (physicians, nurses) may make this evaluation, it is wise to check with patients as they may have a different perspective.

Criterion validity is the strength of a relationship between the scale and a gold standard measure of the same construct. As there is no gold standard for the dimensions of quality of life, we rely on the demonstration of *construct validity*. This is the evidence that the instrument behaves as expected and shows similar relationships (*convergent validity*) and the lack of relationships (*divergent validity*) with other reliable measures for related and unrelated characteristics, respectively.

The next question is Would a subject give the same response at another time if they were experiencing the same HRQoL? This is referred to as *reliability*. If there is a lot of variation (noise) in responses for subjects experiencing the same level of HRQoL, then it is difficult to detect differences between subjects or changes over time. Finally, we ask Does the instrument discriminate among subjects who are experiencing different levels of HRQoL? and Is the instrument sensitive to changes that are considered important to the patient? These characteristics are referred to as *discriminant validity* and *responsiveness*.

Although all the above characteristics are necessary, responsiveness is the most important in a clinical trial as it directly affects the ability to detect changes that occur as the result of an intervention. One of the obvious factors that can affect responsiveness is the *and ceiling effects*. If responses are clustered at either end of the scale, it may not be possible to detect change due to interventions because scores can not get much higher or lower.

2.6.3 Appropriateness

Will the instrument discriminate among subjects in the study and will it detect change in the target population? Ware et al. [1981] suggest two general principles.

1. When studying general populations, consider using positively defined measures. Only some 15% of general population samples will have chronic physical limitations and some 10 to 20% will have substantial psychiatric impairment. Relying on negative definitions of health tells little or nothing about the health of the remaining 70 to 80% of general populations.

2. By contrast, when studying severely ill populations, the best strategy may be to emphasize measures of the negative end of the health status continuum.

Are the questions appropriate and unambiguous for subjects? One can not always assume that a questionnaire that works well in one setting will work well in all settings. For example, questions about the ability to perform the tasks of daily living, which make sense to individuals who are living in their own homes, may be confusing when administered to a patient who has been in the hospital for the past week. Questions about work may be problematic for students, homemakers and retired individuals. Similarly, questions about the amount of time spent in bed provide excellent discrimination for non-hospitalized subjects, but not for a hospitalized patient.

Are the questions appropriate for the subjects across time? In cases where the population is experiencing very different HRQoL over the length of the study, very careful attention must be paid to the selection of the instrument or instruments. Some studies will require difficult choices between the ability to discriminate among subjects during different phases of their disease and treatment. In the adjuvant breast cancer trial (Study 1), the subjects were free of any symptoms or detectable disease and at the time of the pre- and post-treatment assessments, they were much like the general population. During therapy, they were likely to be feeling ill from the side effects of the treatment. In the example, at the time that the study was planned there were very few choices of HRQoL instruments. The compromise was the selection of the Breast Chemotherapy Questionnaire (BCQ), which was very sensitive to chemotherapy side effects but may have been less sensitive to any post-treatment differences.

If an international trial, has the instrument been validated in other languages and cultures? Simple translation is unlikely to be adequate. There are numerous examples where investigators have found problems with certain questions as questionnaires are validated in different languages and cultures. Cognitive testing with subjects describing verbally what they are thinking as they form their responses has been very valuable when adapting a questionnaire to a new language or culture.

2.7 Conduct of HRQoL Assessments

In many clinical trials, the decision to include HRQoL assessments is made at the end of the planning phase. Often, a questionnaire is added to the data collection without any appreciation of the amount of staff time required and with no allocation of additional resources. This generally results in overly ambitious assessment schedules and large amounts of missing data, which make analysis difficult and results open to criticism. Although this behavior has decreased over time, there are still too many trials in which the details of how the HRQoL assessments are to be obtained are missing from the protocol and training materials.

Hopwood et al. [1997] surveyed 29 centers participating in one or more of three randomized trials for lung and head and neck cancer. They observed that there was a very high proportion of preventable missing data. The three most commonly reported problems were that staff were not available, questionnaires were not available and the staff considered the patient to be too ill. Pre-planning and budgeting have the potential to fix the first two problems. Education is needed to address the third.

2.7.1 Order and Place of Administration

The order and place of administration can influence the responses on a questionnaire. The effect is sometimes referred to as the *framing illusion*. Ordering of questions or questionnaires can influence responses. If questions about side effects of a treatment are asked before a global question about health status and overall quality of life, the responses to these later questions will have a stronger correlation with side effects. Sometimes the focusing is deliberate. The first question of the SF-36 asks the respondent to evaluate their health and is not used in the scoring of the eight domain scores; presumably the role of this question is to focus the respondent on their health. The M. D. Anderson Symptom Inventory (MDASI) [Cleeland et al., 2000] used in Study 5 first asks about the severity of symptoms and then the impact on daily living. Focusing the respondent on their disease and treatment may be appropriate when the goals are to compare difference in HRQoL that are directly attributable to the disease. It will not be appropriate when comparing individuals with disease to the general population.

There are a number of other factors that can similarly influence the responses. The place and timing, such as asking patients to complete questionnaire after they have gone through testing or have received news about their disease condition or bringing individuals back to settings (e.g. the hospital) where they have experienced painful procedures or have other negative memories [Noll and Fairclough, 2004], may influence responses. Answering the questionnaire at home may result in different responses than in a hospital/clinic environment [Wiklund et al., 1990]. Smith et al. [2006] demonstrated the influence of the content of an introduction during telephone surveys of Parkinson's disease patients on the responses.

2.7.2   Mode of Administration and Assistance by Third Parties

Methods of administration that have been used successfully in clinical trials include paper-and-pencil self-report, in-clinic face-to-face assessments with trained interviewers and centralized telephone administration with trained interviewers. Paper-and-pencil self-report is the most economical but requires that the patients be available on a regular basis. Interviewer administration is useful when the population has low literacy (children, immigrant populations), physical difficulty with pen-and-pencil forms (advance neurological conditions, hospice patients) or the questionnaire involves complex skip patterns (standard gamble assessments).

Schipper [1990] cautions against administration of an instrument designed for self-administration by a third party, noting several issues. There is evidence that self-report data differs from interview-generated data in ways that cannot be predicted. This is particularly true when there is the potential for the influence of personal relationships and social desirability on the responses. Great care must be taken to ensure that patients do not feel the need to please the clinical investigator with their answers. Similarly, patients may feel reluctant to answer the questions honestly in the presence of family and friends.

It is preferable to use the same mode throughout the study, unless it has been shown that responses are not affected by mode of administration. This advice is balanced by considerations of greater bias that can be introduced if this policy results in more non-response among selected groups of patients (e.g. those who are sicker). Often a compromise is required to balance feasibility and resources with ideal research conditions. Whatever procedures are selected, they should be carefully documented in the protocol and emphasized during training.

2.7.3   Data Collection and Key Personnel

First, it should be absolutely clear who is the key person at each clinical site responsible for administering the HRQoL. This will include, in addition to the usual responsibilities associated with the clinical trial, ensuring that there is someone who knows when the patient will arrive, will make sure the patient receives the questionnaire prior to undergoing diagnostic or therapeutic procedures and has a quiet place to complete the assessment; and is responsible for implementing follow-up procedures when the patient is not available as expected. At the time of the first assessment this key person should communicate the importance to the investigators of obtaining the patient's perspective, review the instructions with the subject, emphasize that there are no correct or incorrect responses, encourage the subjects to provide the best answer they can to every question and remind the patient that they will be asked to repeat the assessment at later dates (if applicable). This person may have the responsibility of reviewing the forms for missing responses, but care needs to be taken to balance confidentiality with the need to minimize missing data. If the assessment consists of an interview, it requires sufficient trained personnel to schedule and conduct the interview.

Second, there needs to be a system that identifies when patients are due for assessments. This may include preprinted orders in the patient's chart that identify which HRQoL assessments should be administered at each clinic visit. This process may be assisted by support from a central data management office where calendars and expectation notices are generated. Stickers on the patient's chart identifying them as part of a study may also be helpful. Other options include flow sheets, study calendars and patient tracking cards [Moinpour et al., 1989].

2.7.4 Avoiding Missing Data

Although analytic strategies exist for missing data, their use is much less satisfactory than initial prevention. Some missing data, such as that due to death, is not preventable. However, both primary and secondary prevention are desirable. In terms of *primary prevention*, missing data should be minimized at both the design and implementation stages of a clinical trial [Fairclough and Cella, 1996a, Young and Maher, 1999]. In most studies, a nurse or research coordinator is responsible for giving the HRQoL questionnaire to the patient. Among these individuals, the reasons for missing data include lack of time and perceived lack of physician support, inadequate protocols, lack of knowledge on justification and rationale for collecting HRQoL data, lack of remainders and lack of adequate sites for questionnaire completion [Young and Maher, 1999]. Thus, clearly specified procedures in the protocol for collecting HRQoL are the first step in minimizing missing data. This should include information on collection procedure if treatment schedule is disrupted and procedures for completion of the questionnaire when the patient requires assistance. Provide a system for prompting nurses/research personnel that a HRQoL assessment is due. Consider alternative methods to obtain follow-up data when patients do not complete questionnaires. Educate patients, research assistants and primary investigators about the importance of collecting these assessments on all patients willing to complete the questionnaire. Point out that reluctance to approach all patients on all occasions will lead to selection bias. The timing and duration of assessment should also be reasonable. Be practical about how often and how long you can follow patients.

Secondary prevention consists of gathering information that is useful in the analysis and interpretation of the results. This includes collection of data on factors that may contribute to missing assessments or predict the missing HRQoL measures. Thus, one should prospectively document reasons for missing data. The classifications that are used should be specified in a manner that helps the analyst decide whether the reason is related to the individual's HRQoL. For example, "Patient refusal" does not clarify this, but reasons such as "Patient refusal due to poor health" and "Patient refusal unrelated to health" will be useful. Other strategies for secondary prevention may include gathering concurrent data on toxicity, evaluations of health status by the clinical staff or HRQoL assessments from a caretaker. Uses of auxiliary data are discussed in later chapters.

Education

Education can be an important part of minimizing missing data. It must start at the investigator level and include research assistants (often nurses) as well the patient. Vehicles for education include the protocol (with strong justifications for the HRQoL assessments), symposia, video and written materials. Videos may be valuable both as training vehicles for research staff and for patients. Although there are often face-to-face training sessions at the initiation of a study, research personnel can change over time. Training tapes directed toward research personnel can deal with procedures in more detail than is possible in the protocol. Examples would include how to handle a patient who is not able to fill in the questionnaire and not letting family or friends assist with the completion of the questionnaire. Training tapes are especially useful for providing positive ways of approaching the patient. Instead of referring to participation as burdensome (e.g. "We have a lot of forms that you'll need to fill out"), the HRQoL assessment can be placed in a positive light [Cella et al., 1993a]:

> We want to know more about the quality of life of people as they go through this treatment and the only way to know is to ask you. In order to do this, we ask that you complete this brief questionnaire. It usually takes about (X) minutes ...

Hopwood et al. [1997] noted that, in three trials for lung and head and neck cancer, staff considering the patient to be too ill to complete the HRQoL assessments was the most commonly cited problem affecting the distribution of questionnaires. However, patient refusal was the least cited problem. It is understandable that study personnel are reluctant to approach patients when they appear to be feeling particularly ill, but to minimize the bias from selecting out these patients, all should be asked to complete the questionnaire. There may be ways of encouraging ill patients, specifically by providing conditions that make it as easy as possible for them to complete the questionnaire. When a patient refuses, of course, that refusal must be respected.

Patient information sheets, which explain to the patient the rationale behind the HRQoL assessments, will minimize missing data. These sheets can contain messages about the importance of the patient's perspective, that there are no "correct" answers to the questions and the reasons it is important to respond to every question and to complete the follow-up questionnaires. In addition to the persuasive information, the fact that patients can refuse without affecting their treatment or their relationship with their doctor should be included.

Data Collection Forms

The data collection forms should be attractive and professional in appearance, using fonts that are large enough to ensure readability (e.g. 12 point characters or greater). Do not use two-sided forms! First, patients will often not look at the back of the page. Second, if forms are copied at the sites, there is a high probability that only the front side will be copied.

Explicit Procedures for Follow-Up

A practical schedule with HRQoL assessments linked to planned treatment or follow-up visits can decrease the number of missing HRQoL assessments. When possible, it is wise to link HRQoL assessments with other clinical assessments (Designs 2 and 3 in Table 2.1). This has several advantages. The availability of the patient increases the likelihood that the HRQoL assessment will be completed. Staff may be more likely to remember when the HRQoL assessment is scheduled if the timing is linked to clinical or laboratory follow-up. Finally, it is possible to link clinical events and laboratory values to the HRQoL assessments for later analysis. Less frequent assessment of HRQoL (Design 1) decreases patient burden slightly but may introduce confusion about the schedule and thus lead to missed assessments. If more frequent assessments of HRQoL (Design 4) are specified in the design, strategies for obtaining the additional assessments must be identified. If the duration of HRQoL assessment continues after therapy is discontinued, this should be clearly stated and protocol flowcharts for treatment and assessments schedules should clearly reflect the difference.

The protocol and training materials should include specific procedures to minimize missing data. It should be clear what are the allowable windows of time for each assessment. The protocol should specify whether or not follow-up by telephone or mail is acceptable. Finally, since missing data will occur it is important to document the reasons for the missing assessment. When constructing the set of possible reasons, the responses should differentiate whether the non-response was likely to be related to the patient's HRQoL.

Documentation of the reasons for missing assessments can be combined with other questions about the conditions under which the HRQoL was administered. For example, What was the site and mode of administration? and Was any assistance given and if so by whom?

2.8   Scoring Instruments

Protocols should include explicit instructions or references to the instructions for creating summary or subscale scores for the HRQoL instruments. References to methodology should be accessible and not in hard-to-obtain manuals or personal communications. If the scoring procedure does not include a strategy for handling missing items, there is the potential for a substantial number of subjects to have missing scores even when they completed the assessment. If there are any proposed variations in the scoring procedure they also should be specified in the protocol. The FACT scales have characteristics that are found in many HRQoL health status measures and will be used to provide a concrete example.

2.8.1   Reverse Coding

The first step is to reverse the scoring of negatively worded questions (Table 2.2). Notice that, in contrast to most of the questions in the Social/Family Well-being section of the FACT (Table 2.3), a higher score is associated with a negative outcome for questions 9 (distant from friends) and 13 (communication is poor). A quick trick to reverse the coding is to add the lowest and highest possible score for the questions and subtract the response from that sum (see Table 2.2). For example, when the range of scores is 0 to 4, the sum is 4. If the responses to questions 9 and 13 were 2 and 3 respectively, the reverse scores are 4-2=2 and 4-3=1.

2.8.2   Scoring Multi-Item Scales

Most HRQoL instruments combine the responses from multiple questions to derive summated scores for the relevant dimensions of HRQoL. The motivation is to increase the reliability of the scores and to facilitate interpretation. The most widely used method of combining responses is the method of *summated ratings* or *Likert summated scales* [Fayers and Machin, 2000]. The total score is obtained by adding the responses from all items. For a scale containing k items, each scored from 0 to r, the summated score will range from 0 to $k \cdot r$. If the scale is scored from 1 to r, the summated score will range from k to $k \cdot r$.

TABLE 2.2 Reverse coding procedure of subtracting response from the sum of the lowest and highest possible responses to obtained reversed score.

Item Range:	Original Responses	0	1	2	3	4
0-4	Calculation	4-0	4-1	4-2	4-3	4-4
	Reversed Score	4	3	2	1	0
Item Range:	Original Responses	1	2	3	4	5
1 -5	Calculation	6-1	6-2	6-3	6-4	6-5
	Reversed Score	5	4	3	2	1

When the possible responses range from 0 to 4, sum is 4. When responses range from 1 to 5 sum is 6.

Because different scales (and even subscales within the same instrument) have a different number of items and a different range of responses, the range of these summated scores will have different ranges, making interpretation more difficult. For example, the emotional well-being score of the FACT (version 2) has a range of 0 to 20; the functional well-being, physical well-being and family social well-being scores have a range of 0 to 28 and the total score has a range of 0-140. It is common practice to standardize the summated scores to range from 0 to 100. This is done by subtracting the lowest possible summated score (S_{min}) from each score (S_i) and then multiplying the result by $100/(S_{max} - S_{min})$.

A much smaller number of HRQoL instruments use factor-analytic weights to construct scales. The source of these weights should be very carefully examined before blindly accepting them. The weights need to be established in very large representative samples of subjects that include all levels of disease (or lack of disease) and expected types of treatment. Fayers and Hand [1997] point out how sensitive the factor structure and resulting weights are to the population from which they were derived. Weights derived from another clinical trial or a selected population are likely to reflect the association of side effects of the specific treatments in that trial rather than the underlying construct.

2.8.3 Item nonresponse

It is not uncommon to have a small proportion (1 to 2%) of the items skipped. The frequency of missing item has been observed to be higher among elderly individuals [Kosinski et al., 2000] and those that are more ill. If the responses from selected patients are excluded from analysis because of missing items, there is a danger of biasing the results. Sometimes skipping an item is inadvertent, but it may also occur because a question is not applicable for that

TABLE 2.3 Sample questions from the Social/Family Well-Being subscale of the Functional Assessment of Cancer Therapy (FACT) questionnaire (Version 3).

Below is a list of statements that other people with your illness have said are important. **By circling one number per line, please indicate how true each statement has been for you during the past 7 days.**

SOCIAL/FAMILY WELL-BEING	not at all	a little bit	some-what	quite a bit	very much
9. I feel distant from my friends	0	1	2	3	4
10. I get emotional support from my family	0	1	2	3	4
11. I get support from my friends and neighbors	0	1	2	3	4
12. My family has accepted my illness	0	1	2	3	4
13. Family communications about my illness is poor	0	1	2	3	4
14. I feel close to my partner (or person who is my main support)	0	1	2	3	4
15. Have you been sexually active during the past year? No __ Yes __ If yes: I am satisfied with my sex life	0	1	2	3	4

subject. Question 13 of the Social/Family Well-being is a good example of a question that is skipped by some subjects. To avoid missing subscale scores because of one or two missing responses, most scales specify exactly how to score the question in the presence of missing items. When a strategy is specified for a particular instrument, that strategy should be used for scoring when reporting the results of a clinical trial unless the new strategy was specified in the protocol as an alternative scoring system.

The most typical strategy, sometimes referred to as the *half rule*, is to substitute the mean of the answered questions for that specific subscale for the missing responses as long as at least half the questions were answered. This strategy works well for scales where there is no particular ordering of the *difficulty* of the questions as in the FACT [Fairclough and Cella, 1996b] and the difficulty of the question does not have a wide range across the subscale items. It should be used cautiously (or not at all) when the questions have a hierarchy,* as when functional well-being is assessed through the ability to do certain activities (Table 2.4). The physical functioning scale of the SF-36 is a good example of a scale where the individual items have a wide range

---

*When questions have a strict hierarchy the scale is referred to as a Guttman scale.

of difficulty. If individuals are *limited a lot* in moderate activities, it is clear that they are also limited a lot in strenuous activities. Similarly, if subjects respond that they can walk a mile without limitations, they will also be able to walk several blocks. Special strategies may need to be specified for these types of questions [Kosinski et al., 2000].

TABLE 2.4 Selected physical function questions from the SF-36 Health Survey that have a roughly hierarchical structure.

The following items are about activities you might do during a typical day. **Does your health now limit you** in these activities? If so, how much?

	Yes, limited a lot	Yes limited a little	No, not limited at all
a) Vigorous activities, such as running, lifting heavy objects, participating in strenuous sports	0	1	2
b) Moderate activities, such as moving a table, pushing a vacuum cleaner, bowling or playing golf	0	1	2
c) Lifting or carrying groceries	0	1	2
d) Climbing several flights of stairs	0	1	2
e) Climbing one flight of stairs	0	1	2
f) Bending, kneeling or stooping	0	1	2
g) Walking more than a mile	0	1	2
h) Walking several blocks	0	1	2
i) Walking one block	0	1	2
j) Bathing or dressing yourself	0	1	2

2.9 Summary

- It is critical to establish explicit research objectives during protocol development. Details should include 1) constructs (domains) (e.g. Fatigue, Physical Well-being, Global HRQoL) underlying the critical hypotheses, 2) population, and 3) time frame relevant to the research questions.

- The HRQoL instruments should be selected carefully, ensuring that they are appropriate to the research question and the population under study. New instruments and questions should be considered only if all other options have been eliminated.

- The frequency and duration of HRQoL assessments should reflect the research objectives and the disease and treatment under study.

- The protocol should include explicit instructions for the conduct of the study to avoid bias and missing data. Educational materials for research staff and patients will be useful.

3

Models for Longitudinal Studies I

3.1 Introduction

In most clinical trials our ultimate goal is to compare the affects of interventions between treatment groups. As the first step we will need to develop a good model for the changes over time within groups defined by treatment or other patient characteristics. In the previous chapter, event- or condition-driven and time-driven designs are briefly described. These designs have corresponding analytic models: a repeated measures model and a growth curve model. In this introduction, I will discuss the choice between the two models. In a repeated measures model, *time* is conceptualized as a categorical variable. Each assessment must be assigned to one category. The remainder of this chapter addresses the analysis of studies with event-driven designs. In a growth curve model, *time* is conceptualized as a continuous variable. The following chapter will describe the analysis of mixed-effects growth curve models.

3.1.1 Repeated Measures Models

Repeated measures models are typically used in longitudinal studies with event-driven designs where there is a strong conceptual identity for each assessment. A good example is the adjuvant breast cancer study (Study 1) where assessments occurred during the three phases of the study: prior to therapy, while on therapy and 4 months after the end of therapy.

Repeated measures models may also be used in some studies with a limited number (two to four) of widely spaced assessments where it is feasible to classify each of the assessments uniquely as one of the repeated measures. For example, in the lung cancer trial study (Study 3), the four categories could be "Pre-therapy," "Early (6 weeks)," "Intermediate (12 weeks)" and "Extended (6 months)." Assignment of assessments to a planned assessment time (landmark event) may become difficult in studies with more numerous or closely timed assessments. If the windows are wide, an individual may have more than one observation within the window, requiring the analyst to discard all but one of the observations occurring within that window. Not only will this reduce the statistical power of the study, but it may also lead to biased estimates depending on how the observations are selected to be discarded. For example, bias may occur if discarded assessments are those delayed when individuals are experiencing toxicity. Using narrow intervals may lead to fewer subjects with data at each landmark. This creates instability of the estimation of both the means and the covariance. In summary, one of the restrictions associated with the choice of a repeated measures model is the necessity of pairing each assessment with a unique landmark event.

The analytic approaches to fit these repeated measures models that will be described in this book are based on maximum likelihood estimation and accommodate both incomplete data and time-varying covariates. In SAS and SPSS, we will use the MIXED procedure and in R we will use the gls function. While the model is not strictly a *mixed-effects model*, it has been strongly associated with that term. In one publication, the reviewers requested that I describe the analysis as "a mixed-effects model that considered assessment identifier (time point) as a categorical factor and used an unstructured variance-covariance matrix to model the covariance structure among each subject's repeated measures." Pinheiro and Bates [2000] state "This extended linear model can be thought of as an extended linear mixed effects model with no random effects."

3.1.2   Growth Curve Models

The term *growth curve models* comes from applications designed to describe changes in height and weight as a function of age. Measurements are taken at different ages for each child in a study. Curves are fit to the data to estimate the typical height or weight for a child as a function of age. The same concept is relevant when we want to describe changes in HRQoL as a function of time. The curves can be defined in many ways but are most often described by a polynomial function or a piecewise linear regression. The simplest example of a growth curve model is a straight line.

Growth curve models are useful in several settings. The first is when the timing of assessments differs widely among individuals. Growth curve models are also useful in studies with a large number of HRQoL assessments, where it is feasible to model changes over time with a smaller number of parameters than is required for a repeated measures model. Finally, analytic approach using a mixed-effects model may be necessary to model HRQoL in the presence of dropout (Chapters 10 and 11).

3.1.3   Selection between Models

In some longitudinal studies, either a repeated measures or growth curve approach is appropriate. But in most studies there will be clear reasons for preferring one or the other of these approaches. Although the schedule for HRQoL assessments is often constrained by practical considerations, such as the timing of patient visits, the research question and the analytic methods

appropriate for that question should be the primary consideration in the selection between the models. Both models can be used to understand how
individuals change over time, how interventions affect that change and how
patient characteristics modify the treatment effects.

Adjuvant Breast Cancer Trial (Study 1)

The adjuvant breast cancer trial is a clear example of a design that requires the
use of a repeated measures model. Each of the three assessments was planned
to measure HRQoL at a different phase of the study. There is variation in the
timing of these landmark events, especially the final assessments, scheduled 4
months after the completion of therapy, which did not occur at the same time
for the two treatment arms (see Figure 1.2). Some post-therapy observations
also occurred earlier than scheduled when a patient discontinued therapy early.
However, the intent of the design was to compare HRQoL when subjects had
been off therapy long enough to recover from the effects of acute toxicity.
Thus, the exact timing of the HRQoL assessment relative to the time they
started therapy is less relevant than the time since completing therapy.

Lung Cancer Trial (Study 3)

The lung cancer trial is a good example of when either a repeated measures
or a growth curve model can be justified. With only four assessments that
are widely spaced in time, it is possible to classify each assessment with a
landmark time. There are no cases where an individual had more than four
assessments and only a few cases where there is some question about whether
an assessment is closer to the 12- or to the 26-week target (Figure 1.3). The
growth curve model is also reasonable as treatment is continous and continues
as long as it is tolerable and effective.

Renal Cell Carcinoma Trial (Study 4)

A growth curve model is the practical choice in the renal cell carcinoma trial,
as the timing of assessments relative to randomization is frequent initially and
becomes more varied as time progresses (see Figure 1.4). Thus, it becomes
increasingly difficult to assign each observation to a landmark time. Forcing
this study into a repeated measures design will also produce unstable estimates
of covariance parameters during the later follow-up periods. It is also likely
in this study, with a maximum of 6 assessments per subject, that a growth
curve model will require less than 6 parameters to describe the trajectory of
the outcome measures over time, in contrast to the 6 parameters that would
be used in a repeated measures model.

3.2   Building Models for Longitudinal Studies

Consider a longitudinal study where n assessments of HRQoL are planned for each subject over the course of the study. We will consistently use h to indicate the hth group, i to designate each unique individual and j to indicate the jth assessment of the ith subject. Thus, y_{hij} indicates the jth observation of HRQoL on the ith individual in the hth group. The indicator of group (h) will often be dropped to simplify notation when it is not necessary to distinguish between groups.

A general linear model for the HRQoL outcomes can be expressed as

$$y_{ij} = x_{0ij}\beta_0 + x_{1ij}\beta_1 + \cdots + \epsilon_{ij} \tag{3.1}$$

or in matrix notation as:

$$Y_i = X_i\beta + \epsilon_i \tag{3.2}$$

where,

Y_i is the *complete data* vector of n planned observations of the outcome for the ith individual, which includes both the *observed data* Y_i^{obs} and *missing data* Y_i^{mis}

X_i is the design matrix of fixed covariates corresponding to the *complete data* (Y_i).

β is the corresponding vector of fixed-effects parameters.

ϵ_i is the vector of residual errors

Σ_i is the covariance of the *complete data* (Y_i) which is a known function of the vector of unknown variance parameters, τ: $\Sigma_i = f(\tau)$.

3.2.1   Advantages of the General Linear Model (GLM)

In this book all of the methods are based on a general linear model (GLM). I have chosen this approach for a number of reasons. Some of the advantages are:

1. **All available data.** The GLMs can use all observations where an outcome (y_{ij}) is measured and the covariates (x_{ij}) are known (observed). This is in contrast with traditional methods such as MANOVA, that delete the entire case when one of the observations is missing. As discussed further in Chapter 6, the assumptions about missing data for GLMs are more liberal than those that analyze only the complete cases.

2. **Time-varying covariates.** The GLMs have a very flexible structure for covariates, allowing different values over the course of time. Again, this is in contrast to MANOVA, which requires characteristics in the

model to either be constant over time or to vary in the same manner for all subjects. This allows us to create innovative models that include indicators of clinical events or measures. A special case is the explanatory variable for time which incorporates the exact timing of mistimed or unequally spaced observations into a growth curve type model.

3. **Flexible covariance structures**. The GLMs allow a wide range of covariance structures, a few of which will be described in this and the following chapter.

3.2.2 Building a General Linear Model

This general linear model can be formed as either a repeated measures model or a growth curve model. The recommended model building process [Diggle et al., 1994, Verbeke and Molenberghs, 1997] starts by defining a fully parameterized model for the means $(X_i\beta)$, then identifying the structure of Σ_i and then finally simplifying the mean structure. This later step may be omitted when the mean structure is not overly complicated (e.g. requiring a large number of parameters) and easily interpreted. Requirements to pre-specify the analysis plan may also limit the reduction steps. The details of the procedure are described in this chapter for repeated measures models and the following chapter for growth curve models.

3.2.3 Statistics Guiding Model Reduction

Likelihood Ratio Tests

Two models, one nested within the other, can be compared with a maximum likelihood (ML) ratio test [Jennrich and Schluchter, 1986] or restricted maximum likelihood (REML) ratio test [Littel et al., 1996, pg 278]. The statistics are constructed by subtracting the values of -2 times the log-likelihood and comparing the statistic with a χ^2 distribution with degrees of freedom equal to the difference in the number of parameters in the two covariance structures. Tests based on the REML are valid as long as the fixed effects in both models are the same. Thus either ML or REML ratio tests are valid when comparing nested covariance structures. However, likelihood ratio tests of the fixed-effects (β's) in nested models must be limited to the use of ML because the restricted likelihood adjustment depends upon the fixed-effects design matrix [Littel et al., 1996, pg 298,502].

To identify nesting, consider whether a set of restrictions on the parameters in one model can be used to define the other model. Typical restrictions are constraining a parameter to be zero ($\beta_a = 0$) or constraining two or more parameters to be equal to each other ($\beta_a = \beta_b = \beta_c$).

Other Statistics

Criteria such as Akaike's Information Criterion (AIC) and the Bayesian Information Criterion (BIC) are useful when comparing non-nested models. These statistics are equal to the -2 log likelihood values with an added penalty that is a function of the number of parameters estimated. The BIC imposes a greater penalty for additional parameters than the AIC, favoring more parsimonious models.

3.3   Building Repeated Measures Models: The Mean Structure

There are two components of a repeated measure model. The first component is the model for the average or means across time $(X_i\beta)$. The second component is the covariance structure $(Var(\epsilon_{ij}))$. Models for the mean structure will be discussed in this section and for the covariance in the following section of this chapter.

3.3.1   Treatment and Time

Repeated measures models for the HRQoL can be conceptualized several ways that are analytically equivalent. The parameters from the repeated measures models are interpreted in the same way that parameters are interpreted in simple regression. Consider a two-factor design with treatment arm and the landmark events as the factors. In the adjuvant breast cancer study we have two treatments and three landmark events: prior to therapy, during therapy and after therapy. There are a number of ways to create a model for this design, all of which will result in exactly the same results for any tests of hypotheses. In the text that follows, four (of many) possible models are presented.

Cell Mean Model

The simplest model for this study is a *cell mean model* with the mean HRQoL score estimated for each of the treatments by time combination (Table 3.1). The equation for the model is:

$$y_{hij} = \mu_{hj} + \epsilon_{hij}, \tag{3.3}$$

where μ_{hj} is the average HRQoL score for the jth measurement of the hth group.

TABLE 3.1 Study 1: repeated measures models in the adjuvant breast cancer trial with two factors, treatment (h) and time (j).

Cell Means Model

Parameters	Treatment Arm	Before Therapy	During Therapy	After Therapy
	CAF	μ_{11}	μ_{12}	μ_{13}
	16-week	μ_{21}	μ_{22}	μ_{23}
	Difference	$\hat{\mu}_{21} - \hat{\mu}_{11}$	$\hat{\mu}_{22} - \hat{\mu}_{12}$	$\hat{\mu}_{23} - \hat{\mu}_{13}$

Reference Row Model

Parameters	Treatment Arm	Before Therapy	During Therapy	After Therapy
	CAF	β_1	β_2	β_3
	16-week	$\beta_1 + \beta_4$	$\beta_2 + \beta_5$	$\beta_3 + \beta_6$
	Difference	β_4	β_5	β_6

Reference Cell Model

Parameters	Treatment Arm	Before Therapy	During Therapy	After Therapy
	CAF	γ_0	$\gamma_0 + \gamma_1$	$\gamma_0 + \gamma_2$
	16-week	$\gamma_0 + \gamma_3$	$\gamma_0 + \gamma_1 + \gamma_4$	$\gamma_0 + \gamma_2 + \gamma_5$
	Difference	γ_3	γ_4	γ_5

Center Point Model

Parameters	Treatment Arm	Before Therapy	During Therapy	After Therapy
	CAF	$\delta_1 - \delta_2/2$	$\delta_3 - \delta_4/2$	$\delta_5 - \delta_6/2$
	16-week	$\delta_1 + \delta_2/2$	$\delta_3 + \delta_4/2$	$\delta_5 + \delta_6/2$
	Difference	δ_2	δ_4	δ_6

Reference Group (Row) Model

An alternative model is a *reference group (row) model* with the mean HRQoL score estimated at each of the three time points for one of the two treatment groups, the reference group. Thus $\beta_1, \beta_2, \beta_3$ are estimates of the means at each of the timepoints for control arm. The remaining parameters estimate the difference between the reference group and the second treatment group $(\beta_4, \beta_5, \beta_6)$. The equation for the model is:

$$y_{hij} = \beta_j * I(time = j) + \beta_{3+j} * I(time = j) * I(tx = 2) + \epsilon_{hij}, \qquad (3.4)$$

where $I(time = j)$ is an indicator variable* that the assessment occurs at the jth measurement, and $I(tx = 2)$ is an indicator for the 2nd treatment group. Note that both this and the cell mean model have the same number of parameters (6) and each parameter in the reference row model can be written as a linear function of the parameters in the cell mean model ($\beta_1 = \mu_{11}, \beta_4 = \mu_{21} - \mu_{11}$. etc.). Thus the models are equivalent and any estimate of differences or hypothesis test will be identical.

Reference Cell Model

A third model is a *reference cell model* with one of the cells selected as a reference and its mean estimated by γ_0. The remaining parameters either estimate the relative difference over time in the reference group (γ_1, γ_2) or the added effect of assignment to the second treatment group at each of the repeated assessments $(\gamma_3, \gamma_4, \gamma_5)$. This model is also equivalent to the previous two models. The equation for this model is:

$$\begin{aligned} y_{hij} = \gamma_0 + \gamma_1 * I(time = 2) + \gamma_2 * I(time = 3) + \\ \gamma_3 * I(tx = 2) + \gamma_4 * I(time = 2) * I(tx = 2) + \\ + \gamma_5 * I(time = 3) * I(tx = 2) + \epsilon_{hij}. \end{aligned} \qquad (3.5)$$

Center Point Model

A fourth model is a a *center point model.* Three of the parameters (δ_1, δ_2, and δ_3) are interpreted as the marginal mean (average score) at each time-point. The remaining three scores (δ_1, δ_2, and δ_3) are the differences between the treatment groups. This model is fit using a *centered* indicator variable. Thus the indicator variable that generally takes on the values of 0 and 1 is transformed to a variable that takes on the values of $-1/2$ and $1/2$.

$$\begin{aligned} y_{hij} = \delta_1 + \delta_2 * (I(time = 1) - 1/2) + \\ \delta_3 + \delta_4 * (I(time = 2) - 1/2) + \\ \delta_5 + \delta_6 * (I(time = 3) - 1/2) + \epsilon_{hij}. \end{aligned} \qquad (3.6)$$

---

*Indicator variables have a value of 1 when the condition is true and 0 when it is false.

3.3.2 Common Baseline

In well-designed[†] randomized trials, the treatment groups are a random sample from the same population. As a result, any observed differences in baseline scores are much more likely to be the result of random variation rather than true underlying differences. Models with a common estimate of the mean scores at baseline both reflect this equivalence, provide a more precise estimate of the mean of the baseline scores and avoid over adjustment of estimates of the changes from the baseline assessment. In the cell mean model, we would add the constraint $\mu_{11} = \mu_{21}$. In the remaining models, we would drop β_4, γ_3 or δ_2 from the models. Details for the implementation are described in the following section.

3.3.3 Change from Baseline

An alternative analysis strategy is to model the change from baseline. This approach has both advantages and limitations. The major limitation occurs when there is missing data. While the models discussed previously include any subject with at least one assessment, analysis of the change from baseline requires that each subject has a baseline assessment and at least one follow-up assessment. As will be discussed in later chapters, this can lead to a selection bias and the randomized groups can no longer be assumed to belong to the same population of subjects. The advantages of randomization are lost and one can not make inferences applicable to an intent-to-treat analysis.

Care must also be taken when interpreting the parameters of the model, especially when covariates have been included in the model. The parameters associated with the covariates will have a very different interpretation than in the previous section. Very careful attention should be paid to how the covariates are coded. For example, if age is included in the model with no modification, we are estimating the difference between treatments in the change from baseline for individuals at birth. This may lead to a very different conclusion than if the covariate was age centered at the average age of participants in the trial. This will be discussed in more detail in Chapter 5.

3.3.4 Covariates

Other explanatory variables (covariates) can be added to the model when needed. An expanded presentation of models that test for moderation (effect modification) is presented in Chapter 5. Here we briefly address covariates that explain a significant proportion of the variation in the outcome, but are independent of the factors of interest in the trial. For example, if the effect of age is independent of treatment and time, but is expected to explain

---

[†] *Well-designed* implies blinded treatment assignment prior to the baseline assessment, adequate sample size and appropriate stratification of the random assignment.

variation in the outcome (Y), we can add age at the time of diagnosis (without interactions) to the model. The equation for the cell mean model is:

$$y_{hij} = \mu_{hj} + \beta_{age}\, x_i(age) + \epsilon_{hij}, \qquad (3.7)$$

where $x_i(age)$ =Age in years at diagnosis - 50. The interpretation of the other parameters (μ_{hj}) will change with the addition of these covariates. To facilitate the interpretation, it is advisable to center continuous covariates at a meaningful point. One option is to use the mean of the covariate for the entire sample. The alternative is to use a value close to that mean that is meaningful. In this example, the average age at diagnosis is approximately (but not exactly) 50 years, so the covariate is centered at that point. The interpretation of μ_{hj} is the expected (or average) HRQoL score for the jth measurement of the hth group for a woman who is 50 years of age. If we used age in years without centering, we would be estimating the mean HRQoL for a woman who is 0 years of age and the estimates of μ_{hj} may be outside the range of possible values. Even when estimates are within the range of possible values, appropriate interpretation of the other parameters is difficult.

More covariates can be added to the model as needed, including those in which there are interactions with treatment, time or both (see Chapter 5). However, there are costs for indiscriminate addition of covariates. Inclusion of covariates with missing values can create bias associated with the deletion of cases with missing values from the study.

3.3.5   Modeling the "Mean" Structure in SAS

In the adjuvant breast cancer study, the datafile BREAST3 has a unique record for each HRQoL assessment. PatID identifies the patient. FUNO identifies the time of the assessment with values of 1, 2 and 3. Trtment identifies the treatment arm.

Cell Mean Model

The first part of the MIXED procedure for a cell means model might appear as:

```
PROC MIXED DATA=BREAST3;
   * Cell Means Model *;
   CLASS FUNO Trtment;
   MODEL BCQ=FUNO*Trtment/NOINT SOLUTION  ddfm=KR;
```

The CLASS statement identifies Trtment and FUNO as categorical variables with two levels of treatment and three levels of time. The term FUNO*Trtment in the MODEL statement creates a design matrix corresponding to the cell means model previously displayed in Table 3.1. An additional term (referred to as the Intercept) is added by default to all models. To create a cell mean model we must suppress this intercept term by the adding NOINT option. The estimates of the means for each treatment by time combination are generated by the SOLUTION option in the MODEL statement:

```
                       Solution for Fixed Effects

                                 Treatment              Standard
Effect            Evaluation       Arm        Estimate    Error
FUNO*Trtment      Pre-Tx         Control       7.6821     0.1260
FUNO*Trtment      Pre-Tx         Experimental  7.5700     0.1266
FUNO*Trtment      During Tx      Control       6.7200     0.1536
FUNO*Trtment      During Tx      Experimental  6.1834     0.1558
FUNO*Trtment      Post-Tx        Control       8.0139     0.1181
FUNO*Trtment      Post-Tx        Experimental  7.9674     0.1212
```

With addition of the age covariate AGE_EVAL, the MIXED statements become:

```
PROC MIXED DATA=BREAST3 Method=ML;
   * Cell Means Model *;
   CLASS PatID FUNO Trtment;
   MODEL BCQ=FUNO*Trtment AGE_EVAL/NOINT SOLUTION  ddfm=KR;
```

Reference Row Model

The reference row model requires indicator variable for the experimental treatment arm. The first set of indicator variables can be created using the CLASS statement in the PROC MIXED procedure, but the second variable (EXP) must be created in a Data step.[‡]. The data step and the initial Proc MIXED statements would appear as:

```
DATA BREAST3B;
   SET BREAST3;
   EXP=(Trtment=2); * Creates indicator variable for Trtment=B *;
PROC MIXED DATA=BREAST3B  Method=ML;
   * Reference Row Model *;
   CLASS PatID FUNO;
   MODEL BCQ=FUNO FUNO*EXP/NOINT SOLUTION;
```

The output appears as follows. Note that the first three estimates are identical to those estimated for the control group using the cell mean model and the second three estimates represent the change from the control to the experimental group.

```
                  Solution for Fixed Effects

                                              Standard
      Effect      Evaluation    Estimate        Error
       FUNO       Pre-Tx         7.6821         0.1260
       FUNO       During Tx      6.7200         0.1536
       FUNO       Post-Tx        8.0139         0.1181
```

[‡]The statement EXP=(Trtment=2); is equivalent to the statements IF Trtment eq 2 THEN EXP=1; ELSE EXP=0;

```
EXP*FUNO     Pre-Tx       -0.1121      0.1786
EXP*FUNO     During Tx    -0.5367      0.2188
EXP*FUNO     Post-Tx      -0.04651     0.1692
```

Reference Cell and Center Point Models with Common Baseline

The reference cell model requires indicator variables for the two followup assessments (T2 and T3) and for the 16-week treatment arm (EXP). For this model we can use the default intercept to create the indicator variable for the reference cell. The DATA step and the initial PROC MIXED statements for the reference cell model would appear as:

```
DATA BREAST3C;
  SET BREAST3;
  EXP=(Trtment=2);     * Indicator for Exp Trtment *;
  EXP_C=EXP-.5;        * Centered Indicator for Exp Trtment *;
  T2=(FUNO eq 2);   * Indicator of FUNO=2 *;
  T3=(FUNO eq 3);   * Indicator of FUNO=3 *;

PROC MIXED DATA=BREAST3C;
  * Reference Cell Model with Common Baseline*;
  CLASS PatID FUNO;
  MODEL BCQ=T2 T3 T2*EXP T3*EXP/ SOLUTION;
```

Effect	Estimate	Standard Error	DF	t Value	Pr > |t|
Intercept	7.6263	0.08938	200	85.32	<.0001
T2	-0.9527	0.1137	180	-8.38	<.0001
T3	0.3585	0.1074	197	3.34	0.0010
T2*EXP	-0.4440	0.1624	181	-2.73	0.0069
T3*EXP	0.01156	0.1426	177	0.08	0.9355

The SAS statements for the center point model are identical except that EXP is replaced by EXP_C. The resulting parameters have the following interpretations: Intercept is the Pre-Tx mean (pooled across groups); T2 and T3 are the changes from Pre-Tx to During Tx and Post-Tx (pooled across groups); and T2*EXP_C and T3*EXP_C are the treatment differences During Tx and Post-Tx.

Effect	Estimate	Standard Error	DF	t Value	Pr > |t|
Intercept	7.6263	0.08938	200	85.32	<.0001
T2	-1.1747	0.08216	177	-14.30	<.0001
T3	0.3643	0.08291	169	4.39	<.0001
T2*EXP_C	-0.4440	0.1624	181	-2.73	0.0069
T3*EXP_C	0.01156	0.1426	177	0.08	0.9355

3.3.6   Modeling the "Mean" Structure in SPSS

We will use the same dataset, Breast3, described at the beginning of the previous section (Section 3.3.5). We will use the MIXED procedure or the *Mixed*

Effects Models option from the *Analyze* menu. For all the models, *Subjects* will be identified by `PatID`, *Repeated* by `FUNO` and *Repeated Covariance Type* will be identified as `Unstructured` in the first screen of options. In the second screen, the *Dependent* variable is identified as `BCQ`. We will select the *ML* option from the *Estimation* menu and *Parameter Estimates* and *Covariance of Residuals* from the *Statistics* menu in the second screen of options.[§]

Cell Mean Model

To create the cell mean model, we need to specify `FUNO` and `Trtment` as *Factors* and then in the *Fixed* menu, select *Factorial* and unselect *Include the Intercept*. The resulting statement is:

```
MIXED BCQ BY FUNO Trtment
  /FIXED=FUNO*Trtment | NOINT SSTYPE(3)
  /METHOD=ML
  /PRINT=R SOLUTION
  /REPEATED=FUNO | SUBJECT(PatID) COVTYPE(UN).
```

The resulting parameters are the same as previously presented in Section 3.3.5.

Reference Row Model

To create a reference row model, we must add an indicator variable for the experimental treatment arm `EXP` to the dataset which is added to the modeling options as a *Covariate* in the second screen. The model for the fixed effects is specified in the *Fixed* menu adding `FUNO` and the interaction of `FUNO` with `EXP` to the model. The resulting syntax is as follows:

```
COMPUTE EXP=(Trtment = 2).
EXECUTE.

MIXED BCQ BY FUNO WITH EXP
  /FIXED=FUNO FUNO*EXP | NOINT SSTYPE(3)
  /METHOD=ML
  /PRINT=R SOLUTION
  /REPEATED=FUNO | SUBJECT(PatID) COVTYPE(UN).
```

The results are the same as displayed in the previous section for `SAS`.

Center Point Model with Common Baseline

To create the cell mean model, we need to create three variables for this model, a centered indicator of the experimental therapy, and indicators for the second and third assessments. The model is built within the *Fixed* menu,

---

[§]SPSS Hint: After using the menu option to specify as much of the syntax as possible, it is recommenced that the user paste the resulting commands into a *Syntax Window* (e.g. a *.sps file), add the additional statements and run the commands from the *Syntax Window*.

first checking the *Include Intercept* and adding the terms for T2, T3, Exp_C*T2, and Exp_C*T3 into the model for the fixed effects.

```
COMPUTE EXP_C=(Trtment = 2)-.5.
COMPUTE T2=(FUNO eq 2).
COMPUTE T3=(FUNO eq 3).
VARIABLE LABELS  EXP_C 'Exp Therapy (centered)'
                 T2    'During Therapy'
                 T3    'Post Therapy'.
EXECUTE.
MIXED BCQ BY FUNO WITH EXP_C T2 T3
  /FIXED= T2 T3 EXP_C*T2 EXP_C*T3 | SSTYPE(3)
  /METHOD=ML
  /PRINT=R SOLUTION
  /REPEATED=FUNO | SUBJECT(PatID) COVTYPE(UN).
```

The parameter associated with `Intercept` is the Pre-Tx mean, `T2` is the average change from Pre-Tx to During Tx, `T3` is the average change from Pre-Tx to Post-Tx, and `T2*EXP_C` and `T3*Exp_C` are the treatment differences During Tx and Post-Tx.

3.3.7   Modeling the "Mean" Structure in R

We will use the same dataset, Breast3, described at the beginning of Section 3.3.5. We will use the `gls` function in the `nmle` library to fit the models.

Cell Mean Model

To create the cell mean model, we need to create two *factor* variables for the treatment groups and the repeated measures:

```
R> Breast3$TrtGrp=factor(Breast3$Trtment)
R> Breast3$FU=factor(Breast3$FUNO)
```

The cell mean model is then formed by crossing the two factors (`TrtGrp:FU`) and suppressing the default intercept (0 or -1) on the model argument of the gls function.

```
R> CMean.Var1 = gls(model=BCQ ~0+ TrtGrp:FU, data=Breast3,
 +                  correlation=corSymm(form= ~1|PatID),
 +                  weights=varIdent(form=~1|FUNO),
 +                  na.action=na.exclude,method="ML")
R> list(CMean.Var1)

Generalized least squares fit by maximum likelihood
  Model: BCQ ~ 0 + TrtGrp:FU
  Data: Breast
  Log-likelihood: -818.4947
```

```
Coefficients:
TrtGrp1:FU1 TrtGrp2:FU1 TrtGrp1:FU2 TrtGrp2:FU2 TrtGrp1:FU3 TrtGrp2:FU3
   7.682032    7.581269    6.718685    6.189271    8.015088    7.947676
```

Center Point Model with Common Baseline

To create a center point model, we need to create three variables for this model:

```
R> Breast$Exp_C=Breast$Trtment-1.5     # Centered Treatment
R> Breast$Time2=0
R> Breast$Time2[Breast$FUNO==2]=1      # Indicator of Time 2
R> Breast$Time3=0
R> Breast$Time3[Breast$FUNO==3]=1      # Indicator of Time 3
```

The center point model is then formed by specifying each term of the model argument of the `gls` function.

```
# Heteroscedastic unstructured covariance
R> CPnt.Var1=gls(model=BCQ~Time2+Time3+Time2:Exp_C+Time3:Exp_C,
 +   data=Breast,
 +   correlation=corSymm(form=~1|PatID), weights=varIdent(form=~1|FUNO),
 +   na.action=na.exclude, method="ML")
R> list(CPnt.Var1)

Generalized least squares fit by maximum likelihood
  Model: BCQ ~ Time2 + Time3 + Time2:Exp_C + Time3:Exp_C
  Data: Breast
  Log-likelihood: -818.6531

Coefficients:
(Intercept)        Time2        Time3 Time2:Exp_C Time3:Exp_C
 7.63197007  -1.17801300   0.34954553 -0.44908859 -0.01259171
```

The parameter associated with `Intercept` is the Pre-Tx mean, `Time2` is the average change from Pre-Tx to During Tx, `Time3` is the average change from Pre-Tx to Post-Tx, and `Time2:EXP_C` and `Time3:Exp_C` are the treatment differences During Tx and Post-Tx.

3.4 Building Repeated Measures Models: The Covariance Structure

The major difference between a univariate regression model for independent observations and a multivariate model for repeated measures is that the assessments for each individual are typically correlated over time, $Var[Y_i] = \Sigma_i$.

Examples of covariance structures include unstructured, Toplitz and compound symmetry (exchangeable) (Table 3.2).

TABLE 3.2 Examples of covariance structures for four repeated measures.

	# Parameters	Structure
Unstructured	10	$\begin{matrix} \sigma_1^2 & \sigma_{12} & \sigma_{13} & \sigma_{14} \\ & \sigma_2^2 & \sigma_{23} & \sigma_{24} \\ & & \sigma_3^2 & \sigma_{34} \\ & & & \sigma_4^2 \end{matrix}$
Heterogeneous Toplitz	7	$\begin{matrix} \sigma_1^2 & \sigma_1\sigma_2\rho_1 & \sigma_1\sigma_3\rho_2 & \sigma_1\sigma_4\rho_3 \\ & \sigma_2^2 & \sigma_2\sigma_3\rho_1 & \sigma_2\sigma_4\rho_2 \\ & & \sigma_3^2 & \sigma_3\sigma_4\rho_1 \\ & & & \sigma_4^2 \end{matrix}$
Heterogeneous Compound Symmetry	5	$\begin{matrix} \sigma_1^2 & \sigma_1\sigma_2\rho & \sigma_1\sigma_3\rho & \sigma_1\sigma_4\rho \\ & \sigma_2^2 & \sigma_2\sigma_3\rho & \sigma_2\sigma_4\rho \\ & & \sigma_3^2 & \sigma_3\sigma_4\rho \\ & & & \sigma_4^2 \end{matrix}$
Toplitz	4	$\begin{matrix} \sigma^2 & \sigma^2\rho_1 & \sigma^2\rho_2 & \sigma^2\rho_3 \\ & \sigma^2 & \sigma^2\rho_1 & \sigma^2\rho_2 \\ & & \sigma^2 & \sigma^2\rho_1 \\ & & & \sigma^2 \end{matrix}$
First-order Autoregressive Moving Average [$ARMA(1,1)$]	3	$\begin{matrix} \sigma^2 & \sigma^2\lambda & \sigma^2\lambda\rho & \sigma^2\lambda\rho^2 \\ & \sigma^2 & \sigma^2\lambda & \sigma^2\lambda\rho \\ & & \sigma^2 & \sigma^2\lambda \\ & & & \sigma^2 \end{matrix}$
Compound Symmetry	2	$\begin{matrix} \sigma^2 & \sigma^2\rho & \sigma^2\rho & \sigma^2\rho \\ & \sigma^2 & \sigma^2\rho & \sigma^2\rho \\ & & \sigma^2 & \sigma^2\rho \\ & & & \sigma^2 \end{matrix}$

Note that structures progress from the least structured at the top of the table to the most structured at the bottom of the table.

3.4.1 Unstructured Covariance

The unstructured covariance is the least restrictive and generally the best choice when the number of repeated measures is small. With only three assessments, this structure has six variance parameters. The variance of the

TABLE 3.3 Number of parameters required to model variance structures with two to seven repeated measures.

Structure	# of Repeated Measures					
	2	3	4	5	6	7
Unstructured	3	6	10	15	21	28
Heterogeneous Toplitz	3	5	7	9	11	13
Heterogeneous Compound	3	4	5	6	7	8
Toplitz	3	3	4	5	6	7
ARMA(1,1)	2	3	3	3	3	3
Compound Symmetry	2	2	2	2	2	2

Note that the number of parameters increases more rapidly for the least structured covariance matrices.

HRQoL measure at each time point $(\sigma_1^2, \sigma_2^2, \sigma_3^2)$ is allowed to be different. The need for this type of flexible structure is illustrated in the adjuvant breast cancer study (Table 3.4) where there is more variation in the HRQoL measure while the subjects are on therapy $(\sigma_2^2 = 2.28)$ than before or after therapy $(\sigma_1^2 = 1.43, \sigma_3^2 = 1.32)$. The covariance of each pair of HRQoL measures $(\sigma_{12}, \sigma_{13}, \sigma_{23})$ is also different. This may be appropriate in many trials, as it is not uncommon for assessments occurring during therapy to be more strongly correlated with each other than with the off therapy assessments.

When the number of repeated measures increases, the number of parameters increases dramatically. For example, as the number increases from 3 to 7 repeated measures the number of parameters increases from 6 to 28 in an unstructured covariance (Table 3.3). In large datasets with nearly complete follow-up, estimation of the covariance parameters is not a problem. But as the dropout increases, especially in smaller studies, it becomes more difficult to obtain stable estimates of all the covariance parameters. In these settings it may be advisable to place restrictions on the covariance structure.

3.4.2 Structured Covariance

There are numerous options for creating alternative covariance structures. In this section I focus on those most likely in trials with HRQoL measures and will start with the least structured and progress to the most structured. To illustrate this, let us rewrite the unstructured covariance matrix displayed in Table 3.2 in terms of the variance parameters and correlations.

$$\Sigma = \begin{bmatrix} \sigma_1^2 & \sigma_{12} & \sigma_{13} & \sigma_{14} \\ & \sigma_2^2 & \sigma_{23} & \sigma_{24} \\ & & \sigma_3^2 & \sigma_{34} \\ & & & \sigma_4^2 \end{bmatrix} = \begin{bmatrix} \sigma_1^2 & \sigma_1\sigma_2\rho_{12} & \sigma_1\sigma_3\rho_{13} & \sigma_1\sigma_4\rho_{14} \\ & \sigma_2^2 & \sigma_2\sigma_3\rho_{23} & \sigma_2\sigma_4\rho_{24} \\ & & \sigma_3^2 & \sigma_3\sigma_4\rho_{34} \\ & & & \sigma_4^2 \end{bmatrix} \quad (3.8)$$

Heterogeneous structures allow the variance $(\sigma_1^2, \sigma_2^2, \sigma_3^2, \sigma_4^2)$ vary across assessments whereas the homogenous structures assume that the variance is equal across assessments ($\sigma_1^2 = \sigma_2^2 = \sigma_3^2 = \sigma_4^2$). The unstructured covariance is a heterogeneous structure.

When HRQoL observations are taken closely in time, the correlation of the residual errors is likely to be strongest for observations that are close in time and weakest for observations that are the furthest apart. In the Toplitz structures, the correlations for all adjacent assessments are equal ($\rho_{12} = \rho_{23} = \rho_{34}$), for all paired assessments that are separated by one assessment ($\rho_{13} = \rho_{24}$), etc. Compound Symmetry assumes that the correlation among all visits is equal ($\rho_{12} = \rho_{23} = \rho_{34} = \rho_{13} = \rho_{24} = \rho_{14}$) regardless of how far apart in time the observations are taken. An autoregressive (AR(1)) structure (not shown) is a very restrictive structure. The covariance decays exponentially as a function of the time separation between the observations ($\rho_2 = \rho_1^2, \rho_3 = \rho_1^3$, etc.) and implies that as the time increases between assessments the correlation will eventually disappear. It is rare that the correlation of HRQoL measures declines this rapidly or ever become completely uncorrelated, even when the observations are far apart in time. The (ARMA(1,1)) provides a slightly more flexible structure with a less rapid decay.¶

More than one covariance structure is likely to provide a reasonable fit to the data. Most structured covariance matrices are nested within the unstructured matrix, as indicated by the restrictions described above and thus can be tested using likelihood ratio tests. The information criteria can be used to provide guidance. Unless the sample size for the study is very large, it is difficult to choose definitively among the various covariance structures. In the breast cancer trial, the estimates of this and the general unstructured covariance are very similar and the differences are unlikely to affect the results of the primary analyses (Table 3.4). The AR(1) structure is included in Table 3.4 to illustrate the rapid decrease in the correlation that generally will not be observed in studies measuring HRQoL.

There are numerous other possible covariance structures that are variations on these described here. Additional options for covariance structures are described in detail in other sources including Jennrich and Schluchter [1986], Jones [1993, chapter 3 and 6], Verbeke and Molenberghs [1997, chapter 3] and in the SAS Proc Mixed documentation [1996].

3.4.3   Building the Covariance Structure in SAS

In the adjuvant breast cancer example, there are only three repeated measures and enough observations to reliably estimate an unstructured covariance (Table 3.4). The unstructured covariance of the repeated measures is defined by the REPEATED statement with TYPE=UN. Selected options for TYPE= are specified in Table 3.2. METHOD=ML is added to the PROC statement to facilitate comparisons between different models. The expanded MIXED procedure assuming an unstructured covariance would appear as:

¶If $\lambda = \rho$, then the ARMA(1,1) is AR(1).

```
PROC MIXED DATA=BREAST3 METHOD=ML;
   title 'Center point Model with Common Baseline';
   title2 'Unstructured (General) Covariance Structure';
   CLASS PatID FUNO;
   MODEL BCQ=T2 T3 T2*EXP_C T3*EXP_C/ SOLUTION  ddfm=KR;
   repeated FUNO/subject=PatID type=un r rcorr;
```

The R and RCORR options request the output of the covariance and correlation matrices for the first subject. (R=2 and RCORR=2 would request the matrices for the second subject; useful if the first subject has incomplete data.)

Estimated R Matrix for PatID 1

Row	Col1	Col2	Col3
1	1.5311	1.1958	0.5889
2	1.1958	2.2412	1.1037
3	0.5889	1.1037	1.3044

Estimated R Correlation Matrix for PatID 1

Row	Col1	Col2	Col3
1	1.0000	0.6455	0.4167
2	0.6455	1.0000	0.6455
3	0.4167	0.6455	1.0000

The correlations estimated for the unstructured covariance range from 0.58 to 0.65, with the smallest correlation between the two observations furthest apart in time. This suggests that the correlation may be slightly decreasing as visits are spaced further apart. The increase in variation during the second assessment (during chemotherapy) suggests heterogeneity of the variance across the assessments.

As a final note, the most frequent error that I encounter when fitting any of these covariance structure occurs when there are more than a single observation associated with one of the landmarks (order categories). In this example, this would occur when a subject has more than one record associated with a value of FUNO. The error message is

```
NOTE: An infinite likelihood is assumed in iteration 0 because
of a nonpositive definite estimated R matrix for Subject XXX.
```

As previously discussed, each landmark can have only one assessment associated with it.

In summary, unless the data is sparse for some of the repeated measures, choosing an unstructured covariance will be the preferred strategy. This structure will always fit the data, though it may not be the most parsimonious. The analysis plan can be easily specified in advance and additional steps are eliminated.

TABLE 3.4 Study 1: Estimated covariance and correlation for the adjuvant breast cancer trial using the SAS or SPSS MIXED Procedure.

Structure	r	AIC	Covariance	Correlation
Unstructured	6	1656.6	1.58 1.32 0.83	1.00 0.70 0.58
TYPE=UN			2.27 1.05	1.00 0.61
COVTYPE(UN)			1.30	1.00
Heterogeneous	4	1658.3	1.57 1.17 0.92	1.00 0.63 0.63
Compound Symmetry			2.19 1.09	1.00 0.63
TYPE=CSH			1.37	1.00
COVTYPE(CSH)				
Homogeneous	2	1671.4	1.70 1.05 1.05	1.00 0.62 0.62
Compound Symmetry			1.70 1.05	1.00 0.62
TYPE=CS			1.70	1.00
COVTYPE(CS)				
Heterogeneous	4	1667.1	1.53 1.20 0.59	1.00 0.65 0.42
Autoregressive			2.24 1.10	1.00 0.65
TYPE=ARH(1)			1.30	1.00
COVTYPE(ARH1)				

r=Number of unique parameters in covariance structure
AIC=Akaike's Information Criterion, smaller values are better.

3.4.4 Building the Covariance Structure in SPSS

The options in SPSS parallel the options in SAS using the same abbreviations to indicate the various structures. For the unstructured covariance, the syntax is:

```
/REPEATED=FUNO | SUBJECT(PatID) COVTYPE(UN)
```

The alternative structures are obtained by modifying the argument of COVTYPE (See Table 3.4).

3.4.5 Building the Covariance Structure in R

The covariance structure is handled in a slightly different way in the gls function of R, with the structure having three components:

$$\Sigma_i = \sigma^2 V_i C_i V_i \tag{3.9}$$

$$Var(e_{ij}) = \sigma^2 [V_i]_{jj}^2 \tag{3.10}$$

$$cor(e_{ij}, e_{ik}) = [C_i]_{jk} \tag{3.11}$$

where C_i is a correlation matrix and V_i is diagonal matrix with one element constrained to be 1 and the rest to be positive values. For repeated measures models, the two most useful structures for C_i will be corSymm and corCompSymm corresponding to a general unstructured correlation matrix and compound symmetry, respectively. V_i allows us to specify whether the variance is homogeneous (constant over time) or heterogeneous.

TABLE 3.5 Study 1: Estimated components of the covariance and correlation for the breast cancer trial using the R function `gls`.

Structure	r	AIC	$\hat{\sigma}$	V_i	Correlation (C_i)		
Unstructured	6	1659.3	1.26	1.00	1.00	0.68	0.60
			1.19			1.00	0.61
			0.91				1.00
Heterogeneous	4	1665.1	1.25	1.00	1.00	0.63	0.63
Compound Symmetry			1.18			1.00	0.63
			0.93				1.00
Homogeneous	2	1693.5	1.30	1.00	1.00	0.62	0.62
Compound Symmetry				1.00		1.00	0.62
				1.00			1.00

r=Number of unique parameters in covariance structure
AIC=Akaike's Information Criterion, smaller values are better.

To generate the general unstructured covariance, we specify `correlation = corSymm(form=~1|PatID)` which indicates that the observations within each patient are correlated but observations between patients are not. To allow the variance to be heterogeneous across assessments, we specify `weights = varIdent(form=~1|FU)`.

```
R> CntrPnt.Var1=gls(model=BCQ ~Time2+Time3+Time2:EXP_C+Time3:EXP_C,
+               data=Breast3,
+               correlation=corSymm(form= ~1|PatID),
+               weights=varIdent(form=~1|FUNO),
+               na.action=na.exclude,method="ML")
R> list(CntrPnt.Var1)

Correlation Structure: General
 Formula: ~1 | PatID
 Parameter estimate(s):
 Correlation:
   1     2
2 0.679
3 0.598 0.608
Variance function:
 Structure: Different standard deviations per stratum
 Formula: ~1 | FUNO
 Parameter estimates:
         1         2         3
1.0000000 1.1885116 0.9140781
```

```
Degrees of freedom: 550 total; 545 residual
Residual standard error: 1.258944
```

While this output looks quite different from the SAS and SPSS output, the results are essentially the same (Table 3.5). The heterogeneous and homogeneous compound symmetry models can be fit by changing the `correlation` and `weights` options:

```
R># Heteroscedastic compound symmetry covariance
R>  CPnt.Var2 = update(CPnt.Var1,corr=corCompSymm(form=~1|PatID))

R># Heteroscedastic compound symmetry covariance
R>  CPnt.Var3 = update(CPnt.Var2,weights=varIdent(form=~1))
```

Note that because these three structures are nested, we can look at the likelihood ratio tests. Again, the results suggest that the general and the heterogeneous compound symmetric structures provide a similar fit, but the homogeneous compound symmetric structure is not appropriate.

```
R># Compare three variance structures
R>  anova(CPnt.Var1,CPnt.Var2,CPnt.Var3)
          Model df     AIC      BIC    logLik    Test  L.Ratio p-value
CPnt.Var1     1 11 1659.306 1706.715 -818.6531
CPnt.Var2     2  9 1658.329 1697.119 -820.1647 1 vs 2  3.02323  0.2206
CPnt.Var3     3  7 1671.360 1701.529 -828.6798 2 vs 3 17.03025  0.0002
```

As noted before, the unstructured general structures will be applicable in almost all trials, unless there are a large number of assessments with sparse data. However, for those who are interested in alternative structures that can be implemented in R, I would recommend Pinheiro and Bates [2000, Chapter 5].

3.5 Estimation and Hypothesis Testing

Although the *cell means model* generates estimates of the means for each treatment, we are usually interested in comparisons of these means. Any hypothesis that can be expressed as a linear combination of the estimated parameters (means) can be tested. For example, to test for differences at each time point the null hypotheses are:

$$H_0 : \mu_{21} = \mu_{11} \quad \text{vs.} \quad H_A : \mu_{21} \neq \mu_{11}$$
$$H_0 : \mu_{22} = \mu_{12} \quad \text{vs.} \quad H_A : \mu_{22} \neq \mu_{12}$$
$$H_0 : \mu_{23} = \mu_{13} \quad \text{vs.} \quad H_A : \mu_{23} \neq \mu_{13}$$

These equations can be rewritten, placing all parameters on one side of the equality:

$$H_0 : \mu_{21} - \mu_{11} = 0 \quad \text{vs.} \quad H_A : \mu_{21} - \mu_{11} \neq 0$$
$$H_0 : \mu_{22} - \mu_{12} = 0 \quad \text{vs.} \quad H_A : \mu_{22} - \mu_{12} \neq 0$$
$$H_0 : \mu_{23} - \mu_{13} = 0 \quad \text{vs.} \quad H_A : \mu_{23} - \mu_{13} \neq 0$$

Thus putting the parameters in exactly the same order as they appear in the SAS, SPSS or R output:

$$H_0 : -1\,\mu_{11} + 1\,\mu_{21} + 0\,\mu_{12} + 0\,\mu_{22} + 0\,\mu_{13} + 0\,\mu_{23} = 0 \qquad (3.12)$$
$$H_0 : \quad 0\,\mu_{11} + 0\,\mu_{21} - 1\,\mu_{12} + 1\,\mu_{22} + 0\,\mu_{13} + 0\,\mu_{23} = 0 \qquad (3.13)$$
$$H_0 : \quad 0\,\mu_{11} + 0\,\mu_{21} + 0\,\mu_{12} + 0\,\mu_{22} - 1\,\mu_{13} + 1\,\mu_{23} = 0 \qquad (3.14)$$

Alternative models such as the *center point with common baseline* generate parameters that reflect the hypotheses of interest, but do not generate estimates for most of the treatment by time combinations. Thus these values may also need to be estimated.

3.5.1 Estimation and Hypothesis Testing in SAS

In Proc MIXED, there are two statements that are particularly useful when constructing estimates or testing hypotheses that are linear functions of the parameters (β), ESTIMATE and CONTRAST. The CONTRAST statement is used for tests that have multiple degrees of freedom.

In the following examples, the option DDFM=KR is added to the MODEL statement. This option calculates the degrees of freedom of test statistics based on the actual design rather than relying on the variable names in the MODEL statement. As an aside, when there are numerous options for a particular aspect of fitting models (in this case determining the denominator degrees of freedom), it is a good indication that none of the options is preferred in all settings. (See the SAS Proc Mixed documentation [SAS, 1996] for further explanation.)

Cell Mean Model

As previously mentioned, the cell mean model automatically generates estimates for each treatment by time combination, but does not provide estimates or tests of treatment differences or changes over time. To estimate and test these treatment differences described above, we would use the ESTIMATE statement. The ESTIMATE statements corresponding to equations 3.12-3.14 would appear as:

```
* Estimates of Treatment Differences *;
ESTIMATE 'Pre-Therapy Diff'      FUNO*Trtment -1 1 0 0 0 0;
ESTIMATE 'During Therapy Diff'   FUNO*Trtment 0 0 -1 1 0 0;
ESTIMATE 'Post-Therapy Diff'     FUNO*Trtment 0 0 0 0 -1 1;
```

The results appear in the output as:

Label	Estimate	Standard Error	DF	t Value	Pr > |t|
Pre-Therapy Diff	0.1121	0.1786	200	0.63	0.5311
During Therapy Diff	0.5367	0.2188	173	2.45	0.0152
Post-Therapy Diff	0.04651	0.1692	168	0.27	0.7838

One might also consider an alternative hypothesis that patients in both treatments experienced a significant decline in HRQoL during therapy. The null hypotheses is:

$$H_0 : \mu_{12} - \mu_{11} = 0 \text{ and } \mu_{22} - \mu_{21} = 0$$

The hypotheses can be tested separately with ESTIMATE statements or jointly with the CONTRAST statement.

```
* Estimates of Change from Pre-therapy to During-therapy *;
ESTIMATE 'Change in Cntl pts'  FUNO*Trtment -1 0 1 0 0 0;
ESTIMATE 'Change in Exp  pts'  FUNO*Trtment 0 -1 0 1 0 0;
* Test Change from Pre-therapy to During-therapy  *;
CONTRAST 'During-Pre Change'   FUNO*Trtment -1 0 1 0 0 0,
                               FUNO*Trtment 0 -1 0 1 0 0;
```

Notice that the CONTRAST statement contains the same syntax for identifying the terms in the hypothesis as the two ESTIMATE statements, but they are separated by a comma. The estimates of change in the outcome measure while on therapy in the control and experimental arms represent declines of approximately 0.6 and 1.1 standard deviations;[||] for the BCQ measure, these are moderate and strong effects respectively [Cohen, 1988].

Label	Estimate	Standard Error	DF	t Value	Pr > |t|
Change in Cntl pts	-0.9621	0.1143	175	-8.42	<.0001
Change in Exp pts	-1.3867	0.1180	179	-11.75	<.0001

Contrasts

Label	Num DF	Den DF	F Value	Pr > F
During-Pre Change	2	177	104.47	<.0001

Center Point with a Common Baseline

In contrast to the cell mean model, the center point model estimates parameters that are the estimates of treatment differences during and post therapy. Since the associated null hypotheses are of the form $\beta = 0$, the tests results are

---

[||] -0.743/1.29 and -1.438/1.29 where $1.29 = \sqrt{\hat{\sigma}_1^2}$ and $\hat{\sigma}_1^2$ is the average baseline variance.

automatically displayed in the `Solution for Fixed Effects`. However, this model does not automatically generate estimates of the means for the treatment groups during or post therapy, nor does it test all hypotheses. So as with the cell mean model we will need to generate some additional estimates and tests.

The procedure is the same as described above. The analyst is advised to construct a table similar to that presented in the beginning of the chapter (Table 3.1) to facilitate this process. For this simple example, it might seem that this is not necessary, but it is a good habit to develop and is extremely useful as the models get more complicated. First, we can use this table to generate the estimates of the means for the treatment groups during and after therapy.

```
* Estimates of Means During and After Treatment *;
  ESTIMATE 'T2 Control' Intercept 1 T2 1 T2*EXP_C -.5;
  ESTIMATE 'T2 Experml' Intercept 1 T2 1 T2*EXP_C  .5;
  ESTIMATE 'T3 Control' Intercept 1 T3 1 T3*EXP_C -.5;
  ESTIMATE 'T3 Experml' Intercept 1 T3 1 T3*EXP_C  .5;
```

Similarly, we can estimate and test the change from baseline to during treatment.

```
* Estimates of Change from Pre-therapy to Post-therapy *;
  ESTIMATE 'Change in Cntl pts'   T2 1 T2*EXP_C -.5;
  ESTIMATE 'Change in Exp pts'    T2 1 T2*EXP_C  .5;
* Test Change from Pre-therapy to Post-therapy  *;
  CONTRAST 'During-Pre Change'    T2 1 T2*EXP_C -.5,
                                  T2 1 T2*EXP_C  .5;
```

3.5.2 Estimation and Hypothesis Testing in SPSS

The `/TEST= ...` option can be used in SPSS to construct estimates or test hypotheses that are linear functions of the parameters (β). The SPSS syntax has many of the same features as just presented for SAS.

Cell Mean Model

As previously mentioned, the cell mean model automatically generates estimates for each treatment by time combination, but does not provide estimates or tests of treatment differences or changes over time. To estimate and test these treatment differences described above, we would use the `TEST=` statement. Thus putting the parameters in exactly the same order as they appear in the output the statements would appear as:

```
/* Cell Mean Model */
MIXED BCQ BY FUNO Trtment
  /FIXED=FUNO*Trtment | NOINT
  /METHOD=ML
  /PRINT=  SOLUTION R
```

```
/REPEATED=FUNO | SUBJECT(PatID) COVTYPE(UN)
/TEST = 'Pre-Therapy Diff'        FUNO*Trtment -1 1 0 0 0 0
/TEST = 'During-Therapy Diff'     FUNO*Trtment 0 0 -1 1 0 0
/TEST = 'Post-Therapy Diff'       FUNO*Trtment 0 0 0 0 -1 1
/TEST= 'Change in Cntl Patients'  FUNO*Trtment -1 0 1 0 0 0
/TEST= 'Change in Exp Patients'   FUNO*Trtment 0 -1 0 1 0 0
/TEST = 'During-Pre Change'       FUNO*Trtment  -1 0 1 0 0 0;
                                  FUNO*Trtment 0 -1 0 1 0 0.
```

Notice that when a test involves multiple degrees of freedom the individual contrasts are separated by a semicolon as in the last test presented above.

Center Point with a Common Baseline

In contrast to the cell mean model, the center point model estimates parameters that are the estimates of treatment differences during and post therapy. Since the associated null hypotheses are of the form $\beta = 0$, the tests results are automatically displayed in the Solution for Fixed Effects. However, this model does not automatically generate estimates of the means for the treatment groups during or post therapy, nor does it test all hypotheses. So as with the cell mean model we will need to generate some additional estimates and tests.

As mentioned previously, the analyst is advised to construct a table similar to that presented in the beginning of the chapter (Table 3.1) to facilitate this process. The SPSS statements would appear as follows:

```
/* Center point with Common Baseline*/
MIXED BCQ BY FUNO WITH EXP_C T2 T3
  /FIXED= T2 T3 EXP_C*T2 EXP_C*T3 | SSTYPE(3)
  /METHOD=ML
  /PRINT=R SOLUTION
  /REPEATED=FUNO | SUBJECT(PatID) COVTYPE(UN)
  /TEST= 'T2 Control'        Intercept 1 T2 1 T2*EXP_C -.5
  /TEST= 'T2 Experml'        Intercept 1 T2 1 T2*EXP_C  .5
  /TEST= 'T3 Control'        Intercept 1 T3 1 T3*EXP_C -.5
  /TEST= 'T3 Experml'        Intercept 1 T3 1 T3*EXP_C  .5
  /TEST= 'Change in Cntl pts'  T2 1 T2*EXP_C -.5
  /TEST= 'Change in Exp pts'   T2 1 T2*EXP_C  .5
  /TEST= 'During-Pre Change'   T2 1 T2*EXP_C -.5;
                               T2 1 T2*EXP_C  .5.
```

3.5.3   Estimation and Hypothesis Testing in R

The functions in R were designed to facilitate the testing of nested models. Tests of nested models can be generated with the anova function. Estimation of linear functions of the parameters is possible with a series of statements that are illustrated below.

Cell Mean Model

As shown in Section 3.3.7, `model=BCQ~0+ TrtGrp:FU` generates the parameter of a cell mean model and the `summary` function displays details of the model.

Linear functions of the parameters, $\hat{\Theta} = C\hat{\beta}$, and univariate tests of the hypothesis $\Theta = 0$ can be constructed as follows: The first step is to create `est.beta`$=\hat{\beta}$ and `var.beta`$=Var(\hat{\beta})$:

```
R> est.beta= as.matrix(CMean.Var1$coef)    # Estimates of Beta
R> var.beta= CMean.Var1$var                # Variance of Estimates
```

Next, we define the linear contrasts, C.

```
R> C1=c(-1, 1, 0, 0, 0, 0)    # Pre-Tx Diff
R> C2=c(0, 0, -1, 1, 0, 0)    # During Tx Diff
R> C3=c(0, 0, 0, 0, -1, 1)    # Post Tx Diff
R> C=rbind(C1, C2, C3)
```

Then we compute $\hat{\theta}$, it variance and standard error, z-statistics and p-values for a 2-sided test.

```
R> est.theta=C %*% est.beta              # Compute theta
R> var.theta=C %*% var.beta %*% t(C)     # Variance
R> se.theta=sqrt(diag(var.theta))        # Standard Error
R> zval.theta=est.theta/se.theta         # Z-statistics
R> pval.theta=(1-pnorm(abs(zval.theta)))*2 # P-value
```

Finally, we put them together with labels and print.

```
R> results=cbind(est.theta,se.theta,zval.theta, pval.theta)
R> dimnames(results)[[2]]=c("Theta","SE","z","p-value")
R> print(results)
```

Again, I have written a function, `estCbeta`, to facilitate this (See Appendix R):

```
R> rownames(C)=c("Pre-Tx Diff","During Tx Diff","Post Tx Diff")
R> estCbeta(C,CMean.Var1$coef,CMean.Var1$var)
                    Theta        SE          z       p-val
Pre-Tx Diff     -0.10076308 0.1797944 -0.5604350 0.57518276
During Tx Diff  -0.52941432 0.2184827 -2.4231404 0.01538698
Post Tx Diff    -0.06741158 0.1711742 -0.3938185 0.69371503
```

If the sample size was much smaller, a simple z-statistic might not be appropriate, but it is more than satisfactory for these examples.

Center Point with a Common Baseline

When hypotheses can be set up as comparisons of nested models, it is relatively easy to perform these tests in R. For example, a test of the treatment differences for the center point model involves removing either one or both of the terms involving EXP_C.

```
R> CPnt.Mn2 = update(CPnt.Var1,model=BCQ~T2+T3+T3:EXP_C)
R> CPnt.Mn3 = update(CPnt.Var1,model=BCQ~T2+T3+T2:EXP_C)
R> CPnt.Mn23 = update(CPnt.Var1,model=BCQ~T2+T3)
```

Then we use the anova function to test a treatment effect during therapy, after therapy, or simultaneously.

```
R> anova(CPnt.Var1,CPnt.Mn23)
             Model df      AIC      BIC   logLik    Test  L.Ratio p-value
  CPnt.Var1      1 11 1667.688 1715.256 -822.8440
  CPnt.Mn23      2  9 1687.613 1726.533 -834.8067 1 vs 2 23.92531  <.0001
R>   anova(CPnt.Var1,CPnt.Mn23)  # Overall Test
           Model df      AIC      BIC   logLik    Test  L.Ratio p-value
CPnt.Var1      1 11 1659.306 1706.715 -818.6531
CPnt.Mn23      2  9 1663.369 1702.158 -822.6845 1 vs 2 8.062832  0.0177
R>   anova(CPnt.Var1,CPnt.Mn2)   # T2 only
           Model df      AIC      BIC   logLik    Test  L.Ratio p-value
CPnt.Var1      1 11 1659.306 1706.715 -818.6531
CPnt.Mn2       2 10 1664.656 1707.755 -822.3278 1 vs 2 7.349348  0.0067
R>   anova(CPnt.Var1,CPnt.Mn3)   # T3 only
           Model df      AIC      BIC   logLik    Test     L.Ratio p-value
CPnt.Var1      1 11 1659.306 1706.715 -818.6531
CPnt.Mn3       2 10 1657.314 1700.413 -818.6571 1 vs 2 0.008048903  0.9285
```

3.6 Summary

- Event-driven designs are generally associated with repeated measures models.

- A maximum likelihood (or restricted maximum likelihood) of estimation method that allows incomplete data and time-varying covariates (e.g. SAS or SPSS MIXED procedure or R gls function) is recommended.

- The recommended model building process starts by defining a fully parameterized model for the means $(X_i\beta)$, then identifying the structure of Σ_i and finally simplifying the mean structure.

- In the majority of settings, this final step will not be required nor feasible if analysis plans must be pre-specified.

- Except when the data are sparse, a general (unstructured) covariance structure is suitable for repeated measures models.

4

Models for Longitudinal Studies II

4.1 Introduction

This chapter focuses on analysis of longitudinal studies using mixed-effect growth-curve models for trials where *time* or other explantory variables are conceptualized as a continuous variable (e.g. time-driven design). Strategies for choosing between repeated measures and growth-curve models for longitudinal studies were discussed in the previous chapter. The most typical approach for modeling growth-curve models uses a *mixed-effects model.*[*] The term *mixed* refers to the mixture of *fixed* and *random* effects:

$$Y_i = \underbrace{X_i\beta}_{\text{Fixed effects}} + \underbrace{Z_i d_i}_{\text{Random effects}} + \underbrace{e_i}_{\text{Residual error}} \tag{4.1}$$

The fixed-effects $(X_i\beta)$ model the *average* trajectory. The fixed-effects are illustrated in Figure 4.1 by the bold line. The *fixed effects* are also referred to as the *mean response*, the *marginal expectation* of the response [Diggle et al., 1994] and the *average evolution* [Verbeke and Molenberghs, 1997, 2000]. The random effects model the variation among individuals relative to the average trajectory. The difference between the bold and dashed lines in Figure 4.1 represent the random effects $(Z_i d_i)$. In the figure there is both variation in the initial values (intercepts) and the rates of change (slopes) among the subjects. The variance of the random effects is also referred to as the between-subjects variation. The final component is the residual error and is represented by the difference between the symbols and the dashed lines. The variance of the residual errors is also referred to as the within-subject variation.

In the remainder of this chapter, two examples will be presented. The first will be the renal cell carcinoma trial (Study 3). I will use this trial in Sections 4.2-4.5 to present the development of a mixed-effects growth-curve model. The second example will be the migraine prevention trial (Study 2) and is presented in Section 4.6. I will use this trial to illustrate an alternative model that will be useful for trials where patients have varied responses to a treatment.

---

[*]Mixed-effect models are also referred to as linear mixed models, random effects models, random-coefficient model, and hierarchical models.

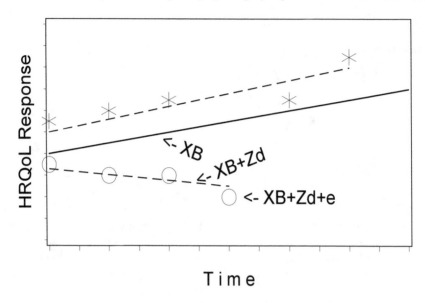

Time

FIGURE 4.1 A simple mixed effects model. The solid line represents the average response across all subjects, $X_i\beta$. The dashed lines represent the trajectories of individual subjects, $X_i\beta + Z_i d_i$. The stars and circles represent the actual observed responses, $X_i\beta + Z_i d_i + e_{ij}$.

4.2　Building Growth Curve Models: The "Mean" (Fixed Effects) Structure

Again we start the process of building a model for the longitudinal data by defining a working model for the means or the average trajectory of the outcome measure. Among the choices are polynomial and piecewise linear models.

4.2.1　Polynomial Models

The most typically taught method of fitting growth curves is to use a polynomial function to describe change. The general form is:

$$Y_{ij}(t) = \beta_0 + \beta_1 t_{ij} + \beta_2 t_{ij}^2 + \beta_3 t_{ij}^3 \cdots + \varepsilon_{ij}. \tag{4.2}$$

The purpose of the polynomial model is to approximate a curve that fits the observed data. There is no biological or theoretical reason that changes in HRQoL over time would follow a such a model. However, polynomial functions can provide a reasonable approximation of the average HRQoL. Figure 4.2 (left) shows how a polynomial model appears in the renal cell carcinoma example. The higher order terms, such as quadratic (t^2) and cubic (t^3) terms, allow the curves to depart from linearity.

The maximum number of terms (including the intercept) allowed to describe the trajectory over time is equal to the number of assessments. In the renal cell carcinoma study, there are 6 planned assessments so the model could include terms as high as t^5. In well-designed trials, more parsimonious models will be adequate to describe the trajectories.

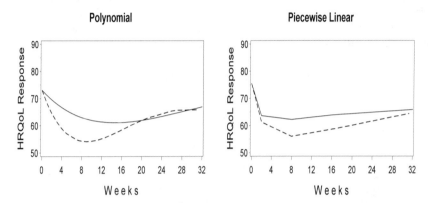

FIGURE 4.2 Study 4: Growth curve models for the FACT-TOI score among patients treated on the renal cell carcinoma trial (Study 4). (Control arm is the solid line and the Experimental arm is the dashed line.)

The major limitation of polynomial models is interpretation when the model contains higher order terms, such as quadratic or cubic. If a test of the equality of the curves is rejected because of differences in the coefficients, it is difficult to say how the curve differ without estimating the difference at specific points in time. An additional limitation of polynomial models is the tendency of the curves to exhibit abrupt changes at the end of the time span to achieve a better fit across the entire time span.

4.2.2 Piecewise Linear Regression

The *piecewise linear regression* model avoids some of the previously mentioned concerns of the polynomial models. The change in HRQoL is modeled as a linear function over short intervals of time. Although we do not expect changes in HRQoL to be strictly linear, it is reasonable to assume that changes are approximately linear over short intervals of time. Figure 4.2 (right) illustrates the use of a piecewise linear model for the renal cell carcinoma study. The general form of the model is:

$$Y_{ij}(t) = \beta_0 + \beta_1 t_{ij} + \beta_2 t_{ij}^{[2]} + \beta_3 t_{ij}^{[3]} + \cdots \varepsilon_{hij},$$
$$t_{hij}^{[c]} = \max(t_{hij} - T^{[c]}, 0) \tag{4.3}$$

In this model, the higher order terms $(t^{[c]})$ allow the curves to depart from linearity. But in contrast to the polynomial model, they model changes in the slope at $T^{[c]}$. Again, the maximum number of terms (including the intercept) is equal to the number of assessments. Figure 4.3 illustrates a model with a single change in the slope.[†] In this model, β_0 is the intercept and β_1 is the initial slope, thus $\beta_0 + \beta_1 t$ describes the initial trajectory. The slope is allowed to change at 8 Weeks by adding a new variable $(t^{[2]}, T^{[2]} = 8)$ indicating the time beyond 8 Weeks. β_2 is the change in the slope relative to β_1 and the sum of the two parameters, $\beta_1 + \beta_2$, describes the rate of change after Week 8.

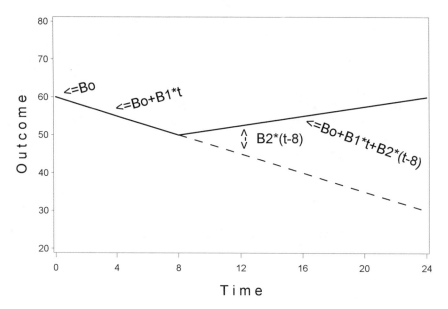

FIGURE 4.3 Study 4: A piecewise linear regression model with a change in the slope at 8 Weeks. $Y_{ij}(t) = \beta_0 + \beta_1 t_{ij} + \beta_{h2} t_{ij}^{[2]} + \varepsilon_{ij}, t_{ij}^{[2]} = max(t_{ij} - 8, 0)$. The intercept is defined by β_0, the initial slope by β_1 and the change in slope after 8 Weeks by β_2, thus the slope after Week 8 is $\beta_1 + \beta_2$.

The selected points of change should correspond to the times when changes

---

[†]These points of change are often referred to as *knots*.

in HRQoL might occur as the result of treatment or some other clinically relevant process. In most trials, this will be the points in time where observations are planned. In the renal cell carcinoma trial, we could consider terms that allow the slope to change at 2, 8, 17 and 34 Weeks.

The first step is to specify a fully parameterized model for the mean. To illustrate, consider the renal cell carcinoma trial (Study 4). We will start with a piecewise linear model that allows changes in the slope at 2, 8, 17 and 34 Weeks and has a common baseline. To construct the piecewise linear regression model, we create four new variables $(t_{ij}^{[2]}, t_{ij}^{[8]}, t_{ij}^{[17]}$ and $t_{ij}^{[34]}, t_{ij}^{[c]} = \max(t_{ij} - c, 0))$ to model possible changes in the slope at 2, 8, 17 and 34 Weeks. For the two treatment groups:

$$Y_{ij} = \beta_0 + \beta_1 t_{ij} + \beta_3 t_{ij}^{[2]} + \beta_5 t_{ij}^{[8]} + \beta_7 t_{ij}^{[17]} + \beta_9 t_{ij}^{[34]}$$
$$+ \cdots \varepsilon_{ij}, \qquad\qquad h = 1 \qquad (4.4)$$

$$= \beta_0 + \beta_2 t_{ij} + \beta_4 t_{ij}^{[2]} + \beta_6 t_{ij}^{[8]} + \beta_8 t_{ij}^{[17]} + \beta_{10} t_{ij}^{[34]}$$
$$+ \cdots \varepsilon_{ij}, \qquad\qquad h = 2 \qquad (4.5)$$

The datafile RENAL3 has a unique record for each HRQoL assessment and is created by merging RENAL1 and RENAL2 by the patient identifier, PatID. TOI2 is the score for the FACT-TOI rescaled so that the possible range is 0 to 100, Weeks identifies the time of the assessment relative to randomization and Trtment identifies the treatment arm.

4.2.3 Modeling the "Mean" Structure in SAS

First to fit the piecewise regression, we create four new variables.

```
DATA RENAL3;
  SET RENAL3;
  * Piecewise regression terms *;
  Week2=MAX(Weeks-2,0);
  Week8=MAX(Weeks-8,0);
  Week17=MAX(Weeks-17,0);
  Week34=MAX(Weeks-34,0);
RUN;
```

An alternative to the above statements is

```
        IF Weeks ge # then Weeks#=Weeks-#; ELSE Weeks#=0;,
```

where # is 2, 8, 17 or 34.

Then we fit the mixed effects model using the MIXED procedure. The first part of the code for this model might appear as:

```
PROC MIXED DATA=WORK.RENAL3 COVTEST IC METHOD=ML;
```

```
CLASS Trtment PatID;
* Piecewise Regression Model with common intercept*;
MODEL TOI=Trtment*Weeks Trtment*Week2 Trtment*Week8
         Trtment*Week17 Trtment*Week34
   /SOLUTION;
```

The CLASS statement identifies two levels of treatment. The terms in the MODEL statement create a design matrix corresponding to the model displayed in equation 4.3. If we wished to relax the assumption of a common baseline, Trtment is added to the MODEL statement along with the NOINT option.

```
* Piecewise Regression Model with separate intercepts*;
MODEL TOI=Trtment Trtment*Weeks Trtment*Week2 Trtment*Week8
         Trtment*Week17 Trtment*Week34
   /NOINT SOLUTION;
```

4.2.4   Modeling the "Mean" Structure in SPSS

First to fit the piecewise regression, we create four new variables.

```
COMPUTE Week2=MAX(Weeks-2,0).
COMPUTE Week8=MAX(Weeks-8,0).
COMPUTE Week17=MAX(Weeks-17,0).
COMPUTE Week34=MAX(Weeks-34,0).
EXECUTE.
```

Then we fit the mixed effects model using the MIXED procedure. The first part of the program for this model might appear as:

```
MIXED TOI2 BY Trtment WITH Weeks Week2 Week8 Week17 Week34
  /FIXED=Trtment*Weeks Trtment*Week2 Trtment*Week8 Trtment*Week17
         Trtment*Week34| SSTYPE(3)
```

Because Trtment follows BY it is treated as a factor, in this case having two levels. The remaining explanatory variables are treated as continuous covariates. If we wished to relax the assumption of a common baseline, Trtment is added to the FIXED= option along with the NOINT option.

```
MIXED TOI2 BY Trtment WITH Weeks Week2 Week8 Week17 Week34
  /FIXED=Trtment Trtment*Weeks Trtment*Week2 Trtment*Week8
         Trtment*Week17 Trtment*Week34| NOINT SSTYPE(3)
```

4.2.5   Modeling the "Mean" Structure in R

To fit the mixed effect growth-curve model, we create several new variables. The first converts the continuous indicator variable of the treatment groups (Trtment) to a variable of the *factor* class (TrtGrp). The remaining four variables will model the changes in the slope. Calculations for Week2 is illustrated below; Week8, Week17, and Week34 are created in like manner.

```
> Renal3$TrtGrp=factor(Renal3$Trtment)   # Creates a CLASS variable
> Week2=Renal3$Weeks-2                    # Week2=Weeks-2
> Week2[Week2<0]=0                        # Negative values set to zero
> Renal3$Week2=Week2                      # Stored in renal3
```

The function lme, from the nlme library of R, fits linear mixed effects models.[‡] It has three required components: fixed=, data=, and random=. fixed= defines $\mathbf{X}_i\beta$ and random= defines $\mathbf{Z}_i d_i$. Note that there is intercept term implied in each of these models. Adding 0 or -1 will suppress the default intercept. na.action=na.exclude excludes observations where variables are missing. method="ML" indicates that maximum likelihood rather than the default REML will be used. This is desirable when comparing models.

```
R> library(nlme)   # Loads functions from the nlme library
```

The following code fits a piecewise linear mixed effects model with a common intercept and changes over time at 2, 8, 17 and 34 weeks with two random effects. The results are stored in PW.Var2.

```
R> PW.full=lme(fixed=TOI2~Weeks:TrtGrp + Week2:TrtGrp + Week8:TrtGrp +
+ Week17:TrtGrp + Week34:TrtGrp,
+ data=Renal3, random=~1+Weeks|PatID, na.action=na.exclude,
+ method="ML")
R> summary(PW.full)
```

The command print(PW.full) displays a short listing of the results and summary(PW.full) displays more information. If we wished to relax the assumption of a common baseline, we would add 0+TrtGrp (suppressing the default intercept).

4.3 Building Growth Curve Models: The Covariance Structure

Because there are multiple assessments on each subject, we expect the assessments for each individual to be correlated over time. For mixed effects models, the covariance of the observations of the ith subject, Y_i, has the general structure:

$$\Sigma_i = Var(Y_i) = Var(Z_i d_i + e_i)$$
$$= Var(Z_i d_i) + Var(e_i)$$
$$= Z_i \mathcal{G} Z_i' + \mathcal{R}_i \qquad (4.6)$$

where $\mathcal{G}$ and $\mathcal{R}_i$ can have various structures. Modeling the covariance will have two components: the random effects, d_i and the residual errors, e_i.

[‡]An alternative function for mixed effects models is lmer from the lme4 library.

4.3.1   Variance of Random Effects ($\mathcal{G}$)

The simplest random-effects model has a single random effect. This model has a random term[§] for each individual where d_{i1} can be interpreted roughly as the average difference between the individual's response and the mean response, $X_i\beta$. This implies the variation between individuals does not change over time and the curves for each individual are parallel.

$$Z_i = [1], \quad \mathcal{G} = Var\left[\, d_{i1} \,\right] = \left[\varsigma_1^2 \right] \tag{4.7}$$

TABLE 4.1 Useful covariance structures for the random effects in a mixed-effects model with two random effects.

	# Parameters	Structure ($\mathcal{G}$)
Unstructured TYPE=UN COVTYPE(UN)	3	$\begin{matrix} \varsigma_1^2 & \varsigma_{12} \\ & \varsigma_2^2 \end{matrix}$
Unstructured (Cholesky Decomposition)* TYPE=FA0(2)	3	$\begin{matrix} \lambda_1^2 & \lambda_{11}\lambda_{21} \\ & \lambda_{21}^2 + \lambda_{22}^2 \end{matrix}$
Uncorrelated TYPE=VC COVTYPE(VC)	2	$\begin{matrix} \varsigma_1^2 & 0 \\ & \varsigma_2^2 \end{matrix}$

SAS: `TYPE=` and SPSS: `COVTYPE( )`
*Not available in SPSS; COVTYPE(FA1) has a different structure.

A more typical model for longitudinal studies has two random effects. The second random effect (d_{i2}) allows variation in the rate of change over time among individuals. This model has a random intercept and random slope for each individual ($Y_i = X_i\beta + d_{i1} + d_{i2}t_i + e_i$). In most examples, the two random effects are allowed to be correlated

$$Z_i = [\mathbf{1}\ t_i], \quad \mathcal{G} = Var\begin{bmatrix} d_{i1} \\ d_{i2} \end{bmatrix} = \begin{bmatrix} \varsigma_1^2 & \varsigma_{12} \\ \varsigma_{21} & \varsigma_2^2 \end{bmatrix}. \tag{4.8}$$

In some trials, we also might expect that there may be variation among individuals responses during the early, later or post- treatment phases. A third random effect (d_{i3}) allows us to incorporate this additional variation.

[§]This term is often referred to as the random intercept, even though in this case the interpretation differs.

$(Y_i = X_i\beta + d_{i1} + d_{i2}t_i + d_{i3}t_i^{[c]} + e_i)$. In theory we can keep adding random effects, but in most cases two or three random effects are sufficient to obtain a good approximation of the covariance structure.

The covariance structures may also differ among the treatment arms. For example, there may be more variation in the rate of change of HRQoL among patients receiving an active treatment than a placebo treatment, thus $\mathcal{G}_h \neq \mathcal{G}_{h'}$.

When the variance of one of the random effects is close to zero, an error message indicating that the covariance of the random effects is not positive definite will often appear. In practice, we might not consider this structure any further. But when we wish to estimate one of the information criteria statistics or fit the model for other purposes, an alternative parameterization to the unstructured variance is the Cholesky factorization or factor analytic structure. In SAS the option is TYPE=FA0(q) where q equals the number of random effects.[¶][‖] For two random effects,

$$\mathcal{G} = \begin{bmatrix} \varsigma_1^2 & \varsigma_{21} \\ \varsigma_{21} & \varsigma_2^2 \end{bmatrix} = \begin{bmatrix} \lambda_1^2 & \lambda_{11}\lambda_{21} \\ \lambda_{11}\lambda_{21} & \lambda_{21}^2 + \lambda_{22}^2 \end{bmatrix} \tag{4.9}$$

where λ_{11}=FA(1,1),λ_{21}=FA(2,1), and λ_{22}=FA(2,2).

4.3.2 Variance of Residual Errors ($\mathcal{R}_i$)

The second part of the variance models the within-subject variation. This structure, $\mathcal{R}_i$, can be as simple as $\sigma^2 I$ when the residual errors, e_{hij}, are uncorrelated. This occurs when most of the systematic variation is explained by the random effects. In some settings, especially those where assessments are close in time, there may exist some autocorrelation of the residual errors [Jones, 1993]. The most common alternative to the simple structure is a first order autoregressive error structure, AR(1), for equally spaced observations or the spatial power structure for unequally spaced observations (Table 4.2). The Toplitz structure relaxes the assumptions of the AR(1) structure, but requires more parameters. Note that these autoregressive structures can be useful when used to model the residual errors in combination with random effects; they are rarely suitable for the repeated measures setting because they do not incorporate the between subject variation that is typical of patient reported outcomes and health status measures.

As a warning, certain structures, such as compound symmetry, cannot be used for modeling $\mathcal{R}_i$. In the case of compound symmetry, both the random effects and $\mathcal{R}$ are modeling the between subject variation. In fact, when $Z_i = [1]$ and $\mathcal{R} = \sigma^2 I$, the covariance structure is the same as compound symmetry when the random effect is omitted.

[¶]This is the default in the R nlme functions.

[‖]SPSS has a version of the factor analytic structure, COVTYPE(FA1), but it has a different

TABLE 4.2 Useful covariance structures for the residual errors, $\mathcal{R}_{hi}$, in a mixed-effects model.

	# Parameters	Structure			
Simple ($\sigma^2 \mathbf{I}$) TYPE=SIMPLE COVTYPE(ID)	1	σ^2	0 σ^2	0 0 σ^2	0 0 0 σ^2
Autoregressive Equal Spacing TYPE=AR(1) COVTYPE(AR1)	2	σ^2	$\sigma^2\rho$ σ^2	$\sigma^2\rho^2$ $\sigma^2\rho$ σ^2	$\sigma^2\rho^3$ $\sigma^2\rho^2$ $\sigma^2\rho$ σ^2
Autoregressive Unequal Spacing* $\delta_{rc} = \lvert t_r - t_c \rvert$ TYPE=SP(POW)(*time_var*)	2	σ^2	$\sigma^2\rho^{\delta_{12}}$ σ^2	$\sigma^2\rho^{\delta_{13}}$ $\sigma^2\rho^{\delta_{23}}$ σ^2	$\sigma^2\rho^{\delta_{14}}$ $\sigma^2\rho^{\delta_{24}}$ $\sigma^2\rho^{\delta_{34}}$ σ^2
Toplitz Equal Spacing TYPE=TOEP COVTYPE(TP)	4	σ^2	$\sigma^2\rho_1$ σ^2	$\sigma^2\rho_2$ $\sigma^2\rho_1$ σ^2	$\sigma^2\rho_3$ $\sigma^2\rho_2$ $\sigma^2\rho_1$ σ^2

SAS: TYPE= and SPSS: COVTYPE( )
* Not an option in SPSS.

Returning to the renal cell carcinoma trial, we examine possible covariance structures. Tables 4.1 and 4.2 illustrate some possible combinations of covariance structures for the random effects and residual errors. In general it is advisable to start with a simple model and build up. I generally start with a model with two random effects and assume that the residual errors are uncorrelated. In our example, the first random effect is always the intercept. We use time, t_{ij}, as the second random effect. In some studies, especially if the trends over time are very non-linear (as in the renal cell carcinoma trial), I will examine the possibility of a third random effect. For the third random effect, we can choose when we believe there will be a change in the variation among patients. For example, we might choose $t_{ij}^{[2]}$, $t_{ij}^{[8]}$, or $t_{ij}^{[17]}$. In this example, a third random effect that allows variation among subjects in the rate of change after 8 weeks provides the better fit. If the variation in the slope is close to zero (usually causing a message that G is not positive definite (SAS) or that tests statistics associated with the parameters can not be computed (SPSS)),

---

structure that does not have the desirable properties of the Cholesky decomposition.

I will drop that random effect. After fitting the random effects portion, I may check for auto-correlation among the residual errors. In practice, once a good random effects model is fit, there is rarely residual autocorrelation unless the assessments are very frequent (e.g. daily or Weekly).

4.3.3 Building the Covariance Structure in SAS

The random effects contribution to the covariance structure is defined by the RANDOM statement. For a model with a single random effect that is homogeneous across groups, the following statement defines Z_i and $\mathcal{G}$:

```
* Single random effect (Equal across groups) *;
RANDOM INTERCEPT /SUBJECT=PatID TYPE=UN;
```

The term INTERCEPT defines $Z_i = [\mathbf{1}]$. Since $\mathcal{G}_h$ is a scalar, it is not necessary to specify the structure. With the TYPE=UN option, the estimate of ς_1^2 is displayed as UN(1,1).

A second random effect, allowing variation in the rate of change over time among subjects, can be added to the random-effects model. The following statement defines a model with two correlated random effects.

```
* Two correlated random effects *;
RANDOM INTERCEPT Weeks/SUBJECT=PatID TYPE=UN;
```

The second random effect is added to the RANDOM statement where Weeks defines $Z_{hi2} = t_{hi}$. TYPE=UN specifies an unstructured covariance of the random effects with 3 covariance parameters, UN(1,1), UN(1,2), UN(2,2), which correspond to ς_1^2, ς_{12} and ς_2^2. Adding a third random effect follows the same pattern.

The residual error contribution to the covariance structure is defined by the REPEATED statement. When this statement is omitted, a simple homogeneous structure is assumed ($\mathcal{R} = \sigma^2 I$) and displayed as Residual. The output for a model with two random effects and uncorrelated homoscedastic residual errors would have the following form:

Covariance Parameter Estimates – Two Random Effects

Cov Parm	Subject	Estimate	Standard Error	Z Value	Pr Z
UN(1,1)	PatID	145.40	20.5751	7.07	<.0001
UN(2,1)	PatID	0.2182	0.6128	0.36	0.7218
UN(2,2)	PatID	0.03464	0.02100	1.65	0.0496
Residual		96.2519	7.1418	13.48	<.0001

Additional random effects can be added. This trial is an example of a study in which there is evidence of a third random effect, in this case associated with the change in slope at Week 8.

Cov Parm	Subject	Estimate	Standard Error	Value	Pr Z
UN(1,1)	PatID	153.72	22.7400	6.76	<.0001
UN(2,1)	PatID	-2.5778	3.2203	-0.80	0.4234
UN(2,2)	PatID	2.4219	0.6137	3.95	<.0001
UN(3,1)	PatID	2.8923	3.8037	0.76	0.4470
UN(3,2)	PatID	-2.8359	0.7146	-3.97	<.0001
UN(3,3)	PatID	3.3700	0.8475	3.98	<.0001
Residual		69.2501	6.5515	10.57	<.0001

In this study, the almost perfect negative correlation of the random effects tells an interesting story, suggesting that those patients who had the most rapid decline in the first 8 weeks (second random effect) had the most rapid improvement after 8 weeks (third random effect) and the individual curves after 8 Weeks would be roughly parallel.

Estimated G Correlation Matrix

Row	Effect	Col1	Col2	Col3
1	Intercept	1.0000	-0.1336	0.1271
2	Weeks	-0.1336	1.0000	-0.9926
3	Week8	0.1271	-0.9926	1.0000

To test a model with autoregressive error structure for the residual variation, we would use the following procedure. Because the observations are unequally spaced we specified this as TYPE=SP(POW)(Weeks) where Weeks is the number of weeks since randomization. Note that Weeks has a unique value for each HRQoL assessment within a particular patient.

```
* Autoregressive structure for unequal spacing of Observations *;
REPEATED /SUBJECT=PatID TYPE=SP(POW)(Weeks);
```

The estimate of the additional parameter ρ is displayed as SP(POW). In this example, the model with three random effects and auto correlation would not converge. When the model was refit with two random effects, the information statistics (AIC and BIC) were larger than for the models without the autocorrelation.

Finally, we can consider whether there is more variation in subjects in one of the treatment groups. By adding GROUP=Trtment to either the REPEATED or the RANDOM statement, we request different estimates of $\mathcal{R}_h$ or $\mathcal{G}_h$ in each treatment arm.

4.3.4   Building the Covariance Structure in SPSS

SPSS has a similar approach with RANDOM= and REPEATED= subcommands. A model with two correlated random effects is specified as:

```
/RANDOM=INTERCEPT Weeks | SUBJECT(PatID) COVTYPE(UN)
```

The labeling of the output is similar to SAS, using UN(1,1) UN(1,2) and UN(2,2) to label the three parameters.

When the residual errors are assumed to be uncorrelated, the REPEATED= subcommand is omitted. With equally spaced observations, the REPEATED= subcommand can be used to test autocorrelation of the residual errors:

```
/REPEATED=FUNO | SUBJECT(PatID) COVTYPE(AR1)
```

4.3.5 Building the Covariance Structure in R

To fit models with two and three random effects, the update allows us to refit the reduced model (PW.full) previously described in Section 4.2.5 changing only the form of $Z_i d_i$.

```
> PW.Var1=update(PW.full,random=~1|PatID)             # 1 random effect
> PW.Var2=update(PW.full,random=~1+Weeks|PatID)       # 2 random effects
> PW.Var3=update(PW.full,random=~1+Weeks+Week8|PatID)# 3 random effects

> anova(PW.Var1,PW.Var2,PW.Var3)                       # Compare models
```

	Model	df	AIC	BIC	logLik	Test	L.Ratio	p-value
PW.Var1	1	13	5206.788	5264.969	-2590.394			
PW.Var2	2	15	5205.484	5272.616	-2587.742	1 vs 2	5.30431	0.0705
PW.Var3	3	18	5177.568	5258.125	-2570.784	2 vs 3	33.91647	<.0001

The anova() function compares nested models. Results are similar to those previously reported where the model with three random effects has the best fit to the data.

Auto correlation of the residuals, where the power is proportional to the time between observations, is added by specifying:

```
> PW.Var2AR=undate(PW.Var2,correlation=corCAR1(form=~Weeks))
> anova(PW.Var2,PW.Var2AR)
```

	Model	df	AIC	BIC	logLik	Test	L.Ratio	p-value
PW.Var2	1	15	5205.484	5272.616	-2587.742			
PW.Var2AR	2	16	5207.484	5279.091	-2587.742	1 vs 2	1.090e-06	0.9992

As before, it was difficult to test autocorrelation for the model with three random effects (results not shown), but clearly in the model with two random effects there is no autocorrelation.

4.4 Model Reduction

The goal in model reduction is not to obtain the most parsimonious model, but to obtain a model that is more easily interpreted than the full model.

In our example, it is theoretically possible to fit a polynomial with terms up to t^5 or a piecewise model with 6 terms. Typically, the shape of the curves changes early in the trial, but becomes approximately linear during the later stages and requires fewer parameters.

The strategy for simplifying the piecewise regression model is straightforward. Because the parameters model the *change* in the slope, failure to reject of a test of $\beta_b = 0$ implies that there is no change in the slope. Note that unlike the parameters of a polynomial model, this test can be performed for any of the parameters describing the trajectory. Thus, a test of change at 17 Weeks ($\beta_7 = 0, \beta_8 = 0$) is highly non-significant ($F_{2,168} = 0.15, p = 0.86$) as was a subsequent test of change at 34 Weeks ($\beta_9 = 0, \beta_{10} = 0$; $F_{2,170} = 0.71, p = 0.49$). When tests are marginal ($p < 0.2$), it is the analyst's decision as to whether to retain these parameters or not. I am generally conservative and retain the parameters.

4.5   Hypothesis Testing and Estimation

Overall Test of Differences between Curves

An overall test of differences between two or more growth curves is straightforward; it is the comparison of the parameters across the H groups. For example, if the growth curve is estimated by a quadratic equation with a common intercept, we would simultaneously test the equality of the β coefficients for linear and quadratic terms. This test does not provide information about when the groups may be experiencing differences in HRQoL, nor whether one group is experiencing better HRQoL than another.

Returning to our example, the overall test of post-randomization differences among the two treatment groups can be constructed by simultaneously comparing the parameters of the two growth curves:

$$H_0 : \beta_1 = \beta_2, \beta_3 = \beta_4, \beta_5 = \beta_6, \tag{4.10}$$

A test of this hypothesis yields $F_{3,172} = 1.75, p = 0.16$, indicating no overall difference between the curves. However, if we had rejected the hypothesis, the obvious question would be how do the curves differ and which group is superior. We could take one of three approaches: construct a summary measure (see Chapter 14), select timepoints of interest or contrast the rates of change within selected intervals.

Area under the Curve

One example of a summary measure is the area under the curve (AUC) which can be written as a linear combination of the parameters of a growth curve model. By contrasting the estimate of the AUC for each treatment group we would be able to say which curve was generally higher or lower.

The equation to generate the estimated AUC can be obtained by integration using a single simple rule: $\int_a^b c^p \partial t = \frac{c}{p} t^{p+1} \big|_a^b$. So

$$AUC(t) = \int_{t=0}^{T} X \hat{\beta} \partial t \tag{4.11}$$

$$= \int_{t=0}^{T} (\hat{\beta}_0 + \hat{\beta}_1 t + \hat{\beta}_3 t^{[2]} + \hat{\beta}_5 t^{[8]}$$

$$= \hat{\beta}_0 t \Big|_{t=0}^{T} + \hat{\beta}_1 \frac{t^2}{2} \Big|_{t=0}^{T} + \hat{\beta}_3 \frac{t^{[2]2}}{2} \Big|_{t^{[2]}=0}^{T-2} + \hat{\beta}_5 \frac{t^{[8]2}}{2} \Big|_{t^{[8]}=0}^{T-8}$$

$$= \hat{\beta}_0 T - 0 + \frac{\hat{\beta}_1}{2} T^2 + \frac{\hat{\beta}_3}{2}(T-2)^2 + \frac{\hat{\beta}_5}{2}(T-8)^2$$

for the first treatment group. If we evaluate this over 6 months (26 Weeks), then

$$AUC(26) = \hat{\beta}_0 * 26 + \hat{\beta}_1 * \frac{26^2}{2} + \hat{\beta}_3 * \frac{24^2}{2} + \hat{\beta}_5 * \frac{18^2}{2}, \quad h = 1$$

$$= \hat{\beta}_0 * 26 + \hat{\beta}_2 * \frac{26^2}{2} + \hat{\beta}_4 * \frac{24^2}{2} + \hat{\beta}_6 * \frac{18^2}{2}, \quad h = 2$$

Note that this is a linear combination of the $\hat{\beta}$s and can be easily estimated. In our example, we obtain estimates of 1648 and 1536 for the standard and experimental treatment groups, suggesting that the scores are higher on average over 26 Weeks in the standard treatment group ($t_{173} = -2.18, p = 0.031$). These AUC estimates are not easily interpreted, but if we divide by T (or 26), the scores of 63.4 and 59.1 can be interpreted as the average score over the 26 Week period and 4.3 points as the average difference between the curves over the entire 26 Weeks.

Contrasts at Specific Points in Time

As an alternative strategy, we may wish to contrast the two treatment groups at pre-specified points in time to represent early and late effects of treatment. In the renal cell carcinoma trial, we might designate 2, 8 and 26 Weeks at the time points of interest:

$$\hat{Y} = \hat{\beta}_0 + \hat{\beta}_1 \underbrace{t}_{2} + \hat{\beta}_3 \underbrace{t^{[2]}}_{0} + \hat{\beta}_5 \underbrace{t^{[8]}}_{0} + \hat{\beta}_9 \underbrace{t^{[32]}}_{0} \quad t = 2 \tag{4.12}$$

$$= \hat{\beta}_0 + \hat{\beta}_1 \underbrace{t}_{8} + \hat{\beta}_3 \underbrace{t^{[2]}}_{6} + \hat{\beta}_5 \underbrace{t^{[8]}}_{0} + \hat{\beta}_9 \underbrace{t^{[32]}}_{0} \quad t = 8 \tag{4.13}$$

$$= \hat{\beta}_0 + \hat{\beta}_1 \underbrace{t}_{26} + \hat{\beta}_3 \underbrace{t^{[2]}}_{24} + \hat{\beta}_5 \underbrace{t^{[8]}}_{18} + \hat{\beta}_9 \underbrace{t^{[32]}}_{0} \quad t = 26 \tag{4.14}$$

TABLE 4.3 Study 4: Piecewise linear regression model for renal cell carcinoma trial with estimates of selected time-specific means and 26 week AUC.

Treatment Group	Standard		Experimental		Difference		
	Est	(s.e.)	Est	(s.e.)	Est	(s.e.)	p-value
Baseline	75.5	(1.1)	75.5	(1.1)			
2 Weeks	63.3	(1.5)	61.7	(1.5)	-1.5	(1.9)	0.42
8 Weeks	61.8	(1.9)	55.8	(2.0)	-6.1	(2.7)	0.023
26 Weeks	64.1	(1.8)	60.6	(1.9)	-3.6	(2.4)	0.11
AUC/26	63.4	(1.5)	59.1	(1.6)	-4.3	(2.0)	0.031
Change 0-2 weeks	-6.1	(0.7)	-6.9	(0.7)			
Change 2-8 weeks	-0.2	(0.3)	-1.0	(0.3)			
Change 8+ weeks	0.12	(0.09)	0.26	(0.07)			

for group 1 and similarly for group 2. The estimates and their differences are summarized in Table 4.3

Rates of Change

For the piecewise linear models, we can generate estimates of the change in the outcome during different periods of time when a piecewise linear model is used. Recall that the parameters of this model associated with $t^{[2]}$ etc. represent the change in the slopes, thus the estimates of the slope for any specific interval is the sum of the parameters.

$$t = 0 \text{ to } 2 \quad \delta Y/\delta t = \hat{\beta}_1 \tag{4.15}$$

$$t = 2 \text{ to } 8 \quad = \hat{\beta}_1 + \hat{\beta}_3 \tag{4.16}$$

$$t = 8 \text{ to } 26 \quad = \hat{\beta}_1 + \hat{\beta}_3 + \hat{\beta}_5 \tag{4.17}$$

for standard therapy and similarly for experimental therapy.

The results can be interpreted as follows: Both groups start with average scores of 75.5 ($\hat{\beta}_0$). There is a rapid decline during the first 2 Weeks, which is slightly less rapid in the patients receiving standard therapy (-6.1 ($\hat{\beta}_1$) vs. -6.9 ($\hat{\beta}_2$) points/Week). This initial rapid decline ceases around Week 2, with estimated rates of decline between Weeks 2 and 8 equal to -0.24 ($\hat{\beta}_1 + \hat{\beta}_3$) and -1.0 ($\hat{\beta}_2 + \hat{\beta}_4$) points/Week in the two arms respectively. After approximately 8 Weeks, HRQoL begins to improve slightly in both arms, +0.13 ($\hat{\beta}_1 + \hat{\beta}_3 + \hat{\beta}_5$) and +0.26 ($\hat{\beta}_2 + \hat{\beta}_4 + \hat{\beta}_6$) points/Week.

4.5.1 Estimation and Testing in SAS

An overall test of post-randomization treatment differences (equation 4.10) can be constructed using a CONTRAST statement, where Trtment*Weeks 1 -1 corresponds to $\beta_1 = \beta_2$, Trtment*Week2 1 -1 to $\beta_3 = \beta_4$, etc.:

```
*** Overall Post Baseline Treatment Effect ***;
CONTRAST 'Overall Diff'   Trtment*Weeks   1 -1,
                          Trtment*Week2   1 -1,
                          Trtment*Week8   1 -1;
```

The corresponding output appears as:

```
              CONTRAST Statement Results
Source                NDF   DDF      F  Pr > F
Overall Diff            3   172   1.75  0.1588
```

The estimates of the means at specific points in time are generated by the ESTIMATE statements. For example, to estimate the predicted values for the two treatment arms at 2, 8 and 26 Weeks (equation 4.12-4.14 for standard treatment arm), as well as the corresponding difference, the statements to be included in the MIXED procedure for the 8 week contrasts are:

```
* Group Specific Estimates at selected times *;
ESTIMATE 'Standard 8 Wks' Intercept 1 Trtment*Weeks 8 0
                                      Trtment*Week2 2 0;
ESTIMATE 'Exprmntl 9 Wks' Intercept 1 Trtment*Weeks 0 8
                                      Trtment*Week2 0 6;
ESTIMATE 'Diff 8 Wks' Trtment*Weeks -8 8  Trtment*Week2 -6 6;
```

To compute the AUC/26 the statements using the DIVSOR option would be:

```
estimate 'Group 1 AUC/26' intercept 26 trtment*Weeks 338 0
              Trtment*Week2 288 0 Trtment*Week8 162 0/divisor=26;
estimate 'Group 2 AUC/26' intercept 26 trtment*Weeks 0 338
              Trtment*Week2 0 288 Trtment*Week8 0 162/divisor=26;
estimate 'Diff AUC/26' trtment*Weeks -338 338
          Trtment*Week2 -288 288 Trtment*Week8 -162 162/divisor=26;
```

4.5.2 Estimation and Testing in SPSS

Addition of the following code tests the overall differences between the curves:

```
/TEST = 'Overall Diff in Curves' Trtment*Weeks -1 1;
                                 Trtment*Week2 -1 1;
                                 Trtment*Week8 -1 1
```

The estimates of the means at specific points in time are generated by the TEST statements. For example, to estimate the predicted values for the two treatment arms at 2, 8 and 26 Weeks (equation 4.12-4.14 for standard treatment arm), as well as the corresponding difference, the statements to be included in the MIXED procedure for the 8 week contrasts are:

```
/TEST ='Standard 8 wks' Intercept 1 Trtment*Weeks 8 0 Trtment*Week2 6 0
/TEST ='Exprmntl 8 wks' Intercept 1 Trtment*Weeks 0 8 Trtment*Week2 0 6
/TEST ='Diff 8 wks' Intercept 1 Trtment*Weeks -8 8 Trtment*Week2 -6 6
```

To compute the AUC/26 the statements, using the DIVSOR option would be:

```
/TEST='Std AUC/26' Intercept 26 Trtment*Weeks 338 0
                   Trtment*Week2 228 0 Trtment*Week8 162 0 DIVISOR=26
/TEST='Exp AUC/26' Intercept 26 Trtment*Weeks 0 338
                   Trtment*Week2 0 228 Trtment*Week8 0 162 DIVISOR=26
/TEST='Diff AUC/26'  Trtment*Weeks -338 338 Trtment*Week2 -228 228
                     Trtment*Week8 -162 162 DIVISOR=26.
```

4.5.3 Estimation and Testing in R

Having identified the covariance structure and reduction of the full model for the fixed effects, dropping the changes at 17 and 34 weeks, we fit PW.Var3r. Testing hypothesis of the form $\beta_a = 0$ or $\beta_a = \beta_b$ is relatively straight forward, as these tests can be formulated as nested models and compared using the anova function. Note that the models without Week17 (PW17.Var3) and without Week34 (PW17.Var3) are not nested and should not be compared directly using the anova function. For example:

```
> summary(PW.Var3) # Examine Standard Errors

> PW17.Var3=update(PW.Var3,fixed=TOI2~Weeks:TrtGrp+Week2:TrtGrp+
+                              Week8:TrtGrp+Week34:TrtGrp)
> PW34.Var3=update(PW.Var3,fixed=TOI2~Weeks:TrtGrp+Week2:TrtGrp+
+                              Week8:TrtGrp+Week17:TrtGrp)
> PW_b.Var3=update(PW.Var3,fixed=TOI2~Weeks:TrtGrp+Week2:TrtGrp+
+                              Week8:TrtGrp)
> anova(PW.Var3,PW17.Var3,PW_b.Var3)
          Model df    AIC      BIC    logLik   Test  L.Ratio p-value
PW.Var3       1 18 5177.568 5258.125 -2570.784
PW17.Var3     2 16 5173.820 5245.427 -2570.910 1 vs 2 0.2524674  0.8814
PW_b.Var3     3 14 5171.300 5233.956 -2571.650 2 vs 3 1.4802727  0.4770
```

Estimation and testing of linear functions of parameters $(\theta = C\beta)$ requires a series of steps. First, we extract the estimates and variance of β:

```
>est.beta = as.matrix(PW_b.Var3$coef$fix)
>var.beta = PW_b.Var3$varFix
```

Then we define C. The following estimates the means at 8 weeks and the AUC over 26 Weeks for the two treatment groups and the difference:

```
> C1=c(1, 8, 0, 6, 0, 0, 0)                        # Cntl 8 weeks
> C2=c(1, 0, 8, 0, 6, 0, 0)                        # Exp 8 weeks
> C3=c(0, -8, 8, -6, 6, 0, 0)                       # Diff 8 weeks
```

```
> C4=c(26, 26*26/2, 0, 24*24/2, 0, 18*18/2, 0)        # Cntl AUC
> C5=c(26, 0, 26*26/2, 0, 24*24/2, 0, 18*18/2)        # Exp AUC
> C6=C5-C4                                             # Diff AUC 26wks
> C7=C6/26                                             # Diff Avg 26wks

> C=rbind(C1,C2,C3,C4,C5,C6,C7)
> rownames(C)=c("Cntl 8wk","Exp 8wk","Diff 8wk",
+   "Cntl AUC","Exp AUC","Diff AUC","Diff Avg")
```

Next we compute the estimates and variances of θ, the standard errors, z-statistics and p-values for a 2-sided test.

```
> est.theta=C %*% est.beta
> var.theta= C %*% var.beta %*% t(C)
> se.theta=diag(sqrt(var.theta))
> zval.theta=est.theta/t(se.theta)
> pval.theta=(1-pnorm(abs(zval.theta)))*2
```

Finally, putting them together with labels and printing:

```
> Theta=cbind(est.theta,t(se.theta),zval.theta,pval.theta)
> dimnames(Theta)[[2]] =c("Theta","SE","z","p-val")
> Theta
               Theta        SE          z       p-val
Cntl 8wk     61.890487  1.941978 31.869823 0.00000000
Exp 8wk      55.829349  2.019748 27.641733 0.00000000
Diff 8wk     -6.061139  2.657614 -2.280669 0.02256802
Cntl AUC   1649.391580 38.988330 42.304751 0.00000000
Exp AUC    1538.206442 40.711263 37.783314 0.00000000
Diff AUC   -111.185138 51.003568 -2.179948 0.02926130
Diff Avg     -4.276351  1.961676 -2.179948 0.02926130
```

I have written a function to facilitate this (see Appendix R). The syntax is:

```
> estCbeta(C,PW_b.Var3$coef$fix,PW_b.Var3$varFix)
```

4.6 An Alternative Covariance Structure

The migraine prevention trial (Study 2) and the osteoarthritis trial (Study 6) provide alternative examples of implementation of a growth curve model. In both trials, we expect that most of the change in the outcome will occur between the baseline and the first follow-up assessment with the curves flattening during the remainder of the trial. In the following section, this is illustrated for Study 2. Study 6 is discussed in Chapter 11.

4.6.1　Model for the Means

In the migraine prevention trial (Study 2) we expect that most of the change in the outcomes will occur between baseline and week 8 (the titration period), and then the curves will be roughly flat from 8 to 26 weeks (the maintenence period). We will, however, fit a piecewise linear model to the data to allow deviations in the model for the means from the expected model.

$$Y_{ij}(t) = \beta_0 + \beta_1 t_{ij} + \beta_{h2} t_{ij}^{[2]} + \beta_3 t_{ij}^{[4]} + \varepsilon_{ij},$$
$$t_{hij}^{[c]} = \max(t_{hij} - T^{[c]}, 0) \tag{4.18}$$

When we fit a model with changes in the slope at 2 and 4 months, we observe that our expectations are roughly correct (Figure 4.4) for all of the MSQ scales, but the composite measure of frequency and severity continues to decline between months 2 and 4.

4.6.2　Model for the Variance

Structure 1

If we take an approach similar to that used for the renal cell carcinoma tria, we would fit a model with three random effects: intercept, initial slope, and change in slope at 2 months (equation 4.19).

$$\varepsilon_{ij}(t) = d_{i1} + d_{i2} t_{ij} + d_{i3} t_{ij}^{[2]} + \epsilon_{ij}, \tag{4.19}$$

The thought behind adding the third random effect was that there would be variation in the initial change during the titration period in the outcome among subjects, but that change would attenuate during the maintenance period. Examination of the correlation of the random effects confirmed that expectation; the second and third random effects were almost perfectly negatively correlated ($\rho < -0.9$)** suggesting that there was variation in the change between baseline and the first follow-up, but not across the three follow-up assessments.

Structure 2

This led to the consideration of an alternative parameterization that allowed between subject variation of the initial assessments and of the follow-up assessments (equation 4.20).

$$\varepsilon_{hij}(t) = d_{i1} x_{ij}^{Base} + d_{i2} x_{ij}^{FU} + \epsilon_{ij}, \tag{4.20}$$

** Estimation procedures for two of the scales (MSQ-RR and MSQ-EF) obtain non-positive definite covariance structures.

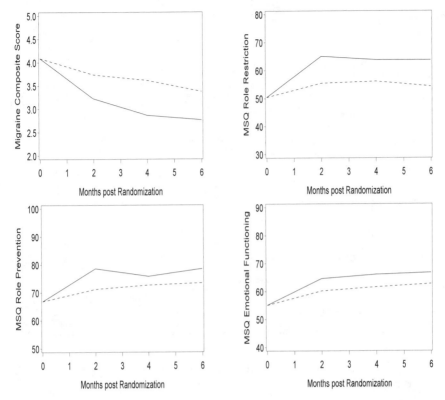

FIGURE 4.4 Study 2: Estimated trajectories in the migraine prevention trial using a piecewise linear model. Placebo (dashed line) and experimental (solid line) arms. Higher scores reflect a poorer outcome for the composite score and better outcomes for the MSQ scales.

where x_{ij}^{Base} is an indicator variable for the baseline assessments and x_{ij}^{FU} for the follow-up assessments ($x_{ij}^{FU}=1-x_{ij}^{Base}$). BIC statistics were smaller across all four measures for this second model when compared to both the model with three random effects and a unstructured repeated measures covariance structure. The correlation between these two random effects ranged from 0.5 to 0.6 indicating those individuals with higher initial scores tended to have higher follow-up scores.

4.6.3 Estimation and Testing

The procedure for estimation and hypothesis testing is the same as previously presented. A number of outcome measures could have been proposed (see Chapter 14) including the average of the maintenence assessments - baseline, the AUC, or the change from baseline to 6 months. If we had chosen the average of the maintenence assessments - baseline, the measure in each treatment group would be:

$$\theta_h = (\underbrace{\beta_0 + 2\beta_{1h}}_{2months} + \underbrace{\beta_0 + 4\beta_{1h} + 2\beta_{2h}}_{4months} + \underbrace{\beta_0 + 6\beta_{1h} + 4\beta_{2h} + 2\beta_{3h}}_{6months})/3$$

$$- \underbrace{\beta_0}_{Baseline} \tag{4.21}$$

$$= (12\beta_{1h} + 6\beta_{2h} + 2\beta_{3h})/3$$

4.7 Summary

- Time-driven designs are associated with mixed effects growth curve models.

    - Both polynomial or piecewise linear models can be used to model the average trajectory over time.

    - One to three random effects typically explain the between-subject variation.

    - The residual errors (within-subject variation) are typically uncorrelated unless observations are very closely spaced.

- The recommended growth-curve model building process starts by defining a fully parameterized model for the means $(X_i\beta)$, then identifying the structure of Σ_i and finally simplifying the mean structure.

- - Piecewise linear models can also be used for continous covariates where the relationship with the outcome may not be linear over the entire range of covariate values.

5

Moderation and Mediation

5.1 Introduction

In clinical trials, the primary research question is generally the effect of treatment on outcomes. Many researchers [Baron and Kenny, 1986, Holmbeck, 1997, Kraemer, 2002, Holmbeck, 2002, Donaldson et al., 2009] argue there is much more that can be learned and understood about for whom and how treatments are effective. This information can improve the next generation of studies. We often pose questions of mediation or moderation in clinical research, though do not formalize objectives and outcomes in terms of these concepts. These same researchers have argued for clear frameworks for these concepts [Baron and Kenny, 1986, Holmbeck, 1997, Kraemer, 2002]. In this chapter, I will present these frameworks and illustrate with several examples.

A *moderator* or *effect modifer* (B) is a variable that specifies conditions under which a given predictor (X) is related to an outcome (Y) [Holmbeck, 2002]. This is illustrated in Figure 5.1. Moderators are typically patient characteristics (age, education, stage of disease). We might expect that age would affect the relationship between disability and QOL. Time and treatment can also be considered moderators. For example, treatment may affect the relationship between time and QOL. Tests of moderation usually appear as interactions in models. A moderator should either be an unchangeable characteristic or be a condition that is measured prior to the intervention and thus not correlated with the predictor[Kraemer, 2002]. The first half of this chapter will illustrate tests of moderation in studies with both simple pre-post designs and more extended longitudinal studies.

A mediation model seeks to identify or confirm the mechanism that underlies an observed relationship between a predictor (e.g., treatment) and an outcome (e.g., sleep disturbance) via the inclusion of a third explanatory variable (e.g., pain), known as a *mediator*. Rather than hypothesizing a direct causal relationship between the predictor (X) and the outcome (Y), a mediation model hypothesizes that predictor affects the mediator, which in turn affects the outcome. The mediator variable, therefore, serves to clarify the nature of the relationship between the predictor and the outcome. This is illustrated in Figure 5.1. In contrast to a moderator, a mediator will be correlated with the predictor [Kraemer, 2002]. For example, an intervention to

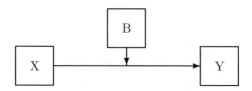

FIGURE 5.1 Example of simple moderation; the moderator (B) affects the relationship between X and Y.

improve sleep quality may do so directly but also indirectly by its reduction of pain [Russell et al., 2009], or anemia may mediate the relationship between treatment and fatigue. Mediation can be demonstrated using regression techniques including structural equation models (SEM). The medical literature abounds with examples in which investigators speculate about the impact of various interventions on quality of life. Some even demonstrate the intervention has a positive impact on both clinical outcomes and measures of HRQoL, but the formal demonstration of mediation is quite rare. The second half of this chapter will illustrate methods demonstrating mediation using regression techniques.

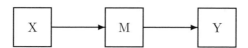

FIGURE 5.2 Example of simple mediation; the independent variable (X) influences the mediator (M) which, in turn, influences the outcome (Y).

In this chapter, I will present several examples of analyses that examine models which include moderators and mediators. The proposed analyses are all forms of regression. I have not attempted to delve into the realm of structural equation models (SEM) or path analysis, which are alternative modeling tools that are very useful when exploring complex relationships among measures.

5.2 Moderation

Before we jump straight into moderation, let's consider the general issue of adding explanatory variables (covariates) to models. My experience is that this is often done without careful thought about either the interpretation of the added parameters or the impact on other parameters. For example, consider the breast cancer trial (Study 1) and the explanatory variable age. There are numerous clinically interesting questions that can be asked:

1. Is there an association of the covariate with the outcome assuming it is constant over time (study period) and treatment? (no moderation of time or treatment effects)

2. Does the association of the covariate with the outcome vary only with time? or Does the covariate modify the impact of time on the outcome (i.e., a covariate by time interaction)?

3. Is the association of the covariate with the outcome modified by treatment arm? or Does the covariate modify the impact of the treatment arm on the outcome?

These are obviously unique questions and require different treatment of covariates in the model.

5.2.1 Moderation across Repeated Measures

First, consider a center point model for treatment and a reference cell for time (Table 5.1) with a common baseline for the breast cancer trial (Study 1). The outcome is the total score for the Breast Chemotherapy Questionnaire (BCQ) which has a possible range of 0 to 10 points. In the absence of covariates, β_0 is interpreted as the average BCQ scores before treatment. β_1 and β_3 are the changes from baseline and β_2 and β_4 are the treatment differences during and after treatment respectively.

$$y_{hij} = \beta_0 + \beta_1 T_2 + \beta_2 T_2 * Tx + \beta_3 T_3 + \beta_4 T_3 * Tx \qquad (5.1)$$
$$+ \epsilon_{hij},$$

where $T_2 = I(time = 2)$, $T_3 = I(time = 3)$, and $Tx = -1/2$ if control, $Tx = 1/2$ if experimental.

Continuous Covariates

If we add age (x_i) without interactions to the model, we are addressing the first question, "Does age have an association with the outcome, BCQ, irrespective of time or treatment?" In the model parameterized as specified in equation 5.2,

TABLE 5.1 Study 1: Repeated measures models that correspond to equations 5.1-5.4.

Center Point Model without covariates (equation 5.1)

Treatment	Before Therapy	During Therapy	After Therapy
Control	β_0	$\beta_0 + \beta_1 - \frac{\beta_2}{2}$	$\beta_0 + \beta_3 - \frac{\beta_4}{2}$
Expmtl	β_0	$\beta_0 + \beta_1 + \frac{\beta_2}{2}$	$\beta_0 + \beta_3 + \frac{\beta_4}{2}$
Difference	0	β_2	β_4

Covariate independent of time or treatment arm (equation 5.2)

Treatment	Before Therapy	During Therapy	After Therapy
Control	$\beta_0 + a_0$	$\beta_0 + \beta_1 - \frac{\beta_2}{2} + a_0$	$\beta_0 + \beta_3 - \frac{\beta_4}{2} + a_0$
Expmtl	$\beta_0 + a_0$	$\beta_0 + \beta_1 + \frac{\beta_2}{2} + a_0$	$\beta_0 + \beta_3 + \frac{\beta_4}{2} + a_0$
Difference	0	β_2	β_4

Covariate dependent on time (equation 5.3)

Treatment	Before Therapy	During Therapy	After Therapy
Control	$\beta_0 + \alpha_0$	$\beta_0 + \beta_1 - \frac{\beta_2}{2} + \alpha_0 + \alpha_1$	$\beta_0 + \beta_3 - \frac{\beta_4}{2} + \alpha_0 + \alpha_2$
Expmtl	$\beta_0 + \alpha_0$	$\beta_0 + \beta_1 + \frac{\beta_2}{2} + \alpha_0 + \alpha_1$	$\beta_0 + \beta_3 + \frac{\beta_4}{2} + \alpha_0 + \alpha_2$
Difference	0	β_2	β_4

Covariate dependent on time and treatment arm (equation 5.4)

Treatment	Before Therapy	During Therapy	After Therapy
Control	$\beta_0 + \alpha_0$	$\beta_0 + \beta_1 - \frac{\beta_2}{2} + \alpha_0 + \alpha_1 - \frac{\alpha_3}{2}$	$\beta_0 + \beta_3 - \frac{\beta_4}{2} + \alpha_0 + \alpha_2 - \frac{\alpha_4}{2}$
Expmtl	$\beta_0 + \alpha_0$	$\beta_0 + \beta_1 + \frac{\beta_2}{2} + \alpha_0 + \alpha_1 + \frac{\alpha_3}{2}$	$\beta_0 + \beta_3 + \frac{\beta_4}{2} + \alpha_0 + \alpha_2 + \frac{\alpha_4}{2}$
Difference	0	$\beta_2 + \alpha_3$	$\beta_4 + \alpha_4$

TABLE 5.2 Study 1: Association of age with BCQ Scores; estimates of the change in BCQ scores with each decade of age. Models 1-3 correspond to equations 5.2 - 5.4

		Pre-Therapy Est (s.e.)	During Therapy Est (s.e.)	Post-Therapy Est (s.e.)
Model 1:		0.17 (0.07)	0.17 (0.07)	0.17 (0.07)
Model 2:		0.20 (0.08)	0.39 (0.10)	0.14 (0.08)
Model 3:	Control	0.20 (0.08)	0.57 (0.12)	0.24 (0.10)
	Experimental	0.20 (0.08)	0.23 (0.11)	0.06 (0.10)

α_0 measures the association of age (x_i) with BCQ (y_{hij}) and is interpreted as the change in the BCQ score for every unit change in age.

$$y_{hij} = \beta_0 + \beta_1 T_2 + \beta_2 T_2 * Tx + \beta_3 T_3 + \beta_4 T_3 * Tx \qquad (5.2)$$
$$+ \alpha_0 x_i$$
$$+ \epsilon_{hij}.$$

The interpretation of β_0 is impacted by the addition of the covariate. This parameter is now the average score when the values of x_i equals 0. If x_i is the age in years of the patient, then these parameters would estimate the expected BCQ score for an infant. This does not make sense and could result in estimates that are outside the range of the measure. For this reason is makes sense to transform or 'center' the covariate at a value that is representative of the study population or the grand-mean for individuals enrolled in the study. In this trial the average age is 47.8 years. For ease of reporting, we might choose to center age at 50 years. In adult studies, it also often facilitates interpretation of parameters if we also rescale the covariate from years to decades. Thus, α_0 is the change in the BCQ score for every decade change in age and β_0 is the expected value prior to therapy for a 50 year old woman. In this example, age is indeed associated with the BCQ scores ($p<0.001$); the BCQ scores increase an estimated 0.17 points with each decade of age (Table 5.2).

To address the second question, "Does the effect of age vary with time irrespective of treatment arm", we add interactions of the covariate with the indicators of the two post baseline assessments. Because time in this case is an indicator of being on or off therapy, the question that we are really addressing is whether the association of age and the BCQ scores varies across the three phases: before, during and after treatment.

$$y_{hij} = \beta_0 + \beta_1 T_2 + \beta_2 T_2 * Tx + \beta_3 T_3 + \beta_4 T_3 * Tx \qquad (5.3)$$
$$+ \alpha_0 x_i + \alpha_1 x_i * T_2 + \alpha_2 x_i * T_3$$
$$+ \epsilon_{hij}.$$

If we parameterize the model in the manner indicated in equation 5.3, α_1 and α_2 measure the change in the relationship between BCQ scores and age during and after therapy relative to before therapy. α_1 reflects the effect of treatment (irrespective of treatment type) on the association between age and time. In the breast cancer trial, the relationship between age and the BCQ scores is the same before or after therapy ($H_0 : \alpha_2 = 0; p = 0.40$), but differs during therapy ($H_0 : \alpha_1 = 0; p = 0.013$). The larger estimate during therapy ($\hat{\alpha}_0 + \hat{\alpha}_1 = 0.39$) than either before ($\hat{\alpha}_0 = 0.20$) or after ($\hat{\alpha}_0 + \hat{\alpha}_2 = 0.14$) therapy indicates that older women do better overall and even more so during therapy than younger women. Note that the same model answers the question as to whether age moderates the effect of time (phase of the study). Specifically, the average change in the BCQ scores from before to during therapy for a 30, 50, and 70 year old woman would be -1.5 points ($\hat{\beta}_1 - 2\hat{\alpha}_1$), -1.2 points($\hat{\beta}_1$), and -0.8 points ($\hat{\beta}_1 + 2\hat{\alpha}_1$) respectively.

For the final question, we add interactions with both time and treatment. The model might appear as defined in equation 5.4.

$$y_{hij} = \beta_0 + \beta_1 T_2 + \beta_2 T_2 * Tx + \beta_3 T_3 + \beta_4 T_3 * Tx \qquad (5.4)$$
$$+ \alpha_0 x_i + \alpha_1 x_i * T_2 + \alpha_2 x_i * T_3 + \alpha_3 x_i * T_2 * Tx + \alpha_4 x_i * T_3 * Tx$$
$$+ \epsilon_{hij}.$$

(Other parameterizations are also valid.) α_3 and α_4 reflect the impact of the specific treatment (control versus experimental) on the relationship between age and the outcome during and after therapy. The impact of the specific treatment on the relationship between age and the scores during therapy is statistically significant ($H_0 : \alpha_3 = 0, p = 0.50$), while the impact on scores post-therapy is nonsignificant ($H_0 : \alpha_4 = 0, p = 0.046$).

These results bring up two issues. The first issue is whether one should include interactions when higher order effects (e.g. main effects in the context of analysis of variance (ANOVA)) are non-significant. Classical textbooks describing ANOVA, often recommend that interactions should not be added to models when main effects are non-significant. In many settings, this recommendation is appropriate as it avoids inflated Type I errors in exploratory analyses. However, any time that specifically identified research question demands an interaction term, it should be maintained.

The second issue is how to present the results of an analysis that has interaction terms in the model. I generally find that tables with parameter estimates are difficult to interpret. When presented with information in this format, I often convert those results into plots. So my recommendation is to supplement the results with a presentation in a graphical format. Figure 5.3 (left figure) represents one possible representation.

Departures from Linear Associations

While many analyses assume that impact of covariates is linear over the entire range of values, in may cases this assumption is unlikely to be true. Figure 5.3

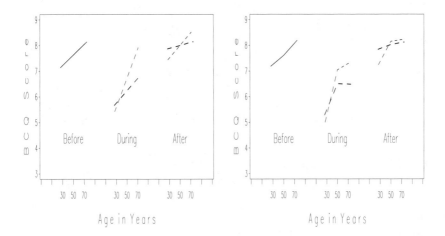

FIGURE 5.3 Study 1: Effects of age. Predicted estimates as a function of treatment arm and age assuming a linear relationship over the entire range of age (left figure, equation 5.4) or below and above 50 years (right figure equation 5.5). Solid line represents the pooled treatment groups, the short and long dashed lines indicate the control and experimental arms respectively. Higher scores reflect less impairment.

(right figure) illustrates a simple extention of the model. In equation 5.5, I have added terms that allow the relationship to change for patients above the age of 50 ($x_i^{50} = max(x_i - 50, 0)$) using the same strategy as in the piecewise linear regression models described in Chapter 4. This choice of a model which allows a departure from linearity is arbitrary, but the results do support the hypothesis that the relationship between age and BCQ scores is not linear across the entire range and that there may be a region where the effect plateaus or declines. If the relationship of age with the outcome is of primary interest, then alternative models that examine the functional form of the relationship may be warranted.

$$y_{hij} = \beta_0 + \beta_1 T_2 + \beta_2 T_2 * Tx + \beta_3 T_3 + \beta_4 T_3 * Tx \qquad (5.5)$$
$$+ \alpha_0 x_i + \alpha_1 x_i * T_2 + \alpha_2 x_i * T_3 + \alpha_3 x_i * T_2 * Tx + \alpha_4 x_i * T_3 * Tx$$
$$+ \alpha_0 x_i^{50} + \alpha_1 x_i^{50} * T_2 + \alpha_2 x_i^{50} * T_3$$
$$+ \alpha_3 x_i^{50} * T_2 * Tx + \alpha_4 x_i^{50} * T_3 * Tx$$
$$+ \epsilon_{hij}.$$

Categorical Covariates

The strategy to test the impact of categorical covariates parallels that of continuous covariates. When the categorical covariates are dichotomous, the concept of "centering" is still appropriate. For example, the extent of disease in breast cancer is often indicated by the number of positive nodes, with 4 or more positive nodes indicating a higher risk. In this study 42.5% of the women had four or more positive nodes. We could either center the covariate so that the estimates of the other parameters reflected this proportion of subjects with 4+ positive nodes or a 50/50 split in the risk factor. Categorical variables that are not dichotomous are more difficult to handle. Race is a good example. In many clinical trials, the majority of subjects identify themselves as white non-Hispanic. In this case, identifying this group as a reference group and testing for interactions with indicators of specific ethnic/racial groups may be an appropriate strategy. However, centering indicator variables for specific subgroups results in estimates of treatment effects that can be interpreted as the average effect for the entire sample.

5.2.2   Change from Baseline

To perform an analysis of the change from baseline, the reference model (equation 5.6) is very similar to that previously defined (equation 5.1) except that the term involving β_0 is dropped and the covariance structure is changed. This is because we choose a model with the baseline assessment as the reference cell, and will not be true for all choices of models. $\beta_1 \cdots \beta_4$ have the same interpretation as before and the estimates are similar. This later result will only be true when there is very little missing data (as is the case in this example) or the missing data are ignorable (see Chapter 6).

$$y_{hij} - y_{hi0} = \beta_0 + \beta_1 T_2 + \beta_2 T_2 * Tx + \beta_3 T_3 + \beta_4 T_3 * Tx \qquad (5.6)$$
$$+ \varepsilon_{hij},$$

If we have chosen an analysis of the change from baseline, we can not answer the first question proposed in the beginning of Section 5.2. We can address the second question with the following model. Note that the term involving α_0 has been dropped. α_1 and α_2 have the same interpretation as before and the estimates are similar.

$$y_{hij} - y_{hi0} = \beta_1 T_2 + \beta_2 T_2 * Tx + \beta_3 T_3 + \beta_4 T_3 * Tx \qquad (5.7)$$
$$+ \alpha_1 x_i * T_2 + \alpha_2 x_i * T_3$$
$$+ \varepsilon_{hij}.$$

We can also address the third question with the following model. α_3 and α_4 have the same interpretation as before and the estimates are similar.

$$y_{hij} - y_{hi0} = \beta_1 T_2 + \beta_2 T_2 * Tx + \beta_3 T_3 + \beta_4 T_3 * Tx \qquad (5.8)$$

$$+ \alpha_1 x_i * T_2 + \alpha_2 x_i * T_3 + \alpha_3 x_i * T_2 * Tx + \alpha_4 x_i * T_3 * Tx$$
$$+ \varepsilon_{hij}.$$

With different parameterizations of the reference model the interpretation of the parameters may be quite different and the analyst is cautioned to be very accurate in the interpretation of the parameters.

5.2.3 Centering Covariates

While it is not absolutely necessary to alway "center" covariates, my experience is that when analysts fail to do so, the results are often misinterpreted [Chuang-Stein and Tong, 1996]. This is particularly true when models contain interaction terms that occur in models testing moderation. The following example illustrates how misinterpretation occurs. Suppose our research question is: Is the impact of treatment on QOL during the treatment phase of the study moderated by age? If we perform an analysis of the first two assessments with uncentered variables where T_2 is an indicator for the assessment during therapy, Exp is an indicator of the experimental therapy, and AGE is age in years. Our model is:

$$y_{hij} = \beta_0 + \beta_1 T_2 + \beta_2 T_2 * Exp \qquad (5.9)$$
$$+ \alpha_0 AGE + \alpha_1 AGE * T_2 + \alpha_3 AGE * T_2 * Exp$$
$$+ \epsilon_{hij}.$$

While this looks like an ANOVA model with main effects and interactions, it does NOT have the same interpretation!

In contrast, if we use centered variables: Tx is a centered indicator of treatment and AGE50 is a centered age variable, our model is:

$$y_{hij} = \beta_0 + \beta_1 T_2 + \beta_2 T_2 * Tx \qquad (5.10)$$
$$+ \alpha_0 AGE50 + \alpha_1 AGE50 * T_2 + \alpha_3 AGE50 * T_2 * Tx$$
$$+ \epsilon_{hij}.$$

This model has the traditional interpretation of main effects and interactions. If misinterpreted, results from the two models appear very different (Table 5.3). In this example, if we take the traditional interpretation, we would conclude that there is a significant treatment effect during therapy in the model with centered covariates ($H_0 : T_2 * Tx = 0$, $p < 0.001$), but would make the opposite conclusion with the model with uncentered covariates ($H_0 : T_2 * Exp = 0, p = 0.17$). Similarly, we might conclude that age modifies the effect of treatment (irrespective of treatment arm) in the centered model ($H_0 : T_2 * Age50 = 0, p = 0.005$) but make the opposite conclusion in the uncentered model ($H_0 : T_2 * Age = 0, p = 0.11$).

To further illustrate the problem, let us first consider a modifier such as gender that is a categorical (dichotomous) variable. If there is an interaction

TABLE 5.3 Study 1: Contrast of two models using centered and uncentered covariates.

	Centered				Uncentered		
	Est	(s.e.)	p		Est	(s.e.)	p
T_2	-1.04	(0.08)	<.001	T_2	-1.61	(0.55)	0.004
T_2*Tx	-0.63	(0.08)	<.001	T_2*Exp	-1.17	(0.78)	0.17
Age50	0.22	(0.07)	0.002	Age	0.22	(0.07)	0.002
T_2*Age50	0.23	(0.08)	0.005	T_2*Age	0.13	(0.11)	0.11
T_2*Tx*Age50	0.11	(0.15)	0.50	T_2*Exp*Age	0.11	(0.15)	0.50

between the modifier (M) and another explanatory variable (X) such as treatment, the relationship might appear as in Figure 5.4 (left side). The two levels of the modifier (M) are labeled A and B; the two levels of the other explanatory variable (X) are labeled EXP and INTL. If we parameterize the model such that the difference between the two treatment groups is estimated considering either A or B to be a reference group we obtain very different estimates, 0.2 and 1.0 respectively. If we center the covariate, the estimates provide a more realistic estimate of the difference. To center a dichotomous variable, we first take a numeric variable that is coded such that the difference between the two groups is 1. Typically the coding is 0 and 1 or 1 and 2. If we then subtract the mean of those values, we would convert them to -.5 and 0.5 if 50% were in each group or -0.25 and 0.75 if 75% were in group B. The estimates of the treatment difference in Figure 5.4 are 0.6 and 0.8 for the two levels of the modifier; these estimates accurately reflecting the treatment difference averaged over all the subjects in the study.

A similar problem occurs when moderators measured by continuous covariates are not centered. Consider a second hypothetical example where the age of the study participants ranges between 40 and 80 years (Figure 5.4 (right side)). If the variable measuring age is uncentered, the estimates of the treatment difference (-0.7) may be quite different than when the centered variable is used (0.8). In the illustration the direction is actually reversed. The procedure for deriving the centered variable is the same with the mean subtracted from the individual's age.

Note that there may be settings where the analyst chooses to establish a reference group and not center a particular covariate. This is appropriate if the meaning/interpretation parameters and associated tests are explicit and clearly communicated.

Centering covariates also alleviates some problems associated with collinearity in linear, quadratic, and higher-order terms.

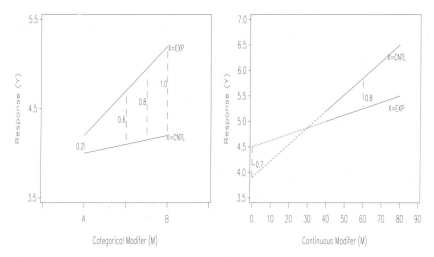

FIGURE 5.4 Hypothetical example to illustrate the problems with uncentered variables.

5.3 Mediation

We may speculate how changes in disease status or symptoms affects HRQoL, however, it is much more satisfying to test hypotheses about the mechanism. We start with a conceptual model that has a clinical/theoretical basis. We can not prove that the model is true, but we can test whether the observed data are consistent with the model. A generic single-mediator model is displayed in Figure 5.5 with two paths. The first is the indirect or mediated path (ab) and the second is the direct or unmediated path (c).

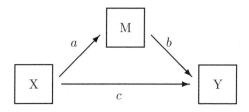

FIGURE 5.5 Simple mediation with a indirect (ab) and direct (c) effect of X on Y. The symbol a represents the relationship between X and M, b the relationship between M and Y and c the relationship between X and Y adjusting for M.

Baron and Kenny [1986] proposed a two-staged approach with four conditions to demonstrate mediation of the effect of X on Y by M:

1. X must be significantly associated with M

2. M must be significantly associated with Y

3. X must be significantly associated with Y

4. the association of X with Y is less after controlling for M

One can assess these conditions using coefficients of the following three regression equations:

$$Y = i_1 + \tau X + e_1 \tag{5.11}$$

$$M = i_2 + aX + e_2 \tag{5.12}$$

$$Y = i_3 + cX + bM + e_3 \tag{5.13}$$

Conditions 1-3 are satisfied when $\tau \neq 0$, $a \neq 0$, and $b \neq 0$ respectively. Condition 4 is satisfied when the coefficient c is smaller than τ (in absolute value) or $|\tau - c| > 0$. MacKinnon et al. [1995] proved that $\tau = ab + c$ for maximum likelihood estimation of equation 5.11-5.13 assuming normality. The interpretation is that the total effect of X on Y (τ) can be divided into two components: the direct effect (c) and the indirect (mediated) effect (ab). A test of the indirect effect, $H_0 : ab = 0$ can be constructed using asymptotic (large sample) theory:

$$z_{ab} = (\hat{a}\hat{b})/\sqrt{\sigma^2_{\hat{a}\hat{b}}} \qquad \sigma^2_{\hat{a}\hat{b}} \approx \sigma^2_{\hat{a}}\hat{b}^2 + \sigma^2_{\hat{b}}\hat{a}^2. \tag{5.14}$$

For small studies ($n < 50$) or those with multiple mediators, this approximation becomes less accurate and a bootstrap analysis is recommended when precision is important.

There is some controversy [MacKinnon et al., 2007] about the necessity of the third condition in settings where there is no direct effect of the predictor on the outcome ($c = 0$). The requirement for the third condition affects the power to detect mediation using this approach.

5.3.1   Mediation with Treatment as the Predictor

This first example illustrates the demonstration of mediation in a randomized trial with treatment assignment as the predictor using univariate data. Consider Study 2, the migraine prevention trial with an active and a placebo treatment arm. The question of interest is the extent that the frequency and severity of migraine attacks mediates the changes in the subscales (role restriction (RR), role prevention(RP) and emotional function (EF)) of the Migraine-Specific Quality of Life Questionnaire (MSQ). The variable MigScore is the product of the square root of the frequency times the average severity. If the frequency is 0 (and the severity is missing), a value of 0 is assigned. To illustrate the methods, we will examine the change from baseline to the average of the available post-baseline assessments.

TABLE 5.4 Study 2: Simple and partial correlations for a simple mediation model; X, M, and Y are the predictor, mediator and outcome.

			Simple Correlations:			
	Trtment	(X)	MigScore	(M)	MSQ_EF	(Y)
Trtment	1.000		-0.165	(1)	0.127	(3)
			$p = 0.0014$		$p = 0.015$	
MigScore					-0.398	(2)
					$p < .001$	
			Partial Correlations (MigScore):			
					MSQ_EF	
Trtment					0.067	(4)
					$p = 0.20$	

(1), (2), (3), and (4) indicate the four conditions previously defined.

Closely related to the regression approach, we can examine simple and partial correlations for evidence of mediation as illustrated in Table 5.4. We note that all four conditions are satisfied: the mediator (MigScore) is correlated with the predictor (Trtment) (Condition 1), MigScore is correlated with the outcome (MSQ_EF) (Condition 2), Trtment is correlated with MSQ_EF (Condition 3), and the correlation of Trtment with MSQ_EF is reduced from 0.127 to 0.067 when controlling for the mediator (Condition 4). Note that examination of the correlations supports the mediation model, but does not directly allow us to quantitate the proportion of the change in the outcome that can be attributed to the direct and mediated effects.

The regression approach for a single mediator begins with estimating the parameters a, b, c, and τ (equations 5.11-5.13). The results are summarized in Table 5.5. Again, we note that the four conditions are satisfied: we reject the hypotheses $a = 0$, $b = 0$ and $\tau = 0$ (Conditions 1-3) and note that $c < \tau$ (Condition 4). The later condition is more formally assessed by testing $ab = 0$ since $\tau - c = ab$. Finally, we note that 50% of the effect of treatment on the change in MSQ_EF is mediated by the change in the frequency and severity of migraines as measured by MigScore.

This regression approach can be extended to multiple mediators. For the purposes of illustration, let's add measures of migraine frequency (MigAtt)

TABLE 5.5 Study 2: Regression approach with single mediator; estimates of parameters and proportion of the effect of treatment on overall QOL that can be attributed to a direct or indirect (mediated) effect.

Regression Models		Estimates	(s.e.)
1: `MSQ_EF` $= \tau*$`Trtment`		$\hat{\tau} = 5.95$	(2.43)
2: `MigScore` $= a*$`Trtment`		$\hat{a} = -0.07$	(0.22)
3: `MSQ_EF` $= c*$`Trtment`		$\hat{c} = 2.95$	(2.95)
$+\ b*$`MigScore`		$\hat{b} = -4.29$	(0.54)

Summary	Estimate	(s.e.)	Proportion
Indirect (mediated)	$\hat{a}\hat{b} = 3.00$	(1.01)	50 %
Direct	$\hat{c} = 2.95$	(2.28)	50 %
Total	$\hat{\tau} = 5.95$	(1.43)	100%

and severity (`MigSev`) to be the mediators. The regression models and parameter estimates are summarized in Table 5.6. We note that the four conditions are satisfied for the measure of frequency (`MigAtt`) and its interaction with severity (`MigScore`), but not for severity alone (`MigSev`): we reject the hypotheses $a_1 = 0, a_3 = 0, b_1 = 0, b_3 = 0$ and $\tau = 0$ (Conditions 1-3) and note that $c < \tau$ (Condition 4).

At this point, several comments are appropriate. First is the issue of causal inference. So far, all we have demonstrated is that the data are consistent with the mediation model. Making a causal inference requires additional conditions including a logical temporal sequence. Second, is the interpretation of the indirect versus direct effects. While we label one of the paths as the *direct effect*, it probably contains two components: the direct effect and the unexplained effect. The later may be either effects of the predictor on the outcome that are mediated by other factors or residual variation because the measure of the mediator(s) is imperfect.

5.3.2 Mediation with Time as the Predictor

While treatment is the most common predictor, other possibilities are possible and can be informative. Consider the single arm trial study of intensive therapy, chemotherapy plus radiation (CXRT), for advanced lung cancer (Study 5) described in Chapter 1. Weekly assessments of symptom severity and interference with daily activity were obtained while on CXRT (first 7 weeks) using the M. D. Anderson Symptom Inventory (MDASI). Higher scores indicate a more negative outcome for all scores. First we note that this overall interference score increases over time while patients are on CXRT; thus the predictor (time) is associated with the outcome (Overall Interference). Next

TABLE 5.6 Study 2: Regression approach with three mediators; estimates of parameters and proportion of the effect of treatment on MSQ_EF QOL that can be attributed to a direct or indirect (mediated) effect.

Regression Models			Estimate	(s.e.)
1:	MSQ_EF	$= \tau$*Trtment	$\hat{\tau} = 5.95$	(2.43)
2a:	MigAtt	$= a_1$*Trtment	$\hat{a}_1 = -0.29$	(0.02)
2b:	MigSev	$= a_2$*Trtment	$\hat{a}_2 = -0.08$	(0.05)
2c:	MigScore	$= a_3$*Trtment	$\hat{a}_3 = -0.70$	(0.22)
3:	MSQ_EF	$= c$*Trtment	$\hat{c} = 2.83$	(2.28)
		$+ b_1$*MigAtt	$\hat{b}_1 = -3.85$	(4.77)
		$+ b_2$*MigSev	$\hat{b}_2 = 0.69$	(4.89)
		$+ b_3$*MigScore	$\hat{b}_3 = -2.96$	(2.36)

Summary	Estimate	(s.e.)	Proportion
Indirect (mediated)- Mig Attacks ($\sqrt{}$)	$\hat{a}_1\hat{b}_1 = 1.10$	(1.41)	18 %
Indirect (mediated)- Mig Severity	$\hat{a}_2\hat{b}_2 = -0.05$	(0.38)	-1 %
Indirect (mediated)- Mig Att*Sev	$\hat{a}_2\hat{b}_2 = 2.07$	(1.77)	35 %
Direct	$\hat{c} = 2.83$	(2.28)	48 %
Total	$\hat{\tau} = 5.95$	(2.43)	100%

we consider models with a single mediator. The procedure is essentially the same as described in the previous section, except because we will use the longitudinal data (rather than a univariate measure on each individual) we need to adjust for correlation of measures on the same subject (see Chapters 3 and 4). In the following example, we add two random effects to the model (intercept and slope).

In this multivariate setting, the relationship $\tau = ab + c$ is only approximately true. This is illustrated in Table 5.7. In single mediation models, pain is associated with 34%, fatigue with 55% and sadness with 38% of the effect of time on overall interference. We can also form models with multiple mediators. Table 5.8 illustrates a model with pain, fatigue, lack of appetite, sore throat and sadness. These five symptoms explain all but 5% of the variation (ignoring the 3% lost in the approximations). Interestingly, in the presence of the other symptoms, pain is no longer associated with the effect of time on interference. Note that this is different than saying pain is not associated with interference; rather that the increases in interference are not attributable to pain in general after accounting for that of the other four symptoms.

TABLE 5.7 Study 5: Regression coefficients for models with a single mediator (pain, fatigue or lack of appetite) between time (predictor) and overall interference (outcome).

	Pain			Fatigue			Lack of Appetite		
	Est	(s.e.)		Est	(s.e.)		Est	(s.e.)	
$\hat{a}$	0.37	(0.062)		0.32	(0.057)		0.41	(0.074)	
$\hat{b}$	0.27	(0.035)		0.46	(0.031)		0.36	(0.029)	
$\hat{a}\hat{b}$	0.10	(0.021)	39%	0.15	(0.028)	58%	0.15	(0.029)	57%
$\hat{c}$	0.15	(0.046)	59%	0.10	(0.038)	40%	0.10	(0.044)	39%
$\hat{\tau}$	0.26	(0.045)	99%	0.26	(0.045)	98%	0.26	(0.045)	97%

5.4   Other Exploratory Analyses

What if the change over time is not linear or the relationship between the moderator and the outcome is not linear? Or we want to examine both the absolute level of interference and the changes over time? The previous models have focused on the coefficients, answering questions such as Is the association of X with Y less after controlling for M? However, we can also examine the variance and answer questions such as Is more of the variation of Y explained by M?

5.4.1   Mediation in Mixed Effects Models

Consider the previous example of the single arm trial of intensive therapy for lung cancer (Study 5), adding post-therapy observations up to 12 weeks total follow-up. If we fit a model in which the change in interference is linear during both the on-therapy and post-therapy periods within two components of variation, between and within subject, the model would appear as:

$$Y_{ij} = \beta_0 + \beta_1 t_{ij} + \beta_2 u_{ij} + d_i + \epsilon_{ij} \tag{5.15}$$

where t_{ij} is the number of weeks since the beginning of therapy and u_{ij} is the number of weeks since the end of therapy (0 if still on-therapy). Thus $\hat{t}_{ij}$ is the estimated change over time while on-therapy, and $\hat{t}_{ij} + \hat{u}_{ij}$ is the estimated change over time after the end of therapy. The between and within subject variation are $Var(d_i)$ and $Var(\epsilon_{ij})$ respectively. d_i can be thought of as the average distance between the predicted trajectory for all the subjects $(\beta_0 + \beta_1 t_{ij} + \beta_2 u_{ij})$ and the ith subject's interference score. ϵ_{ij} is the week-to-week variation and measurement error in the interference scores across the J measurements. The question of interest is how much of the change over time and the variation is explained by the symptom severity. To answer this

TABLE 5.8 Study 5: Regression coefficients for models with a multiple mediator between overall interference and time.

Effect	Mediator	Parameter	Estimate	(s.e.)	
Indirect	Pain	a	0.38	(0.062)	
		b	0.06	(0.031)	
		ab	0.02	(0.012)	8%
	Fatigue	a	0.32	(0.057)	
		b	0.33	(0.031)	
		ab	0.10	(0.021)	41%
	Lack of Appetite	a	0.41	(0.074)	
		b	0.17	(0.027)	
		ab	0.07	(0.017)	27%
	Sad	a	0.07	(0.065)	
		b	0.25	(0.033)	
		ab	0.02	(0.016)	7%
	Sore Throat	a	0.53	(0.081)	
		b	0.04	(0.030)	
		ab	0.02	(0.016)	9%
Direct		c	0.01	(0.033)	3%
Total		τ	0.25	(0.045)	97%

question, we add the symptom severity scores (s_{ijk}) to the model where k indicates the kth symptom.

$$Y_{ij} = \beta_0 + \beta_1 t_{ij} + \beta_2 u_{ij} + \sum_{k=1}^{K} \beta_{(2+k)} s_{ijk} + d_i + \epsilon_{ij} \qquad (5.16)$$

The results are summarized in Table 5.9. Virtually all ($> 90\%$) of the estimated change over time is explained by all fifteen symptoms. Similarly, most of the between subject variation is also explained. Thus, subjects who report more interference than average, are reporting more symptom severity. However, only about half of the week-to-week variation is accounted for by symptom severity. This is not totally unexpected because the residual error contains not only the week-to-week variation in interference but also the measurement error.

5.4.2 Non-Linear Relationships

A second example of an exploratory analysis examines the possibility of a nonlinear relationship between symptoms and interference over the range of symptom scores. Suppose we allow the relationship to change at 2, 5, and 7

TABLE 5.9 Study 5: Proportion of change over time or variation in interference explained by symptom severity. Models include no mediation (none), single symptoms, and multiple (all 15) symptoms.

| | Slope | | | | Variation | | | |
| | On Tx | | Off Tx | | Between | | Within | |
Symptom	Est	%	Est	%	Est	%	Est	%
None	0.282		-0.140		3.43		2.19	
Pain	0.157	44%	-0.060	57%	2.02	41%	1.99	9%
Fatigue	0.099	65%	-0.039	72%	1.45	58%	1.54	30%
Lack of Appetite	0.130	54%	-0.054	61%	2.06	40%	1.79	10%
All fifteen	0.019	93%	-0.005	96%	0.50	86%	1.03	53%

TABLE 5.10 Study 5: Estimated change in overall interference scores with a 1 point change in symptoms severity estimated over distinct ranges of symptom severity.

| | 0-2 | | 2-5 | | 5-7 | | 7-10 | |
Symptom	Est	(s.e.)	Est	(s.e.)	Est	(s.e.)	Est	(s.e.)
Fatigue	0.17	(0.08)	0.47	(0.10)	0.50	(0.10)	0.86	(0.11)
Pain	0.23	(0.07)	0.26	(0.12)	0.30	(0.15)	0.49	(0.18)
Sleep	0.19	(0.07)	0.47	(0.10)	0.50	(0.10)	0.66	(0.15)
Shortness of Breath	0.21	(0.07)	0.40	(0.13)	0.45	(0.21)	0.77	(0.26)
Distress	0.46	(0.14)	0.45	(0.14)	0.50	(0.16)	0.06	(0.18)
Sadness	0.55	(0.08)	0.36	(0.17)	0.34	(0.19)	0.02	(0.21)

points on the symptom scale, noting that the choice of these points is arbitrary other than dividing the symptom scale into 4 roughly equal parts. The regression equation for a model with a single symptom would appear as:

$$Y_{ij} = \beta_0 + \beta_1 t_{ij} + \beta_2 u_{ij} + \beta_3 s_{ij} + \beta_4^{[2]} s_{ij} + \beta_5 s_{ij}^{[5]} + \beta_6 s_{ij}^{[7]} + d_i + \epsilon_{ij}. \quad (5.17)$$

The estimates of the change in interference for each point change in the symptom score would be $\hat{\beta}_3$ over the range of 0-2, $\hat{\beta}_3 + \hat{\beta}_4^{[2]}$ over 3-5, $\hat{\beta}_3 + \hat{\beta}_4^{[2]} + \hat{\beta}_5^{[5]}$ over 5-7, and $\hat{\beta}_3 + \hat{\beta}_4^{[2]} + \hat{\beta}_5^{[5]} + \hat{\beta}_6^{[7]}$ over 7-10. While we would not expect the function to have abrupt changes at these points, we can approximate the shape of the change. Table 5.10 summarizes the results for a few of the symptoms. For these selected symptoms, two patterns emerge. Changes in interference are greater in the upper ranges of fatigue, pain and shortness of breath. One interpretation is that patients may be better able to accommodate increases in these symptoms in the lower range of symptoms severity. In contrast, for distress and sadness the change is greater even in the very low range of severity, though a plateau occurs around scores of 7. This might suggest the importance of scores in the lower range for these symptoms than traditionally indicated as meriting intervention.

5.5   Summary

- Moderators (effect modifiers) are variables that specify conditions under which a given predictor (typically treatment) is related to an outcome. They are generally incorporated into regression models in the form of interactions. The predictor affects the outcome differently depending on the level of the moderator.

- Mediation occurs when predictors (treatment, disease status, time) influence the mediator which, in turn, influences the outcome.

6

Characterization of Missing Data

6.1 Introduction

Missing assessments of HRQoL occur in most longitudinal studies. Because the patients participating in these trials are free-living individuals and often experience disease- and treatment-related morbidity and mortality, missing assessments are inevitable. There are many reasons given for missing assessments (Table 6.1). Missing data may occur for reasons totally unrelated to the subject's current quality of life (a missed appointment due to a snow storm) or may be intimately related (severe episodes of nausea or vomiting). The goal of this chapter is to present methods that characterize the patterns and nature of the missing assessments in longitudinal studies. Strategies for missing responses to individual items of a questionnaire will be discussed later in Chapter 8.

I will use three examples in this chapter. The lung cancer trial (Study 3) illustrates a trial in which the missing data can be characterized for each of the four assessments and is used throughout the chapter. The renal cell carcinoma trials (Study 4) illustates how the metods may be adapted when the timing of assessments becomes more varied. The final example, the migraine prevention trial (Study 2) illustrates different dropout patterns across the two treatment arms.

TABLE 6.1 Examples of "Why subjects fail to complete HRQoL assessments."

Patient misses a specified appointment
Staff forgets to administer questionnaire
Translation not available in patient's language
Patient drops out from study because no longer ill
Patient refuses to complete questionnaire
Patient states he or she is too ill to complete questionnaire
Staff does not approach patient because of health status
Patient dies

6.1.1   Terminology

There is some controversy as to whether an assessment is missing if the assessment was not expected as defined in the protocol either because the patient had died or had been removed from the trial. In this book, I will use the term *missing* to include both attrition and noncompliance where *attrition* refers to death or termination of follow-up as specified in the protocol and *noncompliance* refers to assessments expected according to the guideline of the protocol. Non-compliance reflects deviations from the planned data collection. The combination of non-compliance and attrition impacts the analysis and interpretation of the results. The term *dropout* will refer to the discontinuation of the assessments either as a result of attrition or noncompliance.

6.1.2   Why are Missing Data a Problem?

The first potential problem associated with missing data is loss of power to detect clinically meaningful differences as a result of a reduced number of observations. However, in many large (Phase III/IV) clinical studies, the sample size is often based on differences in a binary outcome such as response or the time to an event such as death. Sample sizes based on these endpoints are often more than sufficient to detect clinically meaningful differences in HRQoL endpoints that are measured on a continuous scale. The loss of power may be an issue in small studies, but the problem can be addressed by increasing the planned sample size of the trial. If the objectives associated with the HRQoL assessment are not of sufficient importance to warrant this increase in sample size, then the investigators should consider omitting the HRQoL assessments altogether rather than burdening patients when the design is inadequate in terms of sample size.

The second and more serious problem is the potential bias of estimates due to missing data. For example, patients who are experiencing poorer HRQoL because of increased morbidity or mortality may be less likely to complete HRQoL assessments. If we ignore the presence of missing data and the analyses are based only on the observed data of patients who are doing well, HRQoL is overestimated. Alternatively, it is possible that individuals will drop out of a study when they are no longer experiencing the signs or symptoms of their disease, in which case HRQoL is underestimated.

6.1.3   How Much Data Can Be Missing?

There are no magic rules about how much missing data is acceptable in a clinical trial. When the proportion of missing assessments is very small (<5%), the potential bias or impact on power may be very minor. In some cases, 10-20% missing data will have little or no effect on the results of the study. In other studies, 10-20% may matter. As the proportion of missing data increase to 30-50%, the conclusions one is willing to draw will be restricted.

The seriousness of the problem depends on the reasons for the missing data, the objectives of the study and the intended use of the results. Results from trials influencing regulatory issues of drug approval or health policy decisions will require more stringent criteria than those used to design future studies. The challenge for the analyst is to provide either a convincing argument that conclusions drawn from the analysis are insensitive to the missing data or clear limits for interpretation of the results. The concepts and tools to do that are the focus of this and the following chapters.

Similar Proportions of Dropout among Intervention Arms

A common question is whether missing data can be ignored if there are similar proportions of missing data across all study arms for the same reason. The answer is often "No." If the goals of the trial are to estimate rates of change in the outcome within groups, the resulting estimates are often dependent on the missing data. The sensitivity of within group estimates to dropout will be illustrated in later chapters. Comparisons between treatment arms are less sensitive to missing data. However, there is always the possibility that this is not a safe assumption and sensitivity analyses, as described in later chapters, are always advisable.

6.1.4 Prevention

Although analytic strategies exist for trials with missing data, they depend on untestable assumptions so their use is much less satisfactory than initial prevention. Some missing data, such as that due to death, is not preventable. However, both primary and secondary prevention are desirable. In terms of primary prevention, missing data should be minimized at both the design and implementation stages of a clinical trial [Fairclough and Cella, 1996a, Young and Maher, 1999]. Some of these strategies are discussed in Chapter 2.

Secondary prevention consists of gathering information that is useful in the analysis and interpretation of the results. This includes collection of auxiliary data that are strongly correlated with the value of the missing HRQoL measures and information about factors that may contribute to the occurrence of missing assessments. Strategies for secondary prevention may include gathering concurrent auxiliary data on toxicity, evaluations of health status by the clinical staff or HRQoL assessments from a caretaker. Use of this type of data is discussed in later chapters.

Prospective documentation of the reasons for missing data is useful. The classifications that are used should be specified in a manner that helps the analyst decide whether the reason is related to the individual's HRQoL. For example, "Patient refusal" does not clarify this, but reasons such as "Patient refusal due to health" and "Patient refusal unrelated to health" will help differentiate missing data that is ignorable from non-ignorable.

6.2   Patterns and Causes of Missing Data

Patterns of missing data consist of terminal dropout (monotone), intermittent (nonmonotone) or mixtures of both. Examples of both patterns are shown in Table 6.2. *Terminal dropout* occurs when no observations are made after a certain point in time. *Intermittent* missing data occurs when an observation is missing but a subsequent observation is observed. Within these two patterns of missing data, the causes of missing data are either related or unrelated to the patient's HRQoL. Similarly, the causes may be planned (by design) or unplanned.

TABLE 6.2 Terminal dropout, intermittent and mixed missing data patterns.

Terminal Dropout (Monotone)					Intermittent (Nonmonotone)					Mixed Pattern				
X	X	X	X	X	X	X	X	-	X	X	X	-	X	-
X	X	X	X	-	X	X	X	-	X	-	X	X	-	-
X	X	X	-	-	X	-	X	X	X	X	-	X	X	-
X	X	-	-	-	-	X	-	-	X	X	-	X	-	-
X	-	-	-	-	X	-	X	-	X	-	X	-	X	-
X=Observe, -=Missing														

In patients with chronic diseases, terminal dropout may occur because a treatment does not work or the patient is no longer experiencing the symptoms that prompted him or her to obtain treatment. In patients with progressive or fatal diseases, such as advanced cancer and AIDS, terminal dropout occurs as a result of progression of disease and death. Intermittent missing data might include missed visits (assessments) due to episodes of severe acute toxicity. Causes such as the weather and staff forgetting are unrelated to the subject's HRQoL, whereas causes such as toxicity are likely to be related to the subject's QoL.

Lung Cancer Trial (Study 3)

In most studies both dropout and intermittent patterns exist but one pattern may predominate. In the lung cancer trial (Table 6.3), the majority of missing data fits the terminal dropout pattern (85% of patients, including complete cases and those with no data). A smaller proportion of subjects (15%) have an intermittent or mixed pattern (intermittent followed by dropout). The predominance of the monotone pattern will influence the choice of methods and the manner in which subsequent analyses will be performed.

However, while these patterns are important, the reasons for the missing data are also very relevant. As previously described (see Table 1.7), death and patient refusal as well as staff oversight contributed to the missing data. The design of this trial specified that assessments were to continue until 6 months, regardless of whether the patient was still receiving the treatment. Death accounted for roughly half of the missing assessments, however, the remaining missing cases are a mixture of those unrelated to the outcome (e.g. administrative), related to the outcome (e.g. health of patient) and for unknown reasons.

TABLE 6.3 Study 3: Patterns of observations in the lung cancer trial.

Pattern	Assessment # 1	2	3	4	N	%
Complete cases	X	X	X	X	139	26.5
Monotone dropout	X	X	X	-	94	17.9
	X	X	-	-	86	16.4
	X	-	-	-	127	24.2
No data	-	-	-	-	3	0.6
Intermittent patterns	X	X	-	X	15	2.9
	X	-	X	X	11	2.1
	X	-	-	X	10	1.9
	-	X	X	X	4	0.8
	-	X	-	X	2	0.4
	-	X	-	X	1	0.2
Mixed patterns	X	-	X	-	18	3.4
	-	X	X	-	3	0.6
	-	X	-	-	12	2.1
	-	-	X	-	1	0.2

X = observed, - = missing.

6.3   Mechanisms of Missing Data

Understanding the missing data mechanism is critical to the analysis and interpretation of HRQoL studies. All analytic methods for longitudinal data incorporate assumptions about the missing data. The robustness of the analytic methods to violations of the assumptions varies. If the assumptions are incorrect, then the resulting estimates will be biased. Thus, examination of available evidence for or against these assumptions is the first major task in the analysis of HRQoL studies.

6.3.1   The Concept

There are three major classes of missing data, differing by whether and how missingness are related to the outcome (e.g. subject's quality of life)[Little and Rubin, 1987]. For example, if HRQoL data are missing because the patient moved out of town or the staff forgot to administer the assessment, the missingness is unrelated to the HRQoL outcome and those assessments are *Missing Completely at Random* (MCAR). At the other extreme, if data are missing because of a positive or negative response to treatment or progression of disease (e.g. increased/decreased symptoms, progressive disease and death), the missingness is likely to be related to the HRQoL outcome and the data are *Missing Not at Random* (MNAR). Intermediate cases are referred to as *Missing at Random* (MAR) where missingness depends on the observed data, generally the most recently observed HRQoL. Table 6.4 presents an overview. The term *ignorable missing data* is often equated with MAR and MCAR and the term *nonignorable missing data* with MNAR. While they are related, the terms are not strictly interchangeable. The distinction as well as formal statistical definitions are presented in Rubin [1987, Chapter 2] and Verbeke and Molenberghs [2000, pages 217-218].

TABLE 6.4 Simple overview of missing data mechanisms.

		Dependent on ...	Independent of ...
Missing Completely at Random	MCAR[†]	Covariates	Observed HRQoL Missing HRQoL
Missing at Random	MAR	Covariates Observed HRQoL	Missing HRQoL
Missing Not at Random	MNAR	Missing HRQoL	
[†] and Covariate-Dependent Dropout			

The remainder of this chapter presents the general concepts of these three mechanisms in more detail and suggests methods for distinguishing among them. The subsequent chapters describe methods of analysis that can be used under the various assumptions.

6.3.2 Notation

Consider a longitudinal study where n_i assessments of HRQoL are planned for each subject over the course of the study. As previously defined, Y_{ij} indicates the jth observation of HRQoL on the ith individual.

Y_i is the *complete data* vector of n_i <u>planned</u> observations of the outcome for the ith individual which includes both the <u>observed</u>(Y_i^{obs}) and <u>missing</u> (Y_i^{mis}) observations of HRQoL.

R_i is a vector of indicators of the missing data pattern for the ith individual where $R_{ij} = 1$ if Y_{ij} is observed and $R_{ij} = 0$ if Y_{ij} is missing.

Note that the term *complete data* is defined as the set of responses that one would have observed if all subjects completed all possible assessments. This is in contrast to the term *complete cases* which is defined as the set of responses on only those subjects who completed all possible assessments ($R_{ij} = 1$ for all possible Y_{ij} from the ith subject). In some of the following chapters, we will differentiate data from these complete cases (Y_i^C) and data from incomplete cases (Y_i^I). Table 6.5 is a summary of terms.

TABLE 6.5 Summary of terms

Complete data	$\mathbf{Y}$	All responses that one would have observed if all subjects had completed all possible assessments.
Observed data	$\mathbf{Y}^{obs}$	All responses that were observed.
Missing data	$\mathbf{Y}^{mis}$	All responses that were not observed.
Complete cases	$\mathbf{Y}^C$	Responses from cases (or subjects) where all possible responses were observed.
Incomplete cases	$\mathbf{Y}^I$	Responses from cases (or subjects) where one or more possible responses is missing.

Example

If a study were planned to have four HRQoL assessments at 0, 4, 13 and 26 weeks and the HRQoL of the ith subject were missing at 4 and 26 weeks, then that subject's data might look like:

$$Y_i = \begin{bmatrix} 78 \\ NA \\ 58 \\ NA \end{bmatrix} \text{ and } R_i = \begin{bmatrix} 1 \\ 0 \\ 1 \\ 0 \end{bmatrix} \text{ or } \begin{matrix} Y_i^{obs} = \begin{bmatrix} 78 \\ 58 \end{bmatrix} \\ \\ Y_i^{mis} = \begin{bmatrix} NA \\ NA \end{bmatrix} \end{matrix}$$

where NA indicates a missing observation. Notice that the vector of the observed data (Y_i^{obs}) contains the first (78) and third (58) observations and the vector of the missing data (Y_i^{mis}) contains the second and fourth observations. The corresponding design matrix for this subject in a model estimating an intercept and a linear trend over time would appear as

$$X_i = \begin{bmatrix} 1 & 0 \\ 1 & 4 \\ 1 & 13 \\ 1 & 26 \end{bmatrix} \text{ and } \begin{matrix} X_i^{obs} = \begin{bmatrix} 1 & 0 \\ 1 & 13 \end{bmatrix} \\ \\ X_i^{mis} = \begin{bmatrix} 1 & 4 \\ 1 & 26 \end{bmatrix} \end{matrix}.$$

Even though the dependent variable (Y_i) is missing at some time points, X_i is fully observed if one assumes that the time of the observation is the planned time of the second and fourth HRQoL assessments.

6.4   Missing Completely at Random (MCAR)

6.4.1   The Concept

The strongest assumption about the missing data mechanism is that the data are missing completely at random (MCAR). The basic assumption is that the reason for a missing HRQoL assessment is entirely unrelated to HRQoL. Examples might include a patient moving or staff forgetting to provide the assessment. Some patients may not be able to participate because translations of the questionnaire are not available in their language.

While some missingness of HRQoL assessments is completely random in clinical trials, it is rare that this assumption holds for the majority of the missing data. Only 0-6% of the missing data in the breast cancer trial (Table 1.4) and 0-15% in the lung cancer trial (Table 1.7) were documented to be missing for reasons likely to be unrelated to the outcome.

6.4.2 Covariate-Dependent Dropout

The missingness may be dependent on patient characteristics measured prior to randomization or treatment assignment (X_i). If, after conditioning on these variables, missingness is unrelated to the outcome it may be considered MCAR. While missing assessments are sometimes associated with covariates, it is rare that they completely explain the missing data mechanism unless the missingness was determined by the study design. It is theoretically possible that dropout could be solely dependent on treatment, but constant within each treatment group irrespective of the outcome (Y_i) [Heyting et al., 1992]. If this assumption is true, then the patients with missing data are a random sample of all patients in each treatment group. However, it is difficult to imagine scenarios where this is true. Dropout related to side effects or lack of effectiveness is likely to affect HRQoL and would not fit this assumption.

6.4.3 Identifying Covariate-Dependent Missingness

The next step in the process of exploring the missing data process is to identify covariates that predict missing observations. There are numerous approaches that one can use. One method is to examine the correlation between an indicator of missing observations (r_{ijk}) and possible covariates. Kendall's τ_b is a useful statistic when one variable is dichotomous, such as the missing data indicator, and the other variables are a mixture of dichotomous, ordered categorical and continuous variables. A second approach is to perform a series of logistic regression analyses to model the probability of a missing assessment. If there are a large number of assessments and a predominately monotone pattern, a Cox proportional hazard model of the time to dropout may be a useful strategy. From a practical standpoint, patient characteristics (covariates) that are related to the subject's HRQoL should be given priority. The reasons for this will become more obvious in the later sections of this chapter and later chapters.

Lung Cancer Trial (Study 3)

In the lung cancer trial, missing assessments were weakly associated with physical characteristics such as older age, performance status and disease symptoms at the time of randomization. Similar results were obtained using either bivariate correlation (Table 6.6) or multivariate logistic regression.

In most studies, because pre-randomization covariates are not directly related to the reasons for dropout, they are likely to be only weakly predictive of missing data. We see this in the lung cancer trial. Although some correlations are statistically significant, none of these covariates individually explains more than 2% of the variation in the likelihood of a missing assessment as indicated by the squared value of the correlation coefficients displayed in Table 6.6. It should be noted that this procedure is an exploratory first step in understanding the missing data mechanism. Because of the number of comparisons, there

TABLE 6.6 Study 3: Association of missing assessments in lung cancer trial with baseline covariates. Correlation measured by Kendall Tau-b. Positive correlations indicate increased likelihood of a missing assessment.

	Assessment			
	Baseline	6 weeks	12 weeks	26 weeks
Male Gender	0.09*	-0.04	-0.01	-0.05
Older age at randomization	-0.02	0.10***	0.06	0.09**
Poorer performance status	-0.03	0.12**	0.13**	0.07
$\geq 5\%$ weight loss prior 6 mo	-0.06	0.07	0.08*	0.07
Primary disease symptoms	0.02	0.04	0.07	0.01
Metastatic disease symptoms	-0.00	-0.00	0.07	0.08
Systemic disease symptoms	-0.03	0.09*	0.07	0.02
Other Chronic Disease	-0.01	0.05	0.02	-0.02
Prior Radiation Therapy	-0.00	0.10*	0.04	0.02
Experimental regimen	0.00	-0.12**	-0.08	-0.06

* $p < 0.05$, ** $p < 0.01$, *** $p < 0.001$

is the possibility of spurious correlations.

6.4.4 Analytic Methods

In general, analytic methods that do not use all the available data require the data to be MCAR. For example, traditional multivariate analysis of variance (MANOVA) utilizes only data on subjects with complete data. The assumption is that these complete cases are a random sample of the larger sample. Similarly, separate univariate analysis of data from each timepoint ignores data obtained at other points in time and requires the data to be MCAR [Murray and Findlay, 1988]. The assumption is that the subjects with observed data at each timepoint are a random sample of all subjects. When this assumption is incorrect, the resulting estimates are likely to be biased. Detailed examples are presented in the following chapter.

6.5 MAR: Missing at Random

6.5.1 The Concept

The assumptions about the missing data mechanism are relaxed slightly when we assume the data are missing at random (MAR). Specifically, the missingness depends on the observed but not the missing data after conditioning on covariates. It is not uncommon for missing HRQoL data to depend on previously observed HRQoL scores. In most cases this is the initial (baseline) or previous HRQoL assessment, but could possibly include subsequent HRQoL assessments. In most settings, individuals who are experiencing better health and HRQoL will generally be more likely to be available for follow-up and more likely to complete the self-assessments required for the evaluation of HRQoL. However there are exceptions, such as individuals who drop out of a trial once their symptoms dissappear.

6.5.2 Identifying Dependence on Observed Data (Y_i^{obs})

Differences between MCAR and MAR can be tested by examining the association of missing data with observed HRQoL scores. Various methods include graphical presentations, formal tests, correlational analyses and logistic regression.

Graphical Approaches

Two examples of a graphical approach are displayed in Figures 6.1- 6.2 for the lung cancer trial. Figure 6.1 displays the average observed FACT-Lung TOI in groups of patients defined by their pattern of missing data. Because the total number of patterns is large and the number of subjects with intermittent or mixed patterns is small (Table 6.3), this plot was simplified by grouping subjects by the time of their last HRQoL assessment. The resulting figure suggests two things: subjects who dropped out earlier had poorer scores at baseline and scores were lower at the time of the assessment just prior to dropout (the last observation). Since missingness depends on previously observed FACT-Lung TOI scores, the data are not MCAR.

Figure 6.2 is a modification of one suggested by Hogan et al. [2004a]. It contrasts the scores just prior to dropout of subjects who drop out (CI without bars at end) with those from subjects with continued follow-up (CI with bars at end); the overall mean is also displayed ($\star$). Subjects clearly have lower scores just prior to dropout.

Formal Tests

Little [1988] proposed a single test statistic for testing the assumption of

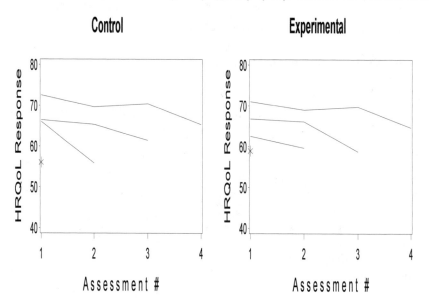

FIGURE 6.1 Study 3: Average FACT-Lung TOI scores for control and experimental arms stratified by time of last assessment.

MCAR vs. MAR. The basic idea is that if the data are MCAR, the means of the observed data should be the same for each pattern of missing data. If the data are not MCAR then the means will vary across the patterns (as is observed in Figure 6.1). This test statistic is particularly useful when there are a large number of comparisons either as a result of a large number of patterns or differences in missing data patterns across multiple outcome variables.

Consider a study designed to obtain J measurements. Let P be the number of distinct missing data patterns (R_i) where $J^{\{p\}}$ is the number of observed assessments in the pth pattern. $n^{\{p\}}$ is the number of cases with the pth pattern, $\sum n^{\{p\}} = N$. Let $M^{\{p\}}$ be a $J^{\{p\}} \times J$ matrix of indicators of the observed variables in pattern P. The matrix has one row for each measure present consisting of 0s and 1s identifying the assessments with non-missing data. For example, in the NSCLC example, if the first and third observation were obtained in the 6th pattern then

$$M^{\{6\}} = \begin{bmatrix} 1\ 0\ 0\ 0 \\ 0\ 0\ 1\ 0 \end{bmatrix}$$

$\bar{Y}^{\{p\}}$ is the $J^{\{p\}} \times 1$ vector of pattern p observed means . $\hat{\mu}$ and $\hat{\Sigma}$ are the ML estimates of the mean and covariance of the pooled data assuming that the missing data mechanism is ignorable. We then multiply these by $M^{\{p\}}$ to select the appropriate rows and columns for the pth pattern. Thus, $\hat{\mu}^{\{p\}} = M^{\{p\}} \hat{\mu}$ is the $J^{\{p\}} \times 1$ vector of ML estimates corresponding to the pth pattern

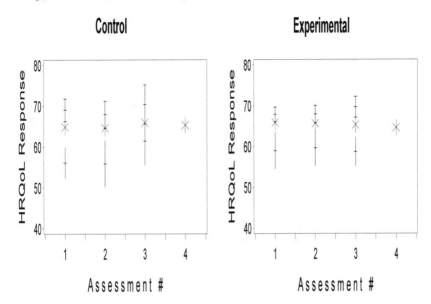

FIGURE 6.2 Study 3: Average FACT-Lung TOI scores for control and experimental arms. Overall mean is indicated by * symbol. Mean and 95% confidence interval (CI) indicated for those who drop out (no bar at end of CI) and do not drop out (bar at end of CI) at the next assessment.

and $\tilde{\Sigma}^{\{p\}} = \frac{N}{N-1} M^{\{p\}} \hat{\Sigma} M^{\{p\}\prime}$ is the corresponding $J^{\{p\}} \times J^{\{p\}}$ covariance matrix with a correction for degrees of freedom. Little's [1988] proposed test statistic,* when Σ is unknown, takes the form:

$$\chi^2 = \sum_{p=1}^{P} n^{\{p\}} (\bar{\mathbf{Y}}^{\{p\}} - \hat{\mu}^{\{p\}})' \tilde{\Sigma}^{\{p\}-1} (\bar{\mathbf{Y}}^{\{p\}} - \hat{\mu}^{\{p\}}) \qquad (6.1)$$

Little shows that this test statistic is asymptotically χ^2 distributed with $\sum J^{\{p\}} - J$ degrees of freedom. In the lung cancer trial, there is considerable evidence for rejecting the hypothesis of MCAR; $\chi^2_{23} = 61.7$, $p < 0.001$ in the control group and $\chi^2_{23} = 76.8$, $p < 0.001$ in the experimental group.

Listing and Schlitten proposed a parametric [1998] and nonparametric [2003] test for monotone patterns of missing data. The test statistic is derived from a comparison of the scores from the last assessment of dropouts to the scores at the same timepoint for those who complete all assessments. If the data are not MCAR then the scores will differ (as is observed in Figure 6.2).

---

*SPSS include this test in the MVA command (see Appendix P). SAS generates all the components in the MI procedure, but not the test.

Analytic Explorations

The next approach examines the association (correlation) between an indicator of missingness or dropout and the observed data. In the NSCLC study, we observe a moderate association between dropout and both the baseline and the most recent HRQoL scores (Table 6.7). The association was strongest for the scales measuring the physical or functional aspects of HRQoL such as functional well-being, physical well-being and lung cancer symptoms, all of which are part of the FACT-Lung TOI.

TABLE 6.7 Study 3: Correlation of missing assessments with baseline or previous HRQoL. Negative correlations indicate increased likelihood of a missing assessment with poorer HRQoL scores.

	Kendall Tau-b Correlation Coefficients			
		Assessment		
	Baseline	6 weeks	12 weeks	26 weeks
Baseline assessment				
Physical Well-being	NA	-0.19^{***}	-0.22^{***}	-0.20^{***}
Functional Well-being		-0.12^{***}	-0.17^{***}	-0.18^{***}
Lung Cancer Subscale		-0.14^{***}	-0.14^{***}	-0.14^{***}
Emotional Well-being		-0.04	-0.11^{**}	-0.03
Social/Family Well-being		0.02	-0.04	-0.05
Previous assessment				
Physical Well-being		-0.19^{***}	-0.18^{***}	-0.17^{***}
Functional Well-being		-0.12^{***}	-0.17^{***}	-0.21^{***}
Lung Cancer Subscale		-0.14^{***}	-0.16^{***}	-0.24^{***}
Emotional Well-being		-0.04	-0.16^{***}	-0.10^{*}
Social/Family Well-being		0.12^{***}	-0.07	-0.05

$^{*}\ p < 0.05,\ ^{**}\ p < 0.01,\ ^{***}\ p < 0.001$

We may also wish to confirm that the missingness depends on the observed data after adjusting for the dependence on covariates. This can be tested by first forcing the baseline covariates into a logistic model and then testing the baseline or previous measures of HRQoL. A variation is described by Ridout [1991] where the approach is to start with the observed data forced into the logistic model, then to test if added covariates can explain the association between dropout and the observed data.

Continuing with the lung cancer trial, we see the same results when using logistic regression models (Table 6.8). For all follow-up assessments, poorer baseline HRQoL, as measured by the FACT-Lung TOI score, is highly predictive of missing data. Similarly, the previous assessment is also highly predictive of missing data. The odds ratios for missing an assessment ranged from 0.63 to 0.74 for each 10 point increase in the FACT-Lung TOI score. These analyses reinforce the evidence that the missingness is dependent on observed HRQoL scores (Y_i^{obs}) and that in the lung cancer trial we can not assume that the observations are MCAR.

TABLE 6.8 Study 3: Odd ratios for missing assessments in lung cancer trial with either baseline or previous FACT-L TOI score. Baseline characteristics are forced into the models (O.R.s for baseline characteristics not shown). O.R. estimated for 10 point difference in FACT-Lung TOI.

	Odds Ratios (95% C.I.)		
	Time of Assessment		
	6 weeks	12 weeks	26 weeks
Baseline score	0.74 (0.64,0.83)	0.72 (0.63,0.83)	0.65 (0.56,0.76)
Previous score	0.72 (0.63,0.83)	0.70 (0.60,0.82)	0.63 (0.52,0.75)

6.5.3 Analytic Methods

In general, analytic methods that assume the missingness is MAR utilize all available HRQoL assessments. When the missing data are *ignorable*, unbiased estimates can be obtained from likelihood based methods using all observed data (Y_i^{obs}) and covariates (X_i) that explain the missing data mechanism. Note that exclusion of part of the observed data or omission of information on covariates in the analysis may result in biased estimates. For example, if missingness is dependent on baseline scores and some individuals are excluded from an analysis of change from baseline differences because they do not have follow-up assessments, the estimates may not be unbiased. Similarly, if missingness is strongly dependent on a covariate and that covariate is ignored, the estimates are biased. Examples of methods assuming *ignorable* missing data are presented in Chapters 3, 4, 5, 7 and 8 in more detail.

6.6 MNAR: Missing Not at Random

6.6.1 The Concept

The final classification for missing data mechanisms, MNAR, has the least restrictive assumptions. In this classification, the missingness is dependent on the HRQoL at the time of the planned assessment. For example, this might occur because assessments that are more likely to be missing when an individual is experiencing side effects of therapy, such as nausea/vomiting or mental confusion. Alternatively, subjects might be less willing to return for follow-up (and more likely to have missing assessments) if their HRQoL has improved as a result of the disappearance of their symptoms.

6.6.2   Identifying Dependence on Unobserved Data (Y_i^{mis})

Because we have not observed the missing HRQoL score, it is not possible to directly test a hypothesis of MNAR versus MAR. The data that we need to test the hypothesis are missing. However, it is possible to gather evidence that suggests the data are MNAR. Specifically, when there are other available measures of the disease or outcomes of treatment that are strongly associated with HRQoL, it may be possible to test for an association between missing observations and these surrogate measures. For example, if missingness is associated with more severe side effects and/or disease progression, then there is a reasonable likelihood that the data are MNAR (Table reftab:MNAREx2). In both cases, missingness may depend on the unobserved value even after conditioning on covariates and observed data. There are three options for indirectly testing for MNAR, none of which are entirely satisfactory.

The first option relies on the assumption of an underlying model for the missing data mechanism. Some of the analytic models such as those described in Chapters 11 and 12 will provide evidence that dropout is MNAR given a particular model. The limitation is that the absence of evidence from one particular model does not prove the null hypothesis of randomness against all alternatives. There are an infinite number of possible models for the non-random mechanism. Just because one model has been tested and there is no evidence of a nonrandom mechanism under that set of assumptions, we can not rule out other mechanisms.

The second option involves identifying observed surrogates for the missing values, such as assessments by a caregiver or evidence of toxicity. While these measures are imperfect, they provide some information about the missing values. Ideally, we want to identify variables associated with the missing HRQoL scores, but we only have access to observed data. Thus, we have to assume that the relationship between the observed HRQoL measures and these events is similar to the relationship between the missing HRQoL measures and these events. This may be a reasonable assumption for the relationship between a caregiver's assessment and the outcome. But it may be a much less realistic assumption between toxicity and the outcome if there is a selection among those experiencing the toxicity such that only those who have less impact on their HRQoL complete the questionnaire. Again, the lack of an identified relation between these additional variables and missingness is NOT proof that the data are not MNAR. Although it may increase the analyst's comfort with that assumption, there is always the possibility that important indicators of the dropout process were not measured in the trial or the analyst failed to identify them.

Evidence for the potential for nonrandom missing data will come from sources outside of the data. Clinicians and caregivers may provide the useful anecdotal information that suggests the presence of nonrandom missing data.

TABLE 6.9 Study 3: lung cancer patient outcomes associated with missing HRQoL among those with a previous assessment.

Assessment	Characteristic	Odds Ratio (95% CI)		p-value
6 weeks	Age†	1.55	(1.22, 1.96)	<0.001
	Performance status	1.21	(0.75, 1.97)	0.42
	Experimental arms of trial	0.64	(0.42, 0.99)	0.046
	Prior FACT-L TOI‡	0.75	(0.65, 0.86)	<0.001
	Neuro toxicity*	0.64	(0.53, 0.79)	<0.001
	PD$^\#$ within 6 cycles	1.61	(1.03, 2.51)	0.37
	Death within 2 months	3.36	(1.80, 6.25)	<0.001
12 weeks	Age†	1.30	(0.99, 1.71)	0.060
	Performance status	1.03	(0.60, 1.74)	0.92
	Experimental arms of trial	1.30	(0.74, 2.29)	0.36
	Prior FACT-L TOI‡	0.77	(0.65, 0.91)	0.002
	Neuro toxicity*	0.79	(0.63, 0.99)	0.041
	PD$^\#$ within 6 cycles	2.60	(1.49, 5.54)	<0.001
	Death within 2 months	5.18	(2.00, 13.4)	<0.001
6 months	Age†	1.51	(1.11, 2.05)	0.008
	Performance status	0.73	(0.42, 1.26)	0.26
	Experimental arms of trial	0.75	(0.42, 1.37)	0.35
	Prior FACT-L TOI‡	0.67	(0.55, 0.80)	<0.001
	Neuro Toxicity*	0.93	(0.73, 1.19)	0.58
	PD$^\#$ within 6 cycles	3.10	(1.54, 6.26)	0.002
	Death within 2 months	1.68	(0.75, 3.73)	0.20

† Age in years at randomization with OR estimated for 10 year difference

‡ OR estimated for 10 point difference in FACT-L TOI

* Maximum NCI Common Toxicity Criteria (CTC) grade, higher score = greater severity

$^\#$ Progressive disease

Lung Cancer Trial (Study 3)

In the lung cancer trial, we have already shown that the missingness depends on both the initial and the most recent HRQoL scores. The question that remains is whether, given the observed HRQoL scores and possibly the baseline covariates, there is additional evidence that missing assessments are more frequent in individuals who are experiencing events likely to impact HRQoL. Obviously, death is a perfect predictor of missingness. We also might expect toxicity, disease progression and nearness to death to impact both HRQoL and missingness.

We can continue with the exploratory approach that utilizes the logistic regression model including measures of toxicity, disease progression and nearness to death. The final step is to determine if these events or outcomes are associated with missingness after adjusting for the covariates and observed HRQoL identified as associated with missingness. After forcing age, performance status, treatment assignment and prior FACT-Lung TOI score into a logistic regression model for missing assessments, progressive disease during the first 6 cycles of therapy and death within 2 months of the planned assessment are strong predictors of missing assessments. This suggests that the data are MNAR. Unexpectedly, missing assessments were less likely among individuals with more toxicity. One possible explanation is that these patients are more likely to have follow-up visits and thus more likely to be available for HRQoL assessments.

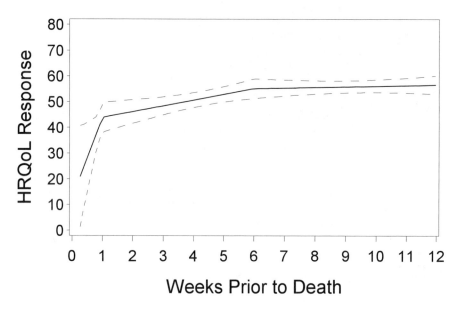

FIGURE 6.3 Study 3: Change in FACT-Lung TOI prior to death.

Other options to explore the relationship of missing data are only limited by the knowledge and thoughtfulness of the analyst. In the lung cancer trial, we can explore the association of observed scores with the proximity to death by plotting scores during the months prior to death backwards from the time of death (Figure 6.3). In this trial we observe a clear relationship with the outcome measure. Fayers and Machin [2000] describe an alternative graphical approach where the origin of the horizontal axis is the date of the last assessment. The HRQoL is then plotted backward in time. The decreasing values of the outcome just prior to dropout suggest that a downward trajectory is likely to continue after dropout.

6.6.3 Analytic Methods

All the analytic methods used to analyze data that are suspected to be MNAR utilize strong untestable assumptions. This concept will be presented in more detail in Chapter 7 and only briefly here. A large number of the analytic methods use auxiliary data, either a surrogate outcome that is measured longitudinally (Y_i^{aux}) or variables that represent the missing data process (M_i). The idea is to convert the analysis back to methods that are appropriate for MAR data; missingness is them assumed to be MAR conditional on the observed data, covariates and the auxiliary data. The analyses presented in Chapters 9-11 all rely on this principle. The methods presented in Chapter 12 rely on strong assumptions about the distribution of the outcome. The validity of all of these analyses can not be tested, so the recommendation is to consider them as sensitivity analyses given a plausible relationship between the outcome and missingness.

6.7 Example for Trial with Variation in Timing of Assessments

Trials that have more assessments or widely varied times of assessment will require variations on the strategies that have been presented in the previous sections of this chapter. When the timing of assessment varies and classifications of assessments into a repeated measures structure is not feasible, some of the methods previously presented, such as the logistic regression models and Little's test, will not be feasible. With a little creativity, one can still explore the relationship of outcomes with the missing data.

In the renal cell carcinoma trial, dropout was classified into three roughly equal groups based on the timing of the last assessment: early dropout (0-5 weeks), mid-period dropout (5-25 weeks) and late dropout/completion. The relationship of observed data with dropout can be displayed utilizing a growth curve model as displayed in Figure 6.4. There is a general trend for subjects remaining on study longer both to start with higher FACT-BRM TOI scores and to maintain higher FACT-BRM TOI scores over time. Again we see that

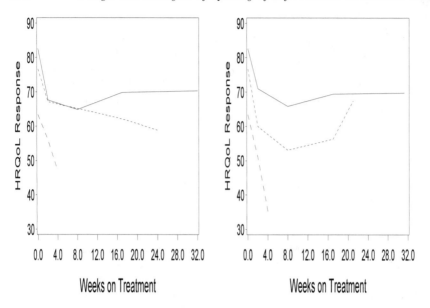

FIGURE 6.4 Study 4: Average FACT-BRM TOI scores for control (left) and experimental (right) arms stratified by time of last assessment. Patients with 25+ weeks of follow-up are represented by the solid line, with between 5 and 25 weeks with the short dashed lines, and with less than 5 weeks with the long dashed lines.

the observed values differ across the groups defined by time of dropout; thus missing assessments are not MCAR.

Using the same classifications, dropout during the early (0-5 weeks) and middle (5-25 weeks) periods can be examined using logistic regression. In both periods, the predictors of dropout are the baseline FACT-BRM TOI scores and the duration of the patient's survival (Table 6.10). The odds of dropout are reduced by about a third in both periods with a 10 point increase in the baseline FACT-BRM TOI scores. The odds are reduced by about half in the early period for every doubling of the survival time.[†] As in the lung cancer trial, the results suggest that dropout depends on observed data and is likely to depend on missing data if we can assume that the measure decreases as death approaches.

[†]Solely for the purposes of this exploratory analysis, censoring of the survival times was ignored. Note that the majority had died (75%) and the minimum follow-up was 2 years, thus the missing information would have only a moderate effect when the length of survival was expressed on a log scale.

TABLE 6.10 Study 4: Predictors of dropout. Results of exploratory multivariate logistic regression models.

Period	Characteristic	OR	(95% C.I.)
< 5 weeks	Baseline FACT-BRM TOI*	0.59	(0.42, 0.84)
vs > 5 weeks	Ln Survival‡	0.32	(0.13, 0.81)
	Ln Time on Tx‡	0.09	(0.03, 0.26)
5-< 25 weeks	Baseline FACT-BRM TOI*	0.84	(0.59, 1.19)
vs 25+ weeks	Ln Survival‡	0.07	(0.02, 0.25)
	Ln Time on Tx‡	0.42	(0.21, 0.86)

* Odd Ratio estimated for 10 point difference in FACT-BRM TOI.

‡ Odds Ratio estimated for doubling of the length of survival or time on treatment (0.693 units on the natural log scale).

6.8 Example with Different Patterns across Treatment Arms

The migraine prevention (Study 2) and the osteoarthritis (Study 6) trials both have a placebo arm and present different patterns of missing data. (Note that in the previous studies, the control arms all consisted of presumably active treatment regimens.) The osteoarthritis trial is described in further detail in Chapter 11; the remainder of this section describes the migraine prevention trial.

In the migraine trial, the experimental arm had more dropout attributed to toxicity (28% vs 15%) which occurred early (median time=7 weeks) but less due to lack of efficacy (6% vs 11%) which occurred later (median time= 14 weeks). Roughly only a half of the patients in each arm complete the trial.

Graphical displays of the mean values by time of dropout (Figure 6.5) and cause of dropout (Figure 6.6) clearly eliminate the possibility that the data are MCAR. The within strata estimates differ more across the strata for the experimental therapy arm than the placebo arm. Patients who drop out due to lack of efficacy have the greatest differences relative to patients who completed the trial.

So what does this suggest with respect to the analysis? First, analytic methods that assume the data is MCAR should be avoided. Second, it is very likely that the missing data are non-ignorable. Thus, some type of sensitivity analysis is highly recommended. Methods that rely on repeated measures type designs or growth curve analyses are all feasible. Concurrent auxiliary data potentially includes measures of frequency and severity of migraine attacks, the time on study and an assessment of the cause of dropout. The potential use

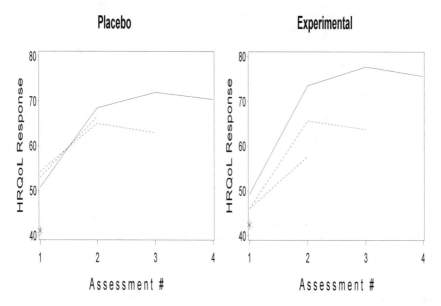

FIGURE 6.5 Study 2: Average MSQ RR scores for placebo (left) and experimental (right) arms stratified by time of last assessment. Patients with 4 assessments are represented by the solid line.

of this auxiliary data will be discussed in later chapters. Finally, Figures 6.5 and 6.6 suggest that the models used in the sensitivity analyses should consider a different relationship between dropout and the response in the two treatment arms.

6.9   Summary

- It is important to understand the missing data patterns and mechanisms in HRQoL studies. This understanding comes from a knowledge of the disease or condition under study and its treatment as well as statistical information.

- MCAR vs. MAR can be tested when the data have a repeated measures structure using the test described by Little [1988] (see Section 6.5.2).

- Graphical techniques are useful when examining the assumption of MCAR for studies with mistimed assessments (Figures 6.1 and 6.4).

- It is not possible to test MAR vs. MNAR without assuming a specific model (see Chapters 11 and 12), however, it may be useful to examine

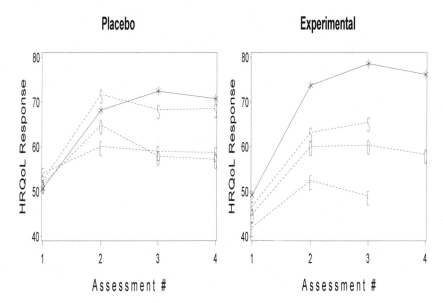

FIGURE 6.6 Study 2: Average MSQ RR scores for placebo (left) and experimental (right) arms stratified by reason for dropout. Patients who completed the study are represented by the solid line and star symbol. Patients who dropped out are represented by dashed lines with E indicating lack of efficacy, S side-effects, and O all other reasons.

the relationship between missing data and other observed outcomes, such as indicators of toxicity and response, that are expected to be related to HRQoL.

- The lack of statistical evidence of MNAR when there is clinical information (based on data or anecdote) that suggests missing data are related to the subject's HRQoL should not be interpreted as sufficient to ignore the missing data.

- A general strategy for missing data is as follows:

  1. Plan the study in a manner that avoids missing data.

  2. Collect auxiliary data that explain variability in the outcome and missing data patterns.

  3. Document the reasons for missing data in a manner likely to distinguish between ignorable and non-ignorable missing data.

  4. Perform sensitivity analyses.

7

Analysis of Studies with Missing Data

7.1 Introduction

In this chapter I will present an overview of methods that are used for the analysis of clinical trials with missing data. The first section covers methods that rely on the assumption that the missing data are missing completely at random (MCAR); I will try to convince you that these methods should always be avoided. The second section reviews methods that assume that the data are ignorable or missing at random (MAR) given covariates and the observed data. In the final section, I will present an overview of models that can be considered when data are suspected to be non-ignorable.

7.2 Missing Completely at Random

It is extremely rare that missing data in clinical trials are solely missing completely at random (MCAR). However, analyses that rely on this assumption continue to appear in the literature. The goal of this section is to identify these methods so that analyst can avoid their use.

The common characteristic of most analytic methods that assume data are MCAR is that they do not use all the available data. When missingness depends on observed data (Y_i^{obs}) and the analytic procedure does not include all available data, the results are biased. Similarly, if dropout is dependent on a covariate (X_i) and the covariate is not included in the analytic model, then the results are also biased. Popular analytic methods such as repeated univariate analyses and MANOVA of complete cases are examples of procedures that exclude observed data; results from these analyses are unbiased only if the missing data are MCAR [Murray and Findlay, 1988]. The magnitude of the bias depends on the amount of missing data and the strength of the association between the missing data (Y_i^{mis}) and the observed data (Y_i^{obs}) or the covariates (X_i).

There is also a misconception that analysis using generalized estimating equations (GEEs) addresses the issues of missing data. These methods actually make stronger assumptions about the missing data. Use of GEEs should be considered when the HRQoL measure has a very strong deviation from normality, transformations are unfeasible and the sample size is so small that the parameter estimates and statistics no longer have a normal distribution. In clinical trials, it is extremely rare that the sample sizes are so small that the estimates and test statistics (not the distribution of scores) are not asymptotically normal.

The safest approach for analysis of studies with missing data is to avoid these methods. Alternative methods include multivariate likelihood methods using *all* the available data, such as mixed-effects models or repeated measures for incomplete data. These are described in the following sections of this chapter and previously in Chapters 3 and 4.

Hypothetical Example

To illustrate the limitations of methods that assume that the data are MCAR, I will generate data from a hypothetical example where the data are actually MAR. This example illustrates how the various methods perform when we know the underlying missing data mechanism. Because all values are known and the example is simple, it is possible to show how the analytic results are affected by the missing data assumptions.

Assume there are 100 subjects with two assessments. The scores are generated from a standard normal distribution ($\mu = 0$, $\sigma = 1$). Three sets of data are generated such that the correlations between the assessments (ρ_{12}) are 0.0, 0.5 and 0.9. Correlations of HRQoL assessments over time in clinical trials are generally in the range of 0.4-0.7. The correlations of 0.0 to 0.9 are outside this range but will serve to illustrate the concepts. All subjects have the first assessment (T1), but 50% are missing the second assessment (T2). This is a larger proportion of missing data than one would desire in a clinical trial, but magnifies the effect we are illustrating. Finally, missing values are generated in two ways. In the first, observations at the second assessment are deleted in a completely random manner that is unrelated to the values at either assessment*. Thus the data are MCAR. In the second, the probability of a missing assessment at the second time point depends on the observed values at the first time point†. Thus the data are MAR conditional on the observed baseline data. The means for these hypothetical data are summarized in Table 7.1. Data from the complete cases is noted as Y^C and data from the cases with any missing data is noted as Y^I. For subjects with both the T1 and T2 assessments, $\bar{y}_1^C$ and $\bar{y}_2^C$ are the averages of the T1 and T2 scores. For subjects with only the T1 assessment, $\bar{y}_1^I$ is the average of the observed T1 scores. $\bar{y}_2^I$ is the average of the deleted T2 scores, which is known only because this is a simulated example.

---

*Uniform selection: $Pr[r_{i2} = 1] = 0.5$
†Probit selection: $Pr[r_{i2} = 1|Y] = \phi(y_{i1})$

TABLE 7.1 Expected means for hypothetical examples with 50% missing data at T2.

		$\rho = 0.0$		$\rho = 0.5$		$\rho = 0.9$	
		MCAR	MAR	MCAR	MAR	MCAR	MAR
Complete cases N=50							
T1	$\bar{y}_1^C$	0.00	0.57	0.00	0.57	0.00	0.57
T2	$\bar{y}_2^C$	0.00	0.00	0.00	0.28	0.00	0.51
Incomplete cases N=50							
T1	$\bar{y}_1^I$	0.00	-0.57	0.00	-0.57	0.00	-0.57
T2	$\bar{y}_2^I$	(0.00)	(0.00)	(0.00)	(-0.28)	(0.00)	(-0.51)
Observed Data							
T1	$\bar{y}_1^{obs}$	0.00	0.00	0.00	0.00	0.00	0.00
T2	$\bar{y}_2^{obs}$	0.00	0.00	0.00	0.28	0.00	0.51

( ) indicates the mean of the deleted or unobserved observations.

7.2.1 Complete Case Analysis (MANOVA)

Limiting the analysis to only those subjects who have completed all assessments was a widely used method of analysis; fortunately its use has decreased dramatically. Complete case analysis is also referred to as case-wise or list-wise deletion. Traditional software for multivariate analysis of variance (MANOVA) automatically limits the analysis to the complete cases. When data are MCAR, the only consequence of choosing this approach is a loss of power due to the reduced number of subjects. However, when the missingness depends on observed HRQoL the results of these analyses are biased.

Case-wise deletion results in an estimate of μ_1 that is the average of only the T1 assessments from the complete cases ($\bar{y}_1^c$) and an estimate of μ_2 that is the average of the T2 assessments ($\bar{y}_2^c$) from the complete cases. Thus, not only are the estimates of the mean at T2 biased when the data are MAR, but so estimates of the baseline (T1) assessment. This is illustrated for the hypothetical example in Table 7.2.

Note that designs that require both a baseline and at least one follow-up assessment can exclude cases and result in bias if a substantial number of cases are excluded.

7.2.2 Repeated Univariate Analyses

One of the most commonly used analytic approaches for data from a study with a repeated measures design is repeated univariate analysis at each time point using test procedures such as the t-test, ANOVA, or Wilcoxon rank sum test. Although simple to implement, this approach has several disadvantages [DeKlerk, 1986, Pocock et al., 1987a, Matthews et al., 1990]. The first is the restrictive assumption of MCAR. If missingness is associated with previous or future observations of HRQoL (MAR), then estimates based on

TABLE 7.2 Estimates of means at T2 ($\hat{\mu}_2$) in hypothetical example. Average of 100 simulations. The expected mean is 0. Estimates in bold face type indicate bias larger than the average standard error of the mean.

	$\rho = 0.5$		$\rho = 0.9$	
	MCAR	MAR	MCAR	MAR
MLE of all observed data	0.00	-0.02	-0.01	-0.02
Complete case (MANOVA)	0.01	**0.28**	0.01	**0.50**
Repeated univariate analyses	0.01	**0.28**	0.01	**0.50**
+ Baseline as a covariate (Naive)[†]	0.01	**0.28**	0.01	**0.50**
+ Baseline as a covariate (Correct)[‡]	0.00	-0.02	-0.01	-0.02

[†]Simple regression with baseline as a covariate; analysis limited to subjects with both assessments.
[‡]Means estimated at average baseline for all subjects.

only the HRQoL assessments at one point in time will be biased. This is illustrated in the hypothetical example for repeated univariate analysis (Table 7.2, second row), where the estimates of $\hat{\mu}_2$ utilize only the data available at T2 from the complete cases ($\bar{y}_2^C$).

$$\begin{bmatrix} \hat{\mu}_1 \\ \hat{\mu}_2 \end{bmatrix} = \begin{bmatrix} \pi\bar{y}_1^C + (1-\pi)\bar{y}_1^I \\ \bar{y}_2^C \end{bmatrix} = \begin{bmatrix} \bar{y}_1 \\ \bar{y}_2^C \end{bmatrix}. \tag{7.1}$$

where π is the proportion of subjects with complete data. Thus when dropout depends on the measure of HRQoL at T1 and responses are correlated ($\rho \neq 0$) there is significant bias in the estimated T2 mean.

There are other disadvantages to the repeated <u>univariate</u> approach. First, the pool of subjects is changing over time. Thus, the inferences associated with each comparison are relevant to a different set of patients. Second, the analyses produce a large number of comparisons that often fail to answer the clinical question but rather present a confusing picture. Further, the Type I error increases as the number of comparisons increase.

Adding Baseline as a Covariate

When repeated univariate analyses are employed, the baseline assessment is often added as a covariate. These analyses are typically performed using simple linear regression techniques and limit each analysis to those individuals with both the baseline and the follow-up assessment. Adjusting for the baseline values fixes the problem only when dropout depends solely on baseline values and not on any of the intermediate outcomes. With extended follow-up, there is likely to be a stronger relationship between dropout and the more recent assessments of HRQoL. Multivariate analyses using all available data as described in the next section provides a more flexible framework. Even when dropout depends only on baseline values, simply adding the baseline value as a covariate in the univariate regression does not fix the bias of the estimation. The problem is that the baseline values of those individuals who do not have a follow-up assessment are ignored.

Consider the hypothetical example where the model is

$$y_{i2} = \beta + y_{i1}\gamma + \epsilon_{i2}. \tag{7.2}$$

If the mean of the T2 scores is estimated using only the baseline data from the subjects with follow-up assessments (y_{i1}^C), then the mean HRQoL scores at T2 will be overestimated because $\bar{y}_1^C$ overestimates the baseline mean, μ_1. This is illustrated in Table 7.2 in the row identified as *Baseline (Naive)*.

$$\hat{\mu}_2 = \hat{\beta} + \bar{y}_1^C \hat{\gamma}. \tag{7.3}$$

In this example the estimates of μ_2 for the hypothetical example are identical to those obtained for the complete case and the univariate analyses without covariates. An alternative model is

$$y_{i2} = \beta + (y_{i1} - \bar{y}_{i1})\gamma + \epsilon_{i2}. \tag{7.4}$$

If $\bar{y}_{i1}$ is calculated using <u>all</u> baseline assessments, the estimates will be unbiased if dropout depends only on the baseline assessment and not intermediate assessments. In the hypothetical example this is designated in Table 7.2 in the row identified as *Baseline (Correct)*.

Procedures that use a *least squares means* (LS means) technique to obtain estimates averaged over nuisance variables (e.g. baseline covariates) generally do not fix the problem. In the context of longitudinal datasets with missing values, the software procedures do not default to the mean of <u>all</u> the baseline assessments, but to the mean of the assessments included in the analysis. The analyst is well advised to check how the LS means are computed in specific software programs.

Change from Baseline

Another frequently misused technique is the <u>univariate</u> analysis of the change from baseline to either a particular assessment or to the last observed assessment. These univariate analyses results in unbiased assessments only if intermediate assessments provide NO information about dropout and the baseline assessment incorporates information from all subjects (including those who do not have a follow-up assessment). Even when the dropout is completely dependent on the baseline values (as in the hypothetical example) the same issues that were addressed in the previous section are relevant (Table 7.3).

TABLE 7.3 Estimates of change from baseline $(\hat{\mu}_2 - \hat{\mu}_1)$ in hypothetical example. Average of 100 simulations. The expected change is 0. Estimates in bold face indicate bias larger than the average standard error.

	$\rho = 0.0$		$\rho = 0.5$		$\rho = 0.9$	
	MCAR	MAR	MCAR	MAR	MCAR	MAR
MLE of all observed data	0.01	0.01	0.01	-0.01	-0.01	-0.01
Complete cases	-0.01	**-0.56**	-0.00	**-0.28**	-0.01	**-0.07**
Regression (Naive)[†]	-0.01	**-0.56**	-0.00	**-0.28**	-0.01	**-0.07**
Regression (Correct)[‡]	0.01	0.01	0.01	-0.01	-0.01	-0.01

[†] Change from baseline analysis limited to subjects with two assessments.

[‡] Includes baseline as a covariate, means estimated at average baseline for all subjects.

7.3 Ignorable Missing Data

If the data are missing at random (MAR), conditional on the observed data Y_i^{obs}, then the method used for the analysis should include all the information from Y_i^{obs}. The maximum likelihood (MLE) and restricted maximum likelihood (REML) methods for the analysis repeated measures models (Chapter 3) and growth curve models (Chapter 4) both accomplish this.

Hypothetical Example

In the hypothetical example, consider a repeated measures model for the two possible assessments,

$$\underbrace{\begin{bmatrix} y_{i1} \\ y_{i2} \end{bmatrix}}_{Y_i} = \underbrace{\begin{bmatrix} 1 & 0 \\ 0 & 1 \end{bmatrix}}_{X_i} \underbrace{\begin{bmatrix} \mu_1 \\ \mu_2 \end{bmatrix}}_{\beta} + \underbrace{\begin{bmatrix} e_{i1} \\ e_{i2} \end{bmatrix}}_{e_i},$$

where the observations on each subject are allowed to be correlated,

$$Var \underbrace{\begin{bmatrix} y_{i1} \\ y_{i2} \end{bmatrix}}_{Y_i} = \underbrace{\begin{bmatrix} \sigma_{11} & \sigma_{12} \\ \sigma_{12} & \sigma_{22} \end{bmatrix}}_{\Sigma_i}.$$

The maximum likelihood estimates of the means (μ_1, μ_2) are

$$\begin{bmatrix} \hat{\mu}_1 \\ \hat{\mu}_2 \end{bmatrix} = \left(\sum X_i' \hat{\Sigma}_i^{-1} X_i \right)^{-1} \sum X_i' \hat{\Sigma}_i^{-1} Y_i.$$

It is difficult to see how the estimates are calculated when written in matrix notation. Consider a special case where all subjects have their first assessment but only a proportion, π, have their second assessment. The resulting estimates of the means are:

$$
\begin{bmatrix} \hat{\mu}_1 \\ \hat{\mu}_2 \end{bmatrix} = \begin{bmatrix} \pi \bar{y}_1^C + (1-\pi)\bar{y}_1^I \\ \bar{y}_2^C + (1-\pi)\frac{\hat{\sigma}_{12}}{\hat{\sigma}_{11}}(\bar{y}_1^I - \bar{y}_1^C) \end{bmatrix}
$$
$$
= \begin{bmatrix} \bar{y}_1 \\ \bar{y}_2^C + (1-\pi)\frac{\hat{\sigma}_{12}}{\hat{\sigma}_{11}}(\bar{y}_1^I - \bar{y}_1^C) \end{bmatrix}. \tag{7.5}
$$

If the variances of Y_1 and Y_2 are equal,

$$
\begin{bmatrix} \hat{\mu}_1 \\ \hat{\mu}_2 \end{bmatrix} = \begin{bmatrix} \bar{y}_1 \\ \bar{y}_2^C + (1-\pi)\hat{\rho}(\bar{y}_1^I - \bar{y}_1^C) \end{bmatrix}. \tag{7.6}
$$

The estimate of the mean at T1 is the simple average of all T1 scores ($\bar{y}_1$), because there are no missing data for the first assessment. With missing data at the second time point (T2), $\hat{\mu}_2$ is not the simple mean of all observed T2 assessments ($\bar{y}_2^C$) but is a function of the T1 and T2 scores as well as the correlation between them. The second term in equation 7.6 ($(1-\pi)\hat{\rho}(\bar{y}_1^I - \bar{y}_1^C)$) is the adjustment of the simple mean ($\bar{y}_2^C$). If we use the information in Table 7.1 for $\rho = 0.5$, we obtain an unbiased estimate:

$$
\hat{\mu}_2 = \bar{y}_2^C + .5\hat{\rho}(\bar{y}_1^I - \bar{y}_1^C) = 0.28 + (0.5)(0.5)(-0.57 - 0.57) = 0.0.
$$

The results are the same for all values of ρ.

The estimates of the T2 means, $\hat{\mu}_2$, using MLE of all available data, are displayed in the first row of Table 7.2. Estimates of change from T1 to T2, $\hat{\mu}_2 - \hat{\mu}_1$, are displayed in Table 7.3. Note that the ML estimates are unbiased for both the MCAR and MAR simulated datasets regardless of the correlation of the assessments over time.

7.3.1 Maximum Likelihood Estimation (MLE)

A more general explanation of the adjustments in the estimates that results from MLE or REML analyses is illustrated using a repeated measures model. Recall that in the previous chapter, we partitioned the complete data, Y_i, into the observed, Y_i^{obs}, and missing Y_i^{mis} assessments. When the complete data have a multivariate normal distribution,

$$
\begin{bmatrix} Y_i^{obs} \\ Y_i^{mis} \end{bmatrix} \sim N \left[\begin{pmatrix} X_i^{obs}\beta \\ X_i^{mis}\beta \end{pmatrix}, \begin{pmatrix} \Sigma^{o,o} & \Sigma^{o,m} \\ \Sigma^{m,o} & \Sigma^{m,m} \end{pmatrix} \right] \tag{7.7}
$$

the expected values of the missing data, conditional on the observed data is

$$
E[Y_i^{mis}|Y_i^{obs}] = E[Y_i^{mis}] + Cov[Y_i^{mis}, Y_i^{obs}]Var[Y_i^{obs}]^{-1}(Y_i^{obs} - E[Y_i^{obs}])
$$
$$
= X_i^{mis}\beta + \Sigma^{m,o}(\Sigma^{o,o})^{-1}(Y_i^{obs} - X_i^{obs}\beta). \tag{7.8}
$$

While this formula seems complicated, the results are not. Consider a subject whose early observations are lower than the average, $Y_i^{obs} < X_i^{obs}\beta$. The term

$[Y_i^{obs} - X_i^{obs}\beta]$ will be negative and if the observations over time are positively correlated $(\Sigma^{m,o}(\Sigma^{o,o})^{-1} > 0)$, the expected value of the missing data conditional on the observed data $(E[Y_i^{mis}|Y_i^{obs}])$ will be less than the unconditional expected value $(X_i^{mis}\beta)$. This is relevant because the algorithms (e.g. EM algorithm, method of scoring, and MCMC) that produce the MLEs in some way incorporate this conditional expectation.

7.3.2 Empirical Bayes Estimates

In the mixed-effects model, the expected value (unconditional expectation) of an observation is

$$E(Y_i) = E(X_i\beta + Z_i d_i + e_i) = X_i\beta. \tag{7.9}$$

Linear functions of the fixed effects are called *estimable functions*. $X_i\beta$ is an estimable function if β is estimable and $X_i\hat{\beta}$ is called the *best linear unbiased estimate* (BLUE) of Y_i.

The conditional expectation of **Y** given the random effects is

$$E(Y_i|d_i) = E(X_i\beta + Z_i d_i + e_i) = X_i\beta + Z_i d_i. \tag{7.10}$$

Linear functions of the fixed and random effects are called *predictable functions*. The *best linear unbiased predictor* (BLUP) of Y_i uses the estimates of β and d_i: $X_i\hat{\beta} + Z_i\hat{d}_i$. The random effects are unobserved and we use the *Empirical Bayes* estimates of the random effects: $\hat{d}_i$ is the expectation of the random effect, d_i, conditional on the observed data Y_i^{Obs}, where

$$E\begin{bmatrix} Y_i \\ d_i \end{bmatrix} = \begin{bmatrix} X_i\beta \\ 0 \end{bmatrix} \tag{7.11}$$

$$Var\begin{bmatrix} Y_i \\ d_i \end{bmatrix} = \begin{bmatrix} \Sigma_i & Z_i D \\ DZ_i & D \end{bmatrix} \tag{7.12}$$

$$E[d_i|Y_i] = 0 + DZ_i\Sigma_i^{-1}(Y_i - X_i\beta) \tag{7.13}$$

Some insight into the estimates obtained from the mixed-effects model is provided by further examination of the BLUPs of the responses for a particular individual, $\hat{Y}_i$. With a bit of algebraic manipulation, we see that the predicted values are a weighted combination of average *population* estimates, $X_i\hat{\beta}$, and observed data, Y_i [Verbeke and Molenberghs, 1997, p 119].

$$\begin{aligned} \hat{Y}_i &= X_i\hat{\beta} + Z_i\hat{d}_i \\ &= X_i\hat{\beta} + Z_i DZ_i'\Sigma_i^{-1}(Y_i^{obs} - X_i\hat{\beta}) \\ &= (I - Z_i DZ_i'\Sigma_i^{-1})X_i\hat{\beta} + Z_i DZ_i'\Sigma_i^{-1}Y_i^{obs} \\ &= (\Sigma_i\Sigma_i^{-1} - Z_i DZ_i'\Sigma_i^{-1})X_i\hat{\beta} + Z_i DZ_i'\Sigma_i^{-1}Y_i^{obs} \\ &= \underbrace{\sigma_w^2 I}_{Within} \Sigma_i^{-1}X_i\hat{\beta} + \underbrace{Z_i DZ_i'}_{Between} \Sigma_i^{-1}Y_i^{obs} \end{aligned} \tag{7.14}$$

Recall that $\Sigma_i = Z_i D Z_i' + \sigma^2 I$, thus $\sigma_w^2 I \Sigma_i^{-1}$ and $Z_i D Z_i' \Sigma_i^{-1}$ are the proportions of the total variance that can be attributed to the within and between subject components of the variance. Thus the predicted values, $X_i \hat{\beta}$, are weighted by the within-subject component and the observed data, Y_i^{obs}, weighted by the between-subject component. When the longitudinal assessments are highly correlated (the between-subject component is large), the observed data tell us more about the missing assessments and the weight on the observed data increases. As the correlation decreases, the BLUPs shrink toward the predicted values.

As before, the algorithms (e.g. EM algorithm [Dempster et al., 1977]) that generate the estimates the mixed-effects parameters, are constructed from these conditional expectations.

7.3.3 Multiple Imputation

Virtually all forms of Multiple Imputation (MI) assumes the data are missing at random given the observed data included in the imputation. Thus, unless surrogate information (data that is strongly correlated with the outcome) is used in the imputation but not in the analysis, the results rarely differ from those obtained using MLE techniques. MI may be helpful when there is missing data in the explanatory variables and a substantial number of subjects would otherwise be eliminated for the analysis. A number of MI techniques will be described in Chapter 9.

7.3.4 Lung Cancer Trial (Study 3)

The sensitivity of results to the assumption of MCAR versus MAR can be illustrated in the lung cancer trial (Example 2). Figure 7.1 illustrates the results from two analyses that assume the missing data are MCAR and one that assumes MAR. Limiting the analysis to the complete cases (designated by C) results in estimates that are 1/3 to 1/2 standard deviations higher than those using all available data (designated by M). The repeated univariate analysis (U) results in estimates that are constant over time, because the analyses are performed on different groups of subjects at each time point with the sickest patients selected out of the sample.

7.3.5 Baseline Assessment as a Covariate

Another strategy for the analysis of repeated measures is to include the baseline assessment in the model as a covariate (X_i) rather than using it as one of the repeated measures. In this model,

$$y_{ij} = x_{ij}\beta_j + y_{i1}\gamma_j + \epsilon_{ij} \quad j = 2 \cdots n_i \tag{7.15}$$

where y_{i1} is the baseline measure for the ith subject. This strategy required that we eliminate the baseline assessment from the dependent variables. It also

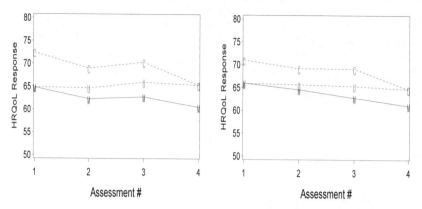

FIGURE 7.1 Study 3: Estimated FACT-Lung TOI scores for control (left) and experimental (right) arms estimated using complete cases (C), repeated univariate analyses (U) and MLE of all available data (M). The standard deviation of the FACT-Lung TOI scores is roughly 16 points.

excludes individuals who do not have both a baseline assessment and at least one follow-up assessment. As a result it makes more restrictive assumptions about missing data and should be used cautiously if there are missing data in either the baseline or early follow-up assessments. In general, this is not a good strategy for randomized clinical trials, but may be useful for observational studies.

7.3.6 Adding Other Baseline Covariates

Dropout is ofen associated with patient characteristics at baseline. The previous discussion would suggest that it will be important to include corresponding covariates in all analysis models. In practice these associations are weak and the inclusion or omission of these baseline covariates rarely makes a difference when the intent is to compare treatment arms in a <u>randomized</u> clinical trial. If the characteristic is not strongly correlated with the HRQoL measure, then its inclusion/exclusion will not affect the results. Even when the characteristic is correlated with the HRQoL measure, much of the covariance with post-randomization measures is explained by the correlation with the pre-randomization baseline measure. Overall, while the association between dropout and baseline characteristics may be statistically significant, they generally do not explain enough of the variation in dropout (see Section 6.4.3) to have an impact on the results. However, it is advisable to perform a sensitivity analysis by repeating the analysis with these covariates.

In randomized trials, the treatment arms should be balanced with respect to these patient characteristics. When there are apparent differences detected in baseline characteristics, two possibilities exist: 1) the differences are real or 2) there is no difference between the groups and a Type I error has occurred. In the first case, it is appropriate to adjust the estimates by inclusion of a covariate in the analysis, but in the second case the differences are ignored. Unfortunately, it is not possible to distinguish the two cases. Again, a sensitivity analysis is advisable.

7.3.7 Final Comments

Exclusion of Subjects

Exclusion of subjects, and thus observed data, from the analysis may occur in subtle ways. It is not uncommon to include only those subjects with a baseline and at least one follow-up assessment in the analysis. This strategy automatically excludes some subjects with observed data because they have only one observation. The assumption is that the reason they do not have at least two assessments is completely random. In practice this is rarely true. Often these are the sickest patients with the poorest HRQoL scores at baseline. In the NSCLC study, only 5% of the subjects are missing all four FACT-Lung TOI scores (Table 7.4). But another 27% of the subjects are excluded if a baseline and at least one follow-up assessment were required for inclusion; 4% because of the requirement for a baseline assessment and 23% because of the requirement for a follow-up assessment.

TABLE 7.4 Study 3: Potential for exclusion of subjects in the lung cancer trial.

	No Taxol		Taxol		Total	
	N (%)		N (%)		N (%)	
No FACT-L TOI data	10 (	5)	16 (	4)	26 (	5)
No Baseline FACT-L TOI	7 (	4)	16 (	4)	23 (	4)
No Follow-up FACT-L TOI	56 (	29)	77 (	20)	133 (	23)
Baseline + at least 1 follow-up	121 (	62)	272 (	71)	393 (	68)
Total Subjects	194 (100)		381 (100)		575 (100)	

Exclusion of Observations

Exclusion of observations from the analysis should be performed very cautiously. In some settings, there is a valid conceptual reason to do so. For example, in the adjuvant breast cancer study (Study 1), four assessments were excluded from the pre-therapy assessments because they occurred after therapy started and two assessments were excluded from the on-therapy assessments because they occurred after therapy had been stopped. In other settings, the artificial attempt to force observations into a repeated measures model may result in the exclusion of observations. If the exclusion is not random or missingness at other occasions depends on the value of these observations, the resulting analyses are biased.

7.4 Non-Ignorable Missing Data

In the past 20 years, there has been an increasing interest in the methods of analysis of studies with nonrandom missing data. Reviews of early methods include Little [1995] and Hogan and Laird [1997b]. Most models can be classified into three approaches to the analysis of longitudinal studies with nonrandom missing data: selection models, mixture models and joint shared-parameter models. These three approaches are not mutually exclusive; the selection models and the mixture models are distinct, but the joint shared-parameter models overlap selection and mixture models. In all these approaches, the joint distribution of the longitudinally measured outcome, Y_i and either the dropout time, T_i^D, or the missing data indicators, R_i, are incorporated into the model.

7.4.1 Selection Models

The term *selection model* was originally used to classify models with a univariate response, y_i, where the probability of being *selected* into a sample depended on the response. In longitudinal studies, the term has been used to describe models where dropout depends on the response. Hogan and Laird [1997b] divide the selection models into *outcome-dependent* selection and *random-effect* selection models. Using the notation presented in the previous chapter,

$$\text{Outcome-dependent selection } f(M_i | Y_i^{obs}, Y_i^{mis}) \qquad (7.16)$$
$$\text{Random effects dependent selection } \quad f(M_i | d_i) \qquad (7.17)$$

where M_i may be the time to dropout T_i^D or a pattern of responses, R_i. In the outcome-dependent selection models, the missing data mechanism (dropout) depends directly on the longitudinal outcome, Y_i. An example of a outcome-dependent selection model is the model proposed by Diggle and Kenward [1994] (see Chapter 12). In the random-effects selection models, dropout depends on then random effects, d_i or the individual trajectories, $\beta_i = \beta + d_i$. This later model is typical of settings where dropout is related to trends over time. An example of a random-effects dependent selection model is the joint model proposed by Schluchter [1992] and DeGruttola and Tu [1994] (see Chapter 11).

In these models, the analyst must specify how dropout depends on the outcome, Y_i, or the random effects, d_i. Because the complete data are not fully observed, we must make untestable assumptions about the form of $f(M_i|\mathbf{Y} \text{ or } d_i)$.

In addition to adjusting the estimates for the missing data, these models allow the investigator to explore possible relationships between HRQoL and explanatory factors causing missing observations. This is particularly interesting, for example, if death or disease progression was the cause of dropout. The criticism of selection models is that the validity of the models for the missing data mechanism is untestable because the model includes unobserved data (Y_i^{mis} or d_i) as the explanatory variable.

7.4.2 Mixture Models

The term *mixture model* originates from the concept of mixing the distributions $f(\mathbf{Y}|\mathbf{M})$ or, more formally, integrating over $f(\mathbf{M})$ to obtain the marginal distribution of the longitudinal outcome. Mixture models factor the joint distribution into the product of $f(\mathbf{Y}|\mathbf{M})$ and $f(\mathbf{M})$. The complete data, $f(Y)$, is characterized as a mixture (weighted average) of the conditional distribution, $f(Y|\mathbf{M})$, over the distribution of dropout times, the patterns of missing data or the random coefficients. The specific form of $\mathbf{M}$ distinguishes the various mixture models where $\mathbf{M}$ is either dropout time, T_i^D, the pattern of missing data, R_i, or a random coefficient, d_i.

$$\text{Pattern mixture} \quad f(Y_i|R_i) \tag{7.18}$$

$$\text{Time-to-event mixture} \quad f(Y_i|T_i^D) \tag{7.19}$$

$$\text{Random effects mixture} \quad f(Y_i|d_i) \tag{7.20}$$

Pattern mixture models are a special case of the mixture models. When $M_i = R_i$, the missingness can be classified into patterns. Chapter 10 presents examples of these models in detail. Where missing data are due to dropout, the distributions, $f(Y_i|T_i^D)$, may be a function of the time to dropout or an associated event. The random-effects mixture, $f(Y_i|d_i)$ is a mixed-effects model where the random-effects model includes the dropout time, T_i^D. Examples include the *conditional linear model* proposed by Wu and Bailey [1989] and the *joint model* proposed by Schluchter [1992] and DeGruttola and Tu [1994] (see Chapter 11).

7.4.3 Final Comments

1. All models for non-ignorable data require the analyst to make strong assumptions.

2. These assumptions cannot be formally tested. Defense of the assumptions must be made on a clinical basis rather than a statistical basis.

3. Lack of evidence of non-ignorable missing data for any particular model does not prove the missing data are ignorable.

4. Estimates are not robust to model misspecification.

7.5   Summary

- Methods that exclude subjects or observations from the analysis should be avoided unless one is convinced that the data are missing completely at random (MCAR). This includes repeated univariate analyses which ignore observations that occur at different times, MANOVA, which deletes cases with any missing assessments and inclusion criteria for the analyses such as requiring both a baseline and at least one follow-up assessment.

- When the proportion of missing data if very small or thought to be ignorable, is advisable to employ likelihood based methods (MLE) that use all of the observed data such as repeated measures models for incomplete data (Chapter 3) or mixed-effects models (Chapter 4).

- When missing data is suspected to be non-ignorable, it is advisable to perform sensitivity analyses using one or more of the methods described in Section 7.4.

8

Simple Imputation

8.1 Introduction to Imputation

There are numerous methods of imputation that are becoming easier to perform with existing software. As a result, there is a danger of using imputation as a quick fix for problems that chould have been prevented with a thoughtful trial design. As we will illustrate in this and the next chapter, all of the methods rely on strong assumptions about the missing data mechanism which are often ignored. In most cases when the assumptions are correct there are direct methods of analysis utilizing all of the available data that produce the same results (see Chapters 3 and 4). If the concern is that the missingness is non-random (MNAR), imputation methods will only be helpful if there is additional auxiliary information. The following quote summarizes the issue:

> It is clear that if the imputation model is seriously flawed in terms of capturing the missing data mechanism, then so is any analysis based on such imputation. This problem can be avoided by carefully investigating each specific application, by making the best use of knowledge and data about the missing-data mechanism, ...
> [Barnard and Meng, 1999]

There are a limited number of situations where imputation is useful in HRQoL research. The first occurs when the respondent skips a small number of items in a questionnaire (Section 8.2). The second occurs when there are multiple explanatory (independent) variables or covariates with very small proportions of missing data individually, but a substantial proportion overall [vanBuuren et al., 1999] (Section 8.5). Missing covariates will result in the deletion of individuals with missing data from any analysis. The concern is that a selection bias occurs when those with incomplete data differ from those with complete data. Missing assessments (entire questionnaire) are a more common problem in HRQoL research. Only when there is auxiliary information such as surrogate variables or strongly correlated clinical data will imputation methods be useful. In Sections 8.3 and 8.4, I will focus on imputation of the HRQoL measures, not because I would recommend simple imputation methods for missing outcome measures, but because it is easier to illustrate the methods and principles.

The choice among methods should be made only after careful consideration of why the observations are missing, the general patterns of change in HRQoL over time, and the research questions being addressed. Without this careful consideration, imputation may increase the bias of the estimates. For example, if missing HRQoL observations are more likely in individuals who are experiencing toxicity as a result of the treatment, the average value from individuals with observations (who are less likely to be experiencing toxicity) will likely overestimate the HRQoL of individuals with missing data.

8.1.1   Simple versus Multiple Imputation

Simple imputation is the process of substituting a single reasonable value for a missing observation. Common simple imputation methods (Table 8.1) include techniques such as last value carried forward (LVCF) and substitution of predicted values from regression based techniques. The most common criticism of simple imputation is that most analyses treat imputed values as if they were observed values. This results in underestimation of the variance of the parameter estimates with the resulting inflation of Type I errors. The problem increases with more missing data; estimates may appear more precise as the proportion of missing data increases. This chapter covers simple imputation techniques and illustrates this concern. Multiple imputation [Rubin and Schenker, 1986, Rubin, 1987] rectifies the above problem by incorporating various compents on uncertainty into the imputation (see Chapter 9).

TABLE 8.1 Examples of simple imputation methods.

Means	Mean of observed data
Predicted Values	Predicted values from univariate or multivariate regression models
Hot Deck	Randomly sampled observation
Ad Hoc	Simple rules
LVCF (LOCF)	Last value (observation) carried forward
MVCF	Minimum value carried forward
Low/High value	A theoretically justified low or high value; possibly the minimum or maximum observed value
δ-adjustments	Subtract a value from the LVCF for subjects who have died.

8.1.2   Imputation in Multivariate Longitudinal Studies

The procedure to implement an imputation scheme will generally seem straightforward when described in terms of a single variable with missing data. However, in practice it is much more complex. There will be numerous variables with missing responses. Clinical trials most often involve longitudinal assessments with multiple measures. Questions start to arise concerning the order of imputing missing values. Should they be imputed sequentially in time or simultaneously? Should relationships between the different outcomes be considered in the ordering? What seems to be a straightforward process can become very complex.

Imputation after Death

One of the most controversial subjects is whether to impute values after death. For preference based (utility) measures this is not an issue as death has a predefined value (usually zero). For other measures the debate continues. I do not propose to resolve the issue, but to point out that most analyses involve some form of implicit imputation of missing data values. In the simplest form, when the result is the mean of the observed data, the implicit imputation is that the missing data have the same mean and variance as the observed data. Arguing that the result only represents the mean for surviving patients limits the inferences that can be made for comparisons across treatment group in the presence of mortality.

Bias toward the Null Hypothesis

One principle of imputation is the need to incorporate information from variables that will be used in later analyses into the imputation procedure. For example, if the intent is to compare two treatment groups, the imputation must either be done separately for each treatment group or an indicator of treatment group included in the imputation model. If this is not done the resulting analysis will be biased toward the null hypothesis. As a simple example, consider a imputation technique that uses the mean of all observed data to impute the missing observations. Using the mean of the entire sample (ignoring treatment group) will result in estimates of means based on the observed and imputed data for each treatment group that are closer together than for the observed data.

8.2 Missing Items in a Multi-Item Questionnaire

First, let us address missing items in a multi-item questionnaire that computes scores using the responses to multiple questions that are all answered on the same scale (e.g. 1-5). The majority of instruments used in HRQoL research employ a procedure that is often referred to as the *half rule*. The procedure is that if the subject completes at least half of the items being used to compute

TABLE 8.2 Example of imputing missing items using the *half rule*. Subjects 2 and 3 have missing responses. The observed responses are indicated in the columns labeled "Obs" and the observed and imputed responses are indicated in the columns labeled "Obs + Imp."

Question #	Subject 1 Observed	Subject 2 Obs	Subject 2 Obs + Imp	Subject 3 Obs	Subject 3 Obs + Imp
1	3	3	3	3	3
2	4	4	4	4	4
3	2	2	2	2	2
4	3	3	3	–	2.75
5	2	2	2	2	2
6	4	4	4	–	2.75
7	2	–	3.0	–	2.75
Average Score	2.86	3.0	3.0	2.75	2.75
Summed Score	20		21		19.25

a score, the mean of the observed responses are substituted for the missing values. This is exactly the same as taking the mean of the observed responses and rescaling that value to have the same potential range as the scale would have if all the items were answered. For example, the social/family well-being scale of the FACT-G has 7 questions with responses that range from 0-4. If all items are answered, the total score is the sum of the responses, but can also be calculated as the mean of the seven responses times 7. Following the half rule, the summated score is also the mean of the responses times 7. To illustrate, consider the three subjects presented in Table 8.2. The first subject completed all items, so her score (the sum of the items) is 20. This is exactly the same as the average multiplied by 7. Subject 2 completed 6 of 7 items. The average of his scores is 3.0, so his total score is 21. Finally, Subject 3 completed only 4 items (more than half). Her average of the 4 items is 2.75, thus her total summed score is 2.75x7=19.25. This particular scale includes one question about sexual activity, making the half-rule particularly useful.

One of the advantages of this method of computing scores in the presence of missing items is that it is simple (can even be done by hand) and only depends on the responses contained in that individual's questionnaire. Thus the score does not depend on the collection of data from other subjects and would not differ from trial to trial. However, one wonders whether this method is the most accurate. Would other regression based methods improve the scores? This answer is surprising and investigators have found it is hard to improve on this simple method with regression based methods [Fairclough and Cella, 1996b]. As more research emerges using item response theory (IRT), this may change. But my suspicions are that the small incremental improvements will only be justifiable when the data are gathered electronically and can be scored electronically.

A final comment: Investigators should be concerned about any individual question that has more than 10% missing responses. For questions about some topics, the lower response rate is expected and unavoidable, such as with questions about sexual activity. It may also indicate that the question is poorly worded or not appropriate for some populations or in some settings. For example, the Breast Chemotherapy Questionnaire (BCQ) used in the breast cancer trial (Study 1), asks questions about how much certain symptoms bother the respondent. It will be difficult to respond to that question if you are not experiencing the symptom. This was particularly a problem when the assessments were prior to or after the completion of therapy. Because of the content of the questions of the BCQ, the instrument is very sensitive to differences that occur during therapy, but is unlikely to be useful for long term follow-up. Another example is an instrument that asks questions specifically about work. If the respondent interprets the question as only referring to paid work, they may not respond to this question, particularly if they are retired, a student or work at home. In the FACT-G, the phrase "including work at home" is added to expand the application of this question although it still may not be applicable for all respondents.

8.3 Regression Based Methods

In this section we are going to consider four regression based methods for simple imputation. First, I will distinguish between the analytic model (equation 8.1) and the imputation model (equation 8.2) using the superscript $(*)$ to distinguish the outcome and explanatory variables included in imputation model

$$\text{Analytic Model } Y_i = X_i\beta + \epsilon_i \tag{8.1}$$

$$\text{Imputation Model } Y_i^* = X_i^*\mathcal{B}^* + \varepsilon_i^* \tag{8.2}$$

Some of the problems with simple imputation cited above are illustrated by examining the results of simple imputation in the lung cancer trial (Study 3) presented in the remainder of this chapter.

8.3.1 Mean Value Substitution

A common simple imputation technique is the substitution of the average value from the individuals who completed the measure of HRQoL for the missing observations. Variables in the analytic model that will be the basis of tests of hypotheses must be included in the imputation model in some form to avoid bias toward the null hypothesis. In the lung cancer trial, the means are estimated separately for each treatment group and the imputation model is the same as the analytic model (using only time and treatment in the analytic model).

The distributions of observed scores and imputed scores at weeks 12 and 26 for the lung cancer trial are displayed in Figure 8.1. The imputed values are centered relative to the observed scores emphasizing the assumption that the missing values are MCAR. This may be valid if the missing data are due to administrative problems, but is hard to justify in most clinical trials. Figure 8.1 emphasizes the distortion of the distributions of observations. In the final section of this chapter, I will illustrate how this impacts estimation of standard errors and severely inflates the Type I error rate (see Section 8.6).

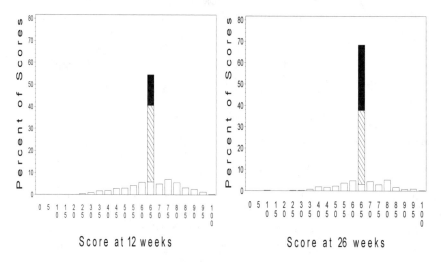

FIGURE 8.1 Study 3: Distribution of observed and imputed values using group means. Imputed values before death are indicated by the shaded area and after death by the solid area.

8.3.2   Explicit Regression Models

In the explicit regression model approach, we identify a regression model to predict the missing observation. The explicit regression approach has the advantage that the regression model used to impute missing observations can readily use auxiliary information about the subject's HRQoL that could not be included in the model used for the ultimate analysis of the clinical trial. This additional information might include indicators of the side effects of treatment and the clinical course of the disease when the therapy succeeds or fails. Alternatively, it could include measures of HRQoL provided by a caregiver when the subject is no longer able to complete self-assessments.

Identification of the Imputation Model

The objective of imputation is to obtain unbiased estimates of the missing observations. In the context of the explicit regression approach, we are looking for a model where the missingness in the imputation model depends only on the observed data (Y_i^*) and covariates in the imputation model (X_i^*). Basically, we are attempting to augment the analytic model with auxiliary information, so that the MAR assumption in the imputation model seems reasonable. The primary candidates for covariates include measures that are strongly correlated with both the measure being imputed and the probability that it is missing. In the lung cancer trial, this suggests adding covariates associated with toxicity, disease progression
indexProgressive disease and the proximity of the patient to death. Recall that * is used to distinguish the covariates and corresponding parameters of the imputation model from those included in the analytic model.

Assuming that the objective of the analysis is the comparison of treatment groups, the following strategy is recommended for identification of the imputation model [vanBuuren et al., 1999]:

1. Identify patient characteristics, measures, and clinical outcomes that are strongly correlated with the HRQoL measure to be imputed. Pay attention to the proportion of variation (R^2) that is explained rather than relying solely on statistical significance.

2. Identify patient characteristics, measures, and clinical outcomes that predict missingness of the HRQoL measures to be imputed.

3. Remove variables from the above lists if they are frequently missing. If X_i^{*mis} includes covariates that are missing, then we will be unable to impute values for Y_i^{mis}.

4. Identify the relationships that will be tested in the analytic model and include the corresponding information in the imputation model regardless of the strength of the relationship in the observed data. These will typically be indicators of the treatment arms in clinical trials. If the sample size is large, develop separate imputation models for each treatment group. Otherwise, force variables identifying the treatment groups into the model. If models are not being developed separately for each treatment group, evaluate interactions between treatment and potential covariates. Failure to do this will bias the treatment comparisons toward the null hypothesis.

When the intent of the analysis extends beyond treatment group comparisons, all important explanatory variables on which inference is planned should be included as explanatory variables in the imputation model to avoid biasing the evidence toward the null hypothesis.

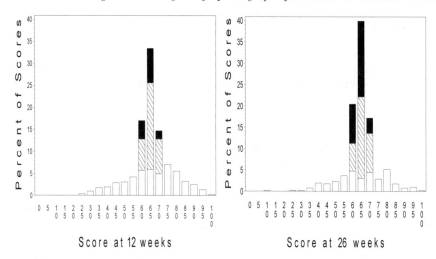

FIGURE 8.2 Study 3: Distribution of observed and imputed values using simple regression with baseline characteristics (treatment group, performance status, prior weight loss, symptoms of primary and systemic disease). Imputed values before death are indicated by the shaded area and after death by the solid area.

Simple Univariate Regression

The parameters of the imputation model for the jth assessment, $\hat{\mathcal{B}}_j^*$, are estimated using the observed data with the model

$$Y_{ij}^{obs} = X_{ij}^{*obs}\mathcal{B}_j^* + \varepsilon_{ij}^*. \tag{8.3}$$

The predicted values are then computed for the missing values:

$$Y_{ij}^{*mis} = X_{ij}^{*mis}\hat{\mathcal{B}}_j^*. \tag{8.4}$$

This approach will result in unbiased estimates if the regression model satisfies the MCAR assumption. In practice this approach will require the luck or foresight to measure the patient characteristics and outcomes (auxiliary) that explain the missing data mechanism.

The distributions of observed scores and imputed scores are displayed in Figures 8.2 and 8.3. The assumptions about the missing data have been relaxed slightly. Adding baseline covariates (Figure 8.2) results in a small amount of variation in the imputed scores and a very small shift in the distribution. The addition of the auxilary outcome information (best response and death within 2 weeks) results in more variation and a perceptible shift downwards of the imputed values (Figure 8.3). We are still assuming that relationships between HRQoL and clinical outcomes such as response and survival are the same for subjects with missing data as for those with observed HRQoL. Note that the range of imputed values is still smaller than the

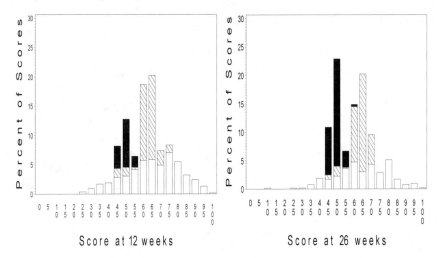

FIGURE 8.3 Study 3: Distribution of observed and imputed values using simple regression with baseline characteristics (treatment group, performance status, prior weight loss, symptoms of primary and systemic disease) and outcome (best response and death within 2 months). Imputed values before death are indicated by the shaded area and after death by the solid area.

range of observed values. The implications of this are discussed later in this chapter (see Section 8.6).

The `SPSS MVA` command with the `REGRESSION` option can be used to output a dataset with the missing values replaced by an imputed value. Random errors are added to Y_{ij}^{*mis} which somewhat mitigates the problems associated with simple imputation, but does not solve it completely [vonHippel, 2004].

Conditional Predicted Values

In the longitudinal setting, the likelihood of missing data often depends on observed data (Y_i^{obs}) such as previous HRQoL assessments. If we wish to obtain unbiased estimates, it is critical that we include the observed data in the imputation procedure. Specifically, we want to predict values of the missing HRQoL scores using the previously observed HRQoL scores from that individual. These conditional estimates are referred to as either Empirical Best Linear Unbiased Predictors (EBLUPs) or Buck's conditional means [Buck, 1960, Little and Rubin, 1987]. (See Section 7.3.3 for more details on EBLUPs.) For both the repeated measures and random-effects model the estimates take the form

$$E[Y_i^{mis}|Y_i^{obs}, \hat{\mathcal{B}}^*] = X_i^{*mis}\hat{\mathcal{B}}^* + \hat{\Sigma}_{mo}\hat{\Sigma}_{oo}^{-1}(Y_i^{obs} - X_i^{*obs}\hat{\mathcal{B}}^*) \quad (8.5)$$

$$Var\begin{bmatrix} Y_i^{mis} \\ Y_i^{obs} \end{bmatrix} = \begin{bmatrix} \Sigma_{mm} & \Sigma_{mo} \\ \Sigma_{om} & \Sigma_{oo} \end{bmatrix}. \quad (8.6)$$

For a mixed-effects model (equation 3.9), the estimates are a special case

$$E[Y_i^{mis}|Y_i^{obs}, \hat{\mathcal{B}}^*, \hat{d}_i^*] = X_i^{*mis}\hat{\mathcal{B}}^* + Z_i^{*mis}\hat{d}_i^* \tag{8.7}$$
$$= X_i^{*mis}\hat{\mathcal{B}}^* + Z_i^{*mis}\hat{D}Z_i^{*obs\prime}\hat{\Sigma}_{oo}^{-1}(Y_i^{obs} - X_i^{*obs}\hat{\mathcal{B}}^*).$$

Note that the observed data (Y_i^{obs}) are now included in the equation used to predict the missing values for each individual. When the observed HRQoL scores for the ith subject are higher (or lower) than the average scores for subjects with similar predicted trajectories, then the difference $(Y_i^{obs} - X_i^{*obs}\hat{\mathcal{B}}^*)$ is positive (or negative). As a result, the imputed conditional predicted value is larger (or smaller) than the imputed unconditional value $(X_i^{*mis}\hat{\beta})$. Further, when HRQoL scores within the same individual are more strongly correlated, the second term, $\hat{\Sigma}_{mo}\hat{\Sigma}_{oo}^{-1}(Y_i^{obs} - X_i^{*obs}\hat{\mathcal{B}}^*)$ in equation 8.5 or $Z_i^{*mis}\hat{d}_i^*$ in equation 8.7, is larger in magnitude and the difference between the conditional and unconditional imputed values will increase.

The entire distribution of observed scores and imputed scores, predicted by multivariate linear regression, are displayed in Figure 8.4. The same set of explanatory variables used to generate the data in Figure 8.3 was used to generate these values. However, the imputed values now include information about the patient's previous HRQoL. As a result the distribution of the imputed values appears to be shifted down and the range of values has greatly expanded.

The imputed values can be obtained using existing software (e.g. SAS Proc Mixed, SPSS Mixed/ Save=PRED(BLUP)). However, the standard errors of estimates using these values will be underestimated(see Section 8.6). The SPSS MVA command with the EM option adds random errors to the expected values which somewhat mitigates the problems associated with simple imputation, but does not solve it completely [vonHippel, 2004].

8.4 Other Simple Imputation Methods

8.4.1 Last Value Carried Forward (LVCF)

Another popular approach is to use the last value (or observation) carried forward (LVCF or LOCF), where the patient's last available assessment is substituted for each of the subsequent missing assessments. Although analyses using LVCF are often reported, the authors rarely justify the use of LVCF or examine the pattern of change in HRQoL as a function of dropout [Raboud et al., 1998]. This approach assumes that the last available response of a patient withdrawing from a study is the response that the patient would have if the patient had remained in the trial. The assumption that HRQoL does not change after dropout seems inappropriate in most studies. Thus, this

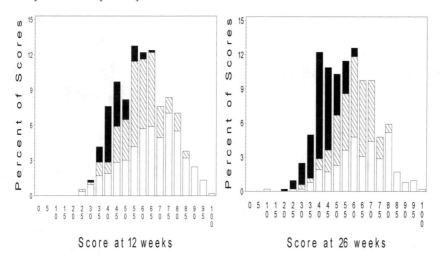

Score at 12 weeks   Score at 26 weeks

FIGURE 8.4 Study 3: Distribution of observed and imputed values using best linear unbiased predictors (BLUPs) from a repeated measures model with baseline characteristics (treatment group, performance status, prior weight loss, symptoms of primary and systemic disease) and outcome (best response and death within two months). Imputed values before death are indicated by the shaded area and after death by the solid area.

approach has limited utility [Gould, 1980, Heyting et al., 1992, Little and Yau, 1996, Revicki et al., 2001] and should be employed with great caution.

Consider a situation where treatment may be associated with toxicity, such as the study of adjuvant therapy for breast cancer previously described. In this study, most women reported poorer HRQoL during therapy than they were experiencing prior to therapy. Thus, carrying forward their previous baseline assessment would create an overly optimistic picture of the HRQoL of subjects on that treatment arm, giving a possible benefit to the therapy with more dropout. As a second example of possible misuse, consider a study where HRQoL is decreasing over time. LVCF could make a treatment with early dropout appear better than a treatment where tolerance to the therapy was higher.

The entire distribution of observed scores and imputed scores is displayed in Figure 8.5 for the lung cancer trial. Imputed scores cover the entire range of possible scores with the distribution of imputed scores much closer to the observed scores. In this trial, we are assuming that a patient's HRQoL is the same after dropout as when the patient completed the last assessment. In this particular setting that does not seem to be a reasonable assumption.

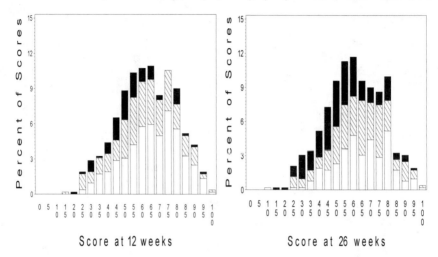

FIGURE 8.5 Study 3: Distribution of observed and imputed values using LVCF. Imputed values before death are indicated by the shaded area and after death by the solid area.

8.4.2 δ-Adjustments

Diehr et al. [1995] describe a variation on LVCF to address the problem of differences in HRQoL between individuals who were able to complete HRQoL assessments and those who were not. In the proposed procedure, a value (δ), is subtracted (or added) to the last observed value. If this value can be justified, then this approach is a useful option in a sensitivity analysis. In Diehr's example, a value of 15 points on the SF-36 physical function scale was proposed, where 15 points is justified as the difference in scores between individuals reporting their health as unchanged versus those reporting worsening [Ware et al., 1993].

8.4.3 Arbitrary High or Low Value

Another example of simple imputation is the substitution of an arbitrarily high or low value for the missing assessments. This is most commonly used when the missing HRQoL data are the result of an adverse event such as death [Fairclough et al., 1999, Raboud et al., 1998]. In some cases a value of 0 is used; in others a value just below the minimum of all observed scores is substituted for the missing data. Both approaches can be partially justified, but neither can be completely defended. One variation that avoids some of the controversy is an analysis based on the ranked HRQoL scores [Fairclough et al., 1999, Gould, 1980, Raboud et al., 1998], for example the Wilcoxon Rank Sum test. Gould [1980] suggests classifying the subjects into four groups. The idea is extended to five groups in Table 8.3.

TABLE 8.3 Strategy for simple imputation of ranks. Assumes that all subjects who completed the study have an observed response (Y_i^{obs}) and all others are missing data.

	Outcome	N	Assumed value	Rank value
1	Died	n_1	$Y_i^{mis} = 0$	Lowest tied rank
2	Withdrawal due to lack of efficacy or for toxicity	n_2	$0 < Y_i^{mis} < min(Y_i^{obs})$	Next lowest tied rank
3	Completed study	n_3	Y_i^{obs}	R_i^{obs}
4	Withdrawal with cure	n_4	$max(Y_i^{obs}) < Y_i^{mis}$	Highest tied rank
5	Withdrawal not related to toxicity or efficacy	n_5	Omitted	

Lowest tied rank $= avg(1, \ldots, n_1)$
Next lowest tied rank $= avg(n_1 + 1, \ldots, n_1 + n_2)$
$R_i^{obs} = n_1 + n_2 +$ Rank of Y_i^{obs} among those who completed the study
Highest tied rank $= avg(n_1 + n_2 + n_3 + 1, \ldots, n_1 + n_2 + n_3 + n_4)$

The strategy for imputing missing data has the advantage that one only has to assume a relative ordering of the HRQoL. For example we are assuming that the HRQoL of subjects who died is poorer than those that remain alive. But even with this seemingly straightforward procedure, it is important to consider the assumptions very carefully. In practice it will not be easy to classify all dropouts into one of the three groups (2, 4 and 5) defined in Table 8.3. Heyting et al. [1992] and Pledger and Hall [1982] describe situations where this strategy may not be appropriate. Also note that when a large proportion of the subjects expire, this approach becomes an approximation to the analysis of survival rather than an analysis of HRQoL.

8.4.4 Hot Deck and Other Sampling Procedures

There is also an entire family of methods based on sampling procedures. The simplest is the *hot deck* in which a value is sampled randomly from the observed data. Variations on this include stratifying the sample on some criteria to produce groups of similar patients or predictive mean matching. These methods are typically employed in multiple imputation (see Section 9.4).

8.5 Imputing Missing Covariates

The exclusion of subjects with missing covariates from analyses may result in selection bias. In most cases, missing covariates (particularly patient characteristics) individually represent a very small proportion (1-2%) of the potential observations. It is only when there are a large number of covariates, each with a small amount of missing data that a problem arises and a more substantial proportion ($> 10\%$) of subjects will be removed from the analysis. When the proportion of missing covariate data is small, the choice of the imputation method will have virtually no impact on the results derived from the analytic model. As the proportion increases, much greater care must be taken. When the proportion is substantial, the first step is to determine if the covariate is absolutely necessary. (Hopefully, the trial design and data management procedures were in place to ensure the capture of vitally important covariates.) If it is determined that the covariate is absolutely necessary, one possible alternative is a missing value indicator. Thus, if the covariate is categorical, one additional category (unknown) would be added. While there has been some criticism of this approach, it will still be appropriate in many settings. For example, the absence of a lab value may indicate that the clinician decided not to obtain the test because the result (normal vs. abnormal) was highly predictable.

If the covariate with missing data is continuous from a symmetric distribution the methods described in Section 8.3.2 may be applicable, remembering that the relationship between the covariate and any other variables in the analytic model needs to be incorporated into the imputation model. If the covariate is dichotomic logistic regression may be appropriate. Predictive mean matching (see Section 9.4) is appropriate for either type of variable.

8.6 Underestimation of Variance

The major disadvantage of simple imputation techniques is the underestimation of the variance of the observations. There are several reasons for the underestimation. First, when we use means or predicted values, we are assuming that there is no variability among the missing observations (i.e. $Var[\epsilon_{hij}] = 0$). Second, we assume that we know the true mean or predicted value (i.e. $Var[\hat{\mu}] = 0$ or $Var[X\hat{\beta}] = 0$) when in fact we have estimated these values.* Finally, we assume that we have observed the HRQoL of all subjects rather than just a subset of the subjects. As a result, test statistics and confidence intervals based on a naive analysis of the observed and imputed data will not be valid.

This is illustrated in the lung cancer trial. Consider the scores at 26 weeks; the estimated standard deviation of the observed data is roughly 15-16 points, where it is calculated as:

$$\hat{\sigma} = \sqrt{\sum_{i=1}^{n}(Y_{hij} - \bar{Y}_{hj})^2/(n-1)}. \qquad (8.8)$$

When we impute values for the missing data using the mean value of the observed data and use a naive estimate of the variance, we add nothing to the squared terms because $Y_{hij}^{mis} - \bar{Y}_{hj} = 0$, but we do increase the apparent number of observations. The effect of this is illustrated in Table 8.4, where the naive estimate of the standard deviation decreases by almost $1/3$ as we increase the apparent number of observations by about 2-fold. In the simple univariate case, the underestimation of the variance is roughly proportional to the amount of missing data. The naive estimate of the variance of y_i is

$$\hat{\sigma}^2 = \frac{\sum^{n^{obs}}(y_i^{obs} - \bar{y}_i^{obs})^2 + n^{mis}(\bar{y}_i^{obs} - \bar{y}_i^{obs})^2}{n^{obs} + n^{mis} - 1}$$
$$= \frac{(n^{obs} - 1)\hat{\sigma}_{obs}^2 + 0}{(n-1)} = \frac{n^{obs} - 1}{n-1}\hat{\sigma}_{obs}^2.$$

When $\hat{\sigma}_{obs}^2 \approx \sigma^2$, then $E[\hat{\sigma}^2] \approx \frac{n^{obs}}{n}\sigma^2$. The standard deviation is underestimated by a factor proportional to the square root of the proportion of missing data. While it is straightforward to adjust the estimate of the variance using mean imputation, it becomes a much more difficult task for other imputation procedures.

The problem with the underestimation of the variance of the observations is compounded when we attempt to estimate the standard errors of means or regression parameters. This in turn affects test statistics and confidence intervals. For example, the naive estimate of the standard error of the mean $(S.E.(\hat{\mu}) = \sqrt{\hat{\sigma}^2/n})$ assumes that we have information on all n individuals, rather than the n^{obs} individuals who completed the HRQoL assessments. In the 6-month estimates for survivors on the NSCLC study, we analyze a dataset with 389 observations when only 191 subjects were observed. The effect is illustrated in Table 8.4, where the naive standard errors are roughly half the true standard errors. For the other simple imputation methods displayed in

---

*The simple imputation performed by the SPSS MVA command addresses the first, but not the second problem [vonHippel, 2004].

Table 8.4, the estimates of the standard deviations are underestimated (for all approaches but LVCF) and thus the standard errors are also underestimated.

The underestimation of standard errors can make a substantial difference in the test statistics inflating the Type I error rate. In the example, t-tests with the standard error in the denominator would be inflated by 30-50%. Consider a small difference of 3 points (1/5 S.D.) in the means of the two groups. With no imputation, the t-statistic for a test of differences utilizing the stardard errors in Table 8.4 is 1.24 (p=0.22). With mean imputation, the t-statistic is now 2.65 (p=0.008), a highly significant difference.

TABLE 8.4 Study 3: Naive estimation of standard deviation (S.D.) and standard error (S.E.) in the lung cancer trial. 26-week estimates for survivors.

Imputation	Therapy	Obs (n)	Mean	S.D. ($\hat{\sigma}$)	S.E. ($\frac{\hat{\sigma}}{\sqrt{n-1}}$)	Ratio[†] of S.E.
None	Std	57	65.0	15.0	1.99	1.00
	Exp	134	64.8	15.7	1.36	1.00
Simple Mean	Std	125	65.0	10.1	0.90	0.45
	Exp	265	64.8	11.1	0.68	0.63
Covariates	Std	125	62.8	11.3	1.01	0.51
	Exp	265	63.6	11.9	0.73	0.54
Conditional	Std	125	61.1	13.1	1.18	0.59
	Exp	265	62.4	13.5	0.83	0.61
LVCF	Std	121	63.9	15.9	1.45	0.73
	Exp	259	64.3	15.6	0.97	0.73

[†] Reference (denominator) is the standard error with no imputation.

8.7 Final Comments

8.7.1 Sensitivity Analysis

Despite the limitations of simple imputation, these methods may be useful as part of a limited analysis of the sensitivity of results. Visual comparison of the means or medians is helpful, but comparisons of test statistics are inappropriate. Several authors have used simple imputation combined with non-parametric analysis to examine the sensitivity of their results to the assumptions made about the missing data. Raboud et al. [1998] used this approach in a study of antimicrobial therapy in patients with HIV to demonstrate the sensitivity of estimates of treatment effects to different rates of dropout and survival.

8.8 Summary

- Simple imputation such as the half rule is useful when a small number of item responses are missing in a questionnaire.

- Simple imputation may be useful when a small proportion of multiple covariates have missing values.

- Simple imputation has very limited usefulness for missing assessments of HRQoL that are intended as outcome measures. The primary limitation of simple imputation is the underestimation of the variance of any estimate and the corresponding inflation of Type I errors.

- Last Value Carried Forward (LVCF), if used, should be well justified and any underlying assumptions verified. This approach will not be conservative in all cases and may in some settings bias the results in favor of a treatment with more dropout associated with morbidity.

- Imputation methods are most useful when auxiliary information exists that can not readily be incorporated into the analytic model.

- Imputation methods may be useful as part of sensitivity analyses to examine the dependence of the results (means but not p-values) on specific assumptions about the HRQoL of individuals with missing observations [vanBuuren et al., 1999].

- Imputation should not be considered either an easy fix or a definitive solution to the problem of missing data; in all cases imputation requires the analyst to make untestable assumptions concerning the missing data.

9

Multiple Imputation

9.1 Introduction

The major criticism of simple imputation methods is the underestimation of the variance (see previous chapter). Multiple imputation [Rubin and Schenker, 1986, Rubin, 1987] rectifies this problem by incorporating both the variability of the HRQoL measure and the uncertainty about the missing observations. Multiple imputation of missing values will be worth the effort only if there is a substantial benefit that cannot be obtained using methods that assume that missing data is ignorable such as maximum likelihood for the analysis of incomplete data (Chapter 3 and 4). As mentioned in the previous chapter, this requires auxiliary information, such as assessments by other observers (caregivers) or clinical outcomes that are strongly correlated with the HRQoL measure. The previous comments about the complexities of actually implementing an imputation scheme when the trial involves both longitudinal data and multiple measures is even more relevant. The following quote summarizes the concern:

> ... multiple imputation is not a panacea. Although it is a powerful and useful tool applicable to many missing data settings, if not used carefully it is potentially dangerous. The existence of software that facilitates its use requires the analyst to be careful about the verification of assumptions, the robustness of imputation models and the appropriateness of inferences. For more complicated models (e.g., longitudinal or clustered data) this is even more important. (Norton and Lipsitz [2001])

9.2 Overview of Multiple Imputation

The basic strategy of multiple imputation is to impute 3 to 20 sets of values for the missing data. Each set of data is then analyzed using complete data methods and the results of the analyses are then combined. The general strategy is summarized in four steps:

Step 1: Selection of the Imputation Procedure

Although the least technical, selection of an appropriate imputation procedure is the most difficult and the most critical step. There are a variety of implicit and explicit methods that can be used for multiple imputation [Rubin and Schenker, 1986]. Explicit methods generally utilize regression models whereas implicit methods utilize sampling techniques. Four specific examples of these strategies are described in the subsequent sections.

There are three desirable properties of an imputation procedure. The first objective is unbiased estimates. This is particularly difficult when there is a suspicion that the missingness depends on the HRQoL of the individual at the time the observation was to be made (MNAR) and is thus non-ignorable. Secondly, the procedure should incorporate the appropriate variation to reflect the randomness of the observations, the loss of information due to the missing observations and the uncertainty about the model used to impute the missing values. Finally, the procedure should not distort the covariance structure of the repeated measurements in longitudinal studies, especially when the analyses involve estimation of changes in HRQoL over time. The challenge is to select an appropriate model and fully understand the assumptions that are being made when that model is implemented. This is the focus of the current chapter.

Step 2: Generation of M Imputed Datasets

Once the model and procedure for imputing the missing observations is selected, the details for implementing the procedure are generally well worked out (see Sections 9.3 through Section 9.5). One of the questions often asked is How many datasets should be imputed? There is no straightforward answer. The recommendations generally range from 3 to 10. As the proportion of missing data increases, the between imputation variance will increase (see Section 9.7) and will become more important in the calculation of the overall variance. Increasing the number of imputed datasets (M) will improve the precision of this estimate. I recommend imputing more (10 or 20) rather than fewer datasets as the additional computational time is a trivial part of the entire analytic effort with modern computing power.

Step 3: Analysis of M Datasets

Each of the M datasets is analyzed using complete data or maximum likelihood methods such as MANOVA or mixed-effects models. Estimates of the primary parameters $(\hat{\beta}^{(m)})$ and their variance $(Var[\hat{\beta}^{(m)}])$ are obtained for each of the M complete datasets. Step 3 is often expanded to include hypothesis testing $(H_0 : \theta = C\beta = 0)$ based on the estimation of secondary parameters $(\hat{\theta}^{(m)} = C\hat{\beta}^{(m)})$ and their variance $(Var[\hat{\theta}^{(m)}])$.

Step 4: Combining Results of M Analyses

The results of the M analyses are then combined by averaging the parameter estimates from each of the M data sets. The variance of these estimates are computed by combining within and between components of the variance of the estimates from the M datasets. As is shown later, it is the combination of the imputation procedures and the computation of the variance estimates that results in the appropriate estimates of variance. Full details for this procedure are presented in Section 9.7.

9.3 Explicit Univariate Regression

In the explicit regression model approach to multiple imputation, we identify a regression model to predict the missing observations. While the imputation model may be similar to the analytic model, it may also include additional terms incorporating auxiliary information that would not be appropriate for the analytic model. Again, it should be emphasized that all the imputation methods assume that missing data is random, conditional on the data incorporated into the model. Addition of auxiliary information into the imputation model may help to satisfy that assumption. A superscript asterisk is used to differentiate the imputation model from the analytic model.

$$\text{Analytic Model } Y_i = X_i\beta + \epsilon_i \tag{9.1}$$
$$\text{Imputation Model } Y_i^* = X_i^*\mathcal{B}^* + \varepsilon_i^* \tag{9.2}$$

This multiple imputation procedure differs from the simple regression techniques described in the previous chapter in two ways. First, because the true parameters of the imputation model are unknown, random error is added to the estimated parameters $(\hat{\mathcal{B}}^*)$. These new values of the parameters $(\beta^{(m)})$ are then used to predict the score for a subject with specific characteristics defined by the covariates $(X^{*(mis)})$. Then, additional random error is added to these values to reflect the natural variability of the individual outcome measures $(Var[Y_i])$.

9.3.1 Identification of the Imputation Model

The explicit regression approach has the advantage that the imputation model can readily use auxiliary information about the subject's HRQoL that could not be included in the model used for the ultimate analysis of the clinical trial. This additional information might include indicators of the side effects of treatment and the clinical course of the disease when the therapy succeeds or fails. Alternatively, it could include measures of HRQoL provided by a caregiver that continue to be obtained when the subject is no longer able to complete self-assessments.

One of the objectives of imputation is to obtain unbiased estimates of the missing observations. In the context of the explicit regression approach, we are looking for a model where the missingness is ignorable after conditioning on the observed data (Y_i^*) and the covariates in the imputation model (X_i^*). Basically, we are attempting to indirectly augment the analytic model with auxiliary information, so that the MAR assumption assuming the imputation model seems reasonable. The primary candidates for covariates include measures that are strongly correlated with both the measure being imputed and the probability that it is missing. In the lung cancer trial (Study 3), this suggests adding covariates associated with toxicity, disease progression and the proximity of the patient to death.

The same strategy outlined in Section 8.3.2 is recommended for identification of the imputation model. To avoid biasing the comparison of treatment groups toward the null hypothesis, it is critical that imputation of post-randomization data be either done separately for each treatment group or include treatment as a covariate.

9.3.2 Computation of Imputed Values

The general procedure for imputing M sets of missing values for univariate data is as follows [Rubin, 1987, Crawford et al., 1995, Little and Yau, 1996]:

1. Estimate the parameters of the regression model $(Y_i^{*obs} = X_i^{*obs}\mathcal{B}^* + \epsilon_i^*)$ using the observed data. Note that Y_i^{*obs} and X_i^{*obs} contain the auxiliary information previously described.

$$\hat{\mathcal{B}}^* = \left(\sum X_i'^{*obs} X_i^{*obs}\right)^{-1} \sum X_i'^{*obs} Y_i^{*obs} \tag{9.3}$$

$$\hat{\sigma}^{2*} = \sum \left(Y_i^{*obs} - \hat{\mathcal{B}}^* X_i^{*obs}\right)^2 / (n^{obs} - p^*) \tag{9.4}$$

where p^* is the number of unknown parameters in $\mathcal{B}^*$.

2. Generate M sets of model parameters $(\beta^{(m)}$ and $\sigma^{2(m)})$ by adding random error to the estimates reflecting the uncertainty of the estimates.

$$\sigma^{2(m)} = \hat{\sigma}^{2*} \times (n^{obs} - p^*)/\mathcal{K}^{(m)} \tag{9.5}$$

$$\beta^{(m)} = \hat{\mathcal{B}}^* + U_\beta \mathcal{Z}_\beta^m \tag{9.6}$$

where

$\mathcal{K}^{(m)}$ is a randomly drawn number from a chi-square distribution with $n^{obs} - p^*$ degrees of freedom,

U_β is the upper triangular matrix of the Cholesky decomposition of the variance of $\hat{\mathcal{B}}^*$ where $U'_\beta U_\beta = Var[\hat{\mathcal{B}}^*]$ and

$$Var[\hat{\mathcal{B}}^*] = \sigma^{2(m)} \left(\sum X_i'^{*obs} X_i^{*obs} \right)^{-1}$$

$\mathcal{Z}_\beta^{(m)}$ is a vector of p^* random numbers drawn from a standard normal distribution.

The *Cholesky* decomposition is also referred to as the *square root* decomposition. In this procedure, we have assumed that the parameters have a normal distribution with variance approximately equal to $\sigma^2 (\sum X_i'^{*obs} X_i^{*obs})^{-1}$. This is a reasonable assumption for large studies, but may not be valid for smaller studies. When there is concern about these assumptions, more complex methods of generating these parameters are required [Schafer, 1997].

3. Generate the imputed values of Y_i^{mis}, for the mth imputation, by adding random error corresponding to the between and within subject variability of the outcome $(Var[Y_i] = \hat{\sigma}^{*2})$.

$$Y_i^{mis(m)} = X_i^{mis} \beta^{(m)} + \sigma^{(m)} \mathcal{Z}_Y^{(m)} \qquad (9.7)$$

where $\mathcal{Z}_Y^{(m)}$ is a random number drawn from a standard normal distribution.

4. The second and third steps are repeated for each of the M datasets.

9.3.3 Practical Considerations

There are two major barriers to implementing this procedure. The first is a small sample. The second is the lack of strong predictors of the HRQoL measure. When the sample size is small, the analyst is unable to obtain precise estimates of the imputation model parameters $(\hat{\mathcal{B}}^*)$. This will result in a wide range of values of $\beta^{(m)}$. Thus, the imputed values may only add noise to the observed data. The lack of strong predictors will have similar consequences. If the variation in the outcome explained by the imputation model is small (the R^2 is small), the values of $\sigma^{2(m)}$ will be large and again the imputed values may only add noise to the observed data. An additional nuisance associated with both problems is that some of the predicted values may lie outside the possible range of values of the HRQoL scale.

The procedure for identifying the imputation model does not specify a cutoff for the significance of potential covariates. This aspect of the model fitting is as much art as it is science. Adding more covariates to the imputation model will improve the procedure by increasing the R^2 and reducing $\sigma^{2(m)}$, thus decreasing the statistical noise added in equation 9.7. This is balanced by adding parameters with large standard errors and increasing the statistical noise added in equation 9.6. Thus, adding covariates that result in small increases in the R^2 is unlikely to improve the imputation procedure even when the statistical significance of a particular parameter is large. Finally, any covariate that will be incorporated into subsequent hypothesis testing (e.g. treatment group) must be retained in order to avoid biasing the results toward the null hypothesis (as previously discussed in Chapter 8).

9.3.4 Extensions to Longitudinal Studies

The above procedure was developed for cross-sectional studies. However, in most clinical trials HRQoL is measured longitudinally. Little and Yau [1996] suggest a sequential procedure for a monotone missing data pattern. The procedure is first to fill in the missing values of the first observation (Y_{i1}), generating M sets of data for the first observation (equation 9.8). The second step is to fill in the missing values of the second observation (Y_{i2}) given the observed (Y_{i1}) or imputed values ($Y_{i1}^{(m)}$) of the first observation (Y_{i1}). Subsequent missing values are imputed using all previously observed and imputed data (equations 9.9 and 9.10). Only one set of new values is generated for each of the M data sets in the second and subsequent steps. The imputation models at each step are:

$$Y_{i1}^{*obs} = X_{i1}^{*obs}\beta_1^* + \varepsilon_{i1}^* \tag{9.8}$$

$$Y_{i2}^{*obs} = X_{i2}^{*obs}\beta_2^{*(m)} + Y_{i1}^{(m)}\beta_{2|1}^{*(m)} + \varepsilon_{i2}^* \tag{9.9}$$

$$Y_{i3}^{*obs} = X_{i3}^{*obs}\beta_3^{*(m)} + Y_{i2}^{(m)}\beta_{3|2}^{*(m)} + Y_{i1}^{(m)}\beta_{3|1}^{*(m)} + \varepsilon_{i3}^* \tag{9.10}$$

$$Y_{i4}^{*obs} = X_{i4}^{*obs}\beta_4^{*(m)} + Y_{i3}^{(m)}\beta_{4|3}^{*(m)} + Y_{i2}^{(m)}\beta_{4|2}^{*(m)} + Y_{i1}^{(m)}\beta_{4|1}^{*(m)} + \varepsilon_{i4}^* \tag{9.11}$$

Statistical software for multiple imputation often requires a repeated measures structure in which each observation can be assigned to a particular time frame. In the lung cancer trial these are the four planned assessments. There are rare exceptions to this requirement (see Section 9.6.3).

9.3.5 Extensions to Multiple HRQoL Measures

In a typical trial involving HRQoL assessments, if one of the HRQoL measures is missing, all of the other measures at that timepoint are usually missing. This complicates the imputation procedures and is part of the quagmire that was mentioned in the previous chapter. The question that the analyst will struggle with is the sequence of filling in both missing observations over time and across the multiple measures. In the lung cancer trial there are five subscales in the FACT-Lung measure. Should the imputation proceed for each measure over time, completely independent of the responses on the other measures? Or if not, how should the sequence proceed. In rare cases there may be a theoretical model that allows the analyst to define the appropriate sequence, but in most cases this will not exist. Despite this, the analyst will have to make choices and defend them. I do not have any recommendations that would be generically applicable across various settings and instruments except to think through what makes conceptual sense and to keep it as simple as possible.

9.3.6 Assumptions

When we impute the missing observations using these models, we are making at least two assumptions that are not testable. First, we are assuming that the relationship between the explanatory variables and HRQoL is the same when individuals complete the HRQoL assessments as when they do not complete the assessments. Basically, we are assuming that $Y_i^{*obs} = X_i^{*obs}\mathcal{B}^* + \varepsilon_i$ and $Y_i^{*mis} = X_i^{*mis}\mathcal{B}^* + \varepsilon_i$ are both true when $\mathcal{B}^*$ is estimated on the basis of the observed data. Second, we are assuming that we have identified *all* the important relevant information such that the missingness no longer depends on the missing HRQoL value (Y_i^{mis}) after conditioning on Y_i^{*obs} and X_i^* (MAR).

Less critical assumptions in this procedure are that the residual errors (ε_i^*) and the parameter estimates $(\hat{\mathcal{B}}^*)$ of the imputation model are normally distributed. The first assumption can be assessed by examining the residual errors (ε_i^*) and the second will be true for studies with moderate sample sizes for which parameter estimates become asymptotically normal.

9.3.7 Lung Cancer Trial (Study 3)

While the procedure described above sounds straightforward, one quickly realizes that there are many choices to be made. The first decision is how to handle the multiple subscales. Should we implement the MI procedure separately for each or in some theoretically plausible sequence? For composite measures, such as the TOI (Treatment Outcome Index), should we impute the components first and then compute the composite or can we directly impute the composite score? In the lung cancer trial, the TOI score is a composite of the physical well-being, the functional well-being and the lung-cancer specific subscales. I present the imputation of the composite score here, primarily because it is less complicated to illustrate the principles and not because I recommend ignoring the individual components.

The covariate (X_{ij}^*) selection process has multiple steps. The selection is a combination of decisions made on a conceptual basis and data exploration (Table 9.1). First, treatment assignment should not have any impact on the baseline (pre randomization) scores and is not included for that model. It is forced into all other models because the intent is to compare the treatment groups even though it was non-significant in the exploratory models. Similarly, treatment outcomes were not considered as predictors of the baseline scores but were considered for all follow-up assessments. Potential covariates with more than 5% missing data were not considered. The second step was to eliminate variables where the correlation with the TOI scores was weak and explained less than 5% of the variation*. Note that eliminating covariates that explain less than 5% ($\rho < 0.22$, $\rho^2 < 0.05$) of the covariance between the TOI scores in the covariate only reduced the R^2 for a model with all of the covariates by 1-3% (Table 9.1). As a final note, when the prior scores where eliminated, the proportion of the total variation that was explained was roughly a cut in half illustrating the importance of addressing the longitudinal nature of the study.

TABLE 9.1 Study 3: Covariate selection for lung cancer trial. The criteria for selection was based on estimates of bivariate R^2 (% of variance explained by the potential covariate). - indicates that covariate was not included. + indicates inclusion.

Potential Covariate	Corr with Obs Score Assessment #				Corr with Miss Ind Assessment #			
	1	2	3	4	1	2	3	4
Treatment Arm		X	X	X	-	+		
Age	-	-	-	+	-	+	-	+
Gender	-	-	-	-	-	-	-	-
Performance status	++	+	-	-	-	+	+	-
Prior radiotherapy	-	+	-	-	-	+	-	-
Weight loss	++	+	-	-	-	-	-	-
Chronic disease	-	-	-	-	-	-	-	-
Primary disease symptoms	+	+	-	-	-	-	-	-
Metastatic symptoms	+	+	+	+	-	-	-	-
Systemic symptoms	++	-	-	+	-	-	-	-
Baseline TOI score		+++	+++	+++		++	++	++
6-week TOI score			+++	+++			++	++
12-week TOI score				+++				++
Cycles of therapy		+++	+++	+		+++	+++	+++
Complete/partial response		+	+	+		++	++	+++
Hematologic toxicity		+	+	-		-	+	+
Neurologic toxicity		-	-	-		++	++	+
Early progressive disease		++	++	++		+	++	++
Survival (log)		+++	+++	+++		+++	+++	+++
R^2 with +, ++, +++ ($R^2 >1\%$)	17%	36%	42%	35%				
R^2 with ++, +++ ($R^2 >5\%$)	16%	35%	41%	32%				
R^2 without prior scores		20%	16%	17%				

X indicates forced into model. - indicates tested but not included,
+ indicates included, $R^2 >1\%$, ++ $R^2 >5\%$, +++ $R^2 >10\%$.

---

*The R^2 for a simple linear regression is equivalent to the square of the Pearson correlation. Thus correlations less than 0.1 (even if statistically significant) would correspond to R^2 values of less than 1%.

After determining the appropriate explanatory variables for the imputation procedure, we have several additional logistical issues. The first is whether to run the imputation procedures separately for each treatment group or to include treatment as a covariate in all imputation models. By taking the second option, we run the risk of missing a potential interaction between one of the covariates and the treatment but gain precision in the estimation of the parameters when the relationships are the same in each treatment group. This later advantage is more important when the sample size is small. Another issue is the question of how to handle the small proportion of subjects with non-monotone missing data patterns. A final decision is how to handle imputed values that are out of the range of the scale. As will be demonstrated later, this is a very minor issue and does not affect the results.

Unfortunately, I cannot provide guidance for these questions that is applicable for all trials, except the following:

- When there are conceptual models underlying the measures and the trial, these should provide the primary guidance.

- Where it is possible to simplify the procedure by ignoring issues that impact only a small proportion of the missing values, do so. For example, if only a small proportion ($< 5\%$) of the data violate a monotone dropout pattern, fill in those missing values using the simplest method, then proceed with your proposed MI procedure. The small proportion of observations that do not fit will have a minimal impact on the results and will simplify both implementation and reporting of the results.

Figure 9.1 displays the observed and imputed scores at the third and fourth assessment. The first feature is the greater variability of the scores when contrasted with those for simple imputation methods (see Chapter 8). As expected in this study, the distribution of the imputed scores is lower than the observed scores. A very small proportion of the scores lie outside the possible range of 0 to 100. Low values (< 0) represent 0.01, 0.03, 0.16 and 1.84% of the scores at each of the four assessments. High values (> 100) represent 0.14, 0.22, 0.19 and 0.26% of the scores respectively. The recommendation is not to replace these out-of-range scores with 0 and 100 (although the software procedures allow this as an option).

9.3.8 Implementation

Implementation in SAS

The SAS MI Procedure implements a variety of MI models. All require that the data for each subject be in a single record. The first step is to create a data set (WORK.ONEREC) with one record per subject containing the four possible FACT-Lung TOI scores (TOI1, TOI2, TOI3, TOI4) and the covariates to be used in the MI procedure.

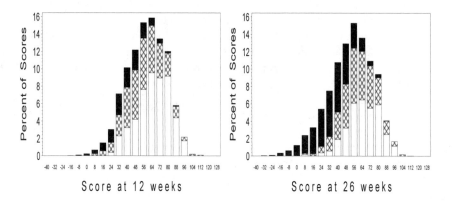

FIGURE 9.1 Study 3: Distribution of observed and multiply imputed values using *Regression*. Imputed values before death are indicated by the shaded area and after death by the solid area.

If the covariates where all observed and the assessment of the TOI scores followed a strictly monotone missing data pattern, the following simple procedure could be used:

```
%let baseline= Wt_LOSS ECOGPS SX_Sys;
proc mi data=work.onerec out=work.regression nimpute=10 /*noprint*/;
  by Trtment;
  var &baseline cycles crpr pd_lt6 ctc_neu ln_surv toi1 toi2 toi3 toi4;
  monotone method=regression;
  run;
```

The MI procedure with a `MONOTONE METHOD=REGRESSION`; statement sequentially imputes missing data using

$$Y_j = \beta_0 + \beta_1 Y_1 + \cdots + \beta_{j-1} Y_{j-1}$$

for the $Y_1, \ldots, Y_j$ identified in the VAR statement with the restriction that the missing data pattern is monotone among the variables for the order specified. The sequential regression of toi1, toi2, toi3, and toi4 can also be tailored:

```
proc mi data=work.onerec out=work.regression nimpute=10 /*noprint*/;
  by Trtment;
  var &baseline cycles crpr pd_lt6 ctc_neu ln_surv toi1 toi2 toi3 toi4;
  monotone reg(toi1=Wt_LOSS ECOGPS SX_Sys);
  monotone reg(toi2=Cycles CRPR PD_lt6 ctc_neu Ln_surv toi1);
  monotone reg(toi3=Cycles crpr PD_lt6 ctc_neu Ln_surv toi1 toi2);
  monotone reg(Toi4=Cycles crpr PD_lt6 ctc_neu Ln_surv toi1 toi2 toi3);
  run;
```

However, in the lung cancer trial (and in most settings) the missing data pattern will not be strictly monotone and the procedure will require an additional step to create a dataset with a monotone pattern. One strategy is to use a technique that does not require a monotone pattern (Section 9.6). When there are a small number of non-monotone missing values, we can fill in the outcome variables (TOI1, TOI2, TOI3, TOI4) as follows:

```
proc mi data=work.onerec out=work.temp nimpute=10 /*noprint*/;
  by Trtment;
  mcmc impute=monotone;
  var &baseline cycles pd_lt6 ln_surv toi1 toi2 toi3 toi4;
  run;
```

This creates a new dataset comprised of 10 sets of data that have a monotone pattern. We can now use the regression procedure to impute the remaining missing values. To do this we are going to rename the variable that identifies these 10 sets from _IMPUTATION_ to _M_ and sort the data by imputation number and treatment group.

```
proc sort data=work.temp out=work.monotone(rename=(_imputation_=_m_));
  by Trtment _imputation_;
  run;
```

From this point on, we are going to impute only one set of values for each of the 10 sets generated in the first step. There are two changes to the procedure; the imputation number (_M_) is added to the BY statement and the number of imputations is changed to 1.

```
proc mi data=work.monotone out=work.regression nimpute=1 /*noprint*/;
  by Trtment _m_;
  var &baseline cycles crpr pd_lt6 ctc_neu ln_surv toi1 toi2 toi3 toi4;
  monotone reg(toi1=Wt_LOSS ECOGPS SX_Sys);
  monotone reg(toi2=Cycles CRPR PD_lt6 ctc_neu Ln_surv TOI1);
  monotone reg(toi3=Cycles crpr PD_lt6 ctc_neu Ln_surv TOI1 TOI2);
  monotone reg(Toi4=Cycles crpr PD_lt6 ctc_neu Ln_surv TOI1 TOI2 TOI3);
  run;
```

Implementation in SPSS

The SPSS MULTIPLE IMPUTATION command implements this procedure when the data have a strictly monotone structure. Details of the procedure for non-monotone data are presented in Section 9.6. When data is strictly monotone, the procedure is identical except that METHOD=FCS is replaced by METHOD=MONOTONE SCALEMODEL=LINEAR.

9.4 Closest Neighbor and Predictive Mean Matching

There are many variations on the explicit regression model approach to multiple imputation. Both closest neighbor [Rubin, 1987, vanBuuren et al., 1999] and predictive mean matching [Rubin and Schenker, 1986, Heitjan and Landis, 1994] have the advantage that it is not possible to impute a value that is out of range for the HRQoL scale. They are also more likely to be robust to deviations from the normality assumptions.

9.4.1 Closest Neighbor

The initial steps for the closest neighbor procedure are the same as those for the explicit regression procedure. M sets of parameter estimates for the imputation model are generated as previously described (equations 9.3 to 9.6). The difference is in the third and fourth step.

3. Predicted values are generated for subjects with both observed and missing data:

$$E[Y_i^{obs(m)}] = X_i^{obs}\beta^{(m)} \tag{9.12}$$

$$E[Y_{i'}^{mis(m)}] = X_{i'}^{mis}\beta^{(m)} \tag{9.13}$$

4. For each subject (i') with a missing observation, the subject with the closest predicted value, $E[Y_i^{obs(m)}]$, is selected and that subject's actual observed value, Y_i^{obs}, is the imputed value for subject i'.

5. Repeat steps 2-4 for M data sets.

9.4.2 Predictive Mean Matching

A similar procedure with some variation is *predictive mean matching*.

1. In the initial step of predictive mean matching [Rubin and Schenker, 1986, Heitjan and Landis, 1994], M bootstrap samples are generated from the subjects with observed data. This consists of sampling N^{obs} subjects at random with replacement.

2. The parameters of the imputation model ($\hat{\beta}^{(m)}$) are then estimated within each of the M samples.

3. Predicted values are generated for both the cases with observed and the cases with missing data (equations 9.12 and 9.13).

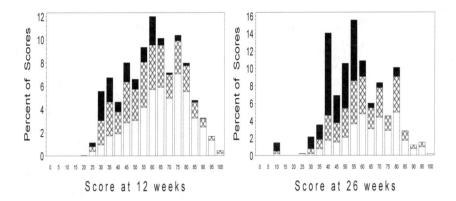

FIGURE 9.2 Study 3: Distribution of observed and multiply imputed values using *Predictive Mean Matching*. Imputed values before death are indicated by the shaded area and after death by the solid area.

4. The five nearest matches among the subjects with observed data are identified for each subject with missing data and one of the five is selected at random. The observed value of the HRQoL measure from that subject is the imputed value.

Figure 9.2 displays the distribution of scores for this procedure. All of the scores are within the range of the observed data. The imputed values are again shifting the distribution toward the lower scores as we would expect given the characteristics of these patients. Note that the distribution of the imputed scores has a ragged shape. This suggests that a limited number of observations are available for sampling for certain ranges of the predicted means and these values are being repeatedly sampled; this is referred to as the *multiple donor* problem.

Implementation in SAS

This procedure can be implemented in SAS, by replacing REG with REGPMM in the MONOTONE statements described in Section 9.3.8.

Implementation in SPSS

The SPSS MULTIPLE IMPUTATION command implements this procedure using only the closest match when the data have a strictly monotone structure. Details of the procedure for non-monotone data are presented in Section 9.6. When data is strictly monotone, the procedure is identical except that METHOD=FCS is replaced by METHOD=MONOTONE SCALEMODEL=PMM.

9.5 Approximate Bayesian Bootstrap (ABB)

An alternative to explicit model-based imputation is implicit or sampling-based imputation. One commonly used method is the approximate Bayesian bootstrap (ABB). This was proposed initially for ignorable missing data from simple random samples [Rubin and Schenker, 1986, Rubin, 1987, Rubin and Schenker, 1991] and focuses on the patient characteristics and outcomes that predict missingness rather than the score. The idea is to identify subgroups within the sample of subjects who have a similar *propensity* to have a missing value and then sample values from these groups to replace the missing values. It is a variation on the original concept proposed by Rosenbaum and Rubin [1984] where they defined a *propensity score* as the conditional probability of receiving a particular treatment given a set of observed patient characteristics (covariates). The concept is modified here to predict the probability that an observation is missing [Lavori et al., 1995].

The procedure is as follows:

1. Create an indicator variable, R_{ij}, to identify missing values (see Section 6.3.2).

2. Fit a logistic regression model for the probability that a subject has a missing value for the jth measure as a function of a set of observed patient characteristics. Calculate the predicted probability (propensity score) that each subject would have missing values, given the set of covariates.

3. Based on the propensity score, divide the subjects into K groups (generally 5 groups).

4. Impute missing values using an approximate Bayesian bootstrap (ABB) procedure in each group. The ABB procedure is as follows. Consider a set of n subjects within the same group, where a score was observed for n_{obs} and missing for n_{mis} subjects ($n = n_{obs} + n_{mis}$). For $m = 1, \ldots, M$, first randomly select a set of n_{obs} possible values with replacement from the n_{obs} values. Then choose n_{mis} observations at random with replacement from each of the M potential samples.

9.5.1 Practical Considerations

The practical considerations are similar to those previously mentioned. The sample size needs to be large to implement the procedure. To guard against biasing the results toward the null hypothesis, the imputation procedures must be done within treatment groups when the objective of the subsequent

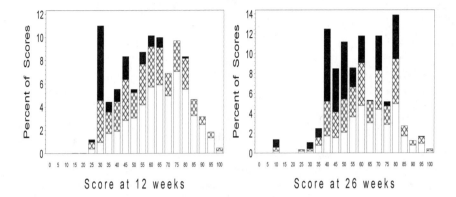

FIGURE 9.3 Study 3: Distribution of observed and multiply imputed values using the *Approximate Baysian bootstrap* (ABB). Imputed values before death are indicated by the shaded area and after death by the solid area.

analysis is to compare treatment groups. Strategies will need to be developed to address multiple measures over longitudinal data.

Finally, when the model that predicts missingness closely fits the data, the stratum with the highest propensity for missing data will have too few or no observed values. It then becomes necessary to reduce the number of strata producing more heterogenous groups for the sampling step.

This procedure can be implemented in SAS using the procedures outlined in Section 9.3.8, replacing REG in the MONOTONE statement with PROPENSITY. Note that in this example the number of groups for the third and forth assessment had to be reduced to 4 and 2 respectively, because for one of the treatment groups, there were no observed values in the group with the highest propensity for missing data.

```
proc mi data=work.monotone out=work.abb nimpute=1 /*noprint*/;
  by Trtment _m_;
  var &baseline cycles crpr pd_lt6 ctc_neu ln_surv toi1 toi2 toi3 toi4;
  monotone propensity(toi1=Wt_LOSS ECOGPS SX_Sys);
  monotone propensity(toi2=Cycles CRPR PD_lt6 ctc_neu Ln_surv TOI1);
  monotone propensity(toi3=Cycles crpr PD_lt6 ctc_neu Ln_surv TOI1 TOI2
          /ngroups=4);
  monotone propensity(Toi4=Cycles crpr PD_lt6 ctc_neu Ln_surv TOI1 TOI2
          Toi3/ngroups=2);
  run;
```

9.5.2   The Assumptions

The critical assumption of the ABB procedure is that the data are *missing at random* conditional on a set of propensity scores derived from covariates (X) and previously observed values of the outcome. However, when the propensity scores are used to define strata, the missing data are assumed to occur *completely at random* within the strata defined by the propensity score. This is a strong assumption which is difficult to justify for HRQoL studies where there is a strong association between missing data and clinical outcomes. Increasing the number of strata defined by the propensity scores would improve the likelihood that this assumption is correct. But this may also result in strata with too few subjects available for drawing the imputed values.

A critical issue with this procedure occurs because the procedure ignores the correlation of the measures across the repeated assessments. Thus it is inappropriate for any analysis of the data involving relationships among the repeated measures, such as change over time. This is apparent when estimating the covariance among the repeated measures or when estimates of longitudinal change are of interest.

9.5.3   A Variation for Non-Ignorable Missing Data

To deal with non-ignorable missing data, Rubin and Schenker [1991] suggest independent draws of the n_{obs} possible values, where the probability of sampling an observation is proportional to some function of Y (e.g. Y^2 or $\sqrt{Y}$) to increase the proportion of large or small values of Y. Another approach that would increase the probability of drawing a smaller (or larger) value to replace the missing observation is to randomly draw k (usually 2 or 3) observations and take the minimum (or maximum) of the k draws. vanBuuren et al. [1999] suggest a *delta-adjustment* where a predetermined constant is subtracted from the imputed value. Unfortunately, the difficult choice among these possible approaches cannot be made on the basis of the observed data or any statistical tests. In practice, testing a range of choices as part of a sensitivity analysis is appropriate.

9.6   Multivariate Procedures for Non-Monotone Missing Data

Multiple imputation techniques for non-monotone missing data rely on data augmentation techniques. Most methods assume that each of the variables has a multivariate normal distribution. The general idea is that missing values are filled in with initial estimates, then the parameters of the model are estimated, new values are generated from the distributions defined by the parameters, and this process is repeated. A detailed description of this method is beyond the scope of this book and the interested reader is referred to Schafer [1997].

The assumption of a multivariate normal distribution has implications for non-normal data. Normalizing transformations (such as a log transformation of the survival times in the lung cancer trial) should be utilized when possible. When dichotomous (and other non-normal) variables are included as an explanatory variable rather than one of the variables to be imputed, the consequences of violating the multivariate normal assumptions should be minimal especially in moderate to large datasets. Use of these procedures for missing dichotomous variables should be performed very cautiously.

The SAS MI procedure, SPSS command, and the R pan function all use data augmentation techniques, but are distinctly different. SAS nad SPSS utilize a repeated measures framework and R a mixed effects model.

9.6.1 Implementation in SAS

The SAS procedure uses a Markov Chain Monte Carlo (MCMC) algorithm. The data which includes both the variables to be imputed and predictors is formed into a N by p matrix, Y^* where N is the number of subjects. Repeated measures are included as separate columns of Y^*. The imputation model is:

$$Y^* \sim N(\mu^*, \Sigma^*)$$

Because the MCMC procedure relaxes the requirement for a monotone missing data pattern, the imputation can be performed in one step.

```
proc mi data=work.onerec out=work.mcmc nimpute=20 /*noprint*/;
  by Trtment;
  var WT_loss ECOGPS SX_Sys cycles crpr pd_lt6 ctc_neu
      ln_surv toi1 toi2 toi3 toi4;
  mcmc IMPUTE=FULL;
  run;
```

The distribution of the resulting data displayed in Figure 9.4 are very similar to those obtained using the regression method (Figure 9.1). This should not be surprising as both methods assume normality and the data from the lung cancer trial have mostly a monotone missing data pattern.

9.6.2 Implementation in SPSS

The SPSS MULTIPLE IMPUTATION command implement a similar strategy as in the previous section, although the SPSS procedure sequentially estimates the missing values. The first step is to transform the data so that there is one record for each subject.

```
GET FILE='C: .... \Lung3.sav'.
DATASET NAME Lung3.
```

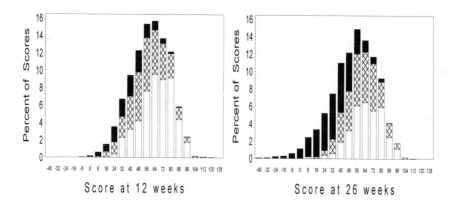

FIGURE 9.4 Study 3: Distribution of observed and multiply imputed values using Markov Chain Monte Carlo (MCMC). Imputed values before death are indicated by the shaded area and after death by the solid area.

```
/* Transpose data to one record  per subject */
SORT CASES BY PatID FUNO.
SPLIT FILE BY PatID.
CASESTOVARS
  /ID=PatID
  /INDEX=FUNO
  /AUTOFIX
  /GROUPBY=VARIABLE.
SPLIT FILE OFF.

COMPUTE Ln_Surv=LN(MAX(.1,SURV_DUR)).
EXECUTE.
```

Then the imputation procedure is implemented separately in each treatment group, generating a dataset `imputedData` with the original data (`IMPUTATION_=0`) and the imputed datasets (`IMPUTATION_=1 ...`).

```
/* Imputation is performed within each treatment group */
SORT CASES BY ExpTx.
SPLIT FILE BY ExpTX.

/* Descriptive Stats */
DATASET ACTIVE Lung3.
MULTIPLE IMPUTATION WT_loss ECOGPS SX_Sys cycles crpr pd_lt6 ctc_neu
  ln_surv FACT_T2.1 FACT_T2.2 FACT_T2.3 FACT_T2.4
  /IMPUTE METHOD=NONE
  /MISSINGSUMMARIES VARIABLES.
```

```
/* MCMC Imputation */
DATASET DECLARE imputedData.
DATASET ACTIVE Lung3.
MULTIPLE IMPUTATION WT_loss ECOGPS SX_Sys cycles crpr pd_lt6 ctc_neu
   ln_surv FACT_T2.1 FACT_T2.2 FACT_T2.3 FACT_T2.4
   /IMPUTE METHOD=FCS NIMPUTATIONS=10
   /IMPUTATIONSUMMARIES  MODELS DESCRIPTIVES
   /OUTFILE IMPUTATIONS = imputedData.
```

The resulting dataset is again restructured for the longitudinal analysis.

```
/* Restructure Files */
DATASET ACTIVE imputedData.
VARSTOCASES
   /INDEX=FUNO(4)
   /MAKE FACT_T2 FROM FACT_T2.1 to FACT_T2.4
   /MAKE MONTHS FROM MONTHS.1 to MONTHS.4.
```

9.6.3   Implementation in R

The R procedure uses a Gibbs sampler algorithm [Schafer, 1997]. The imputation model is the standard mixed effects model:

$$Y^* \sim N(X_i^*\beta + Z_i^*b_i, Z_i\Psi Z_i^{*\prime} + \Sigma^* I)$$

The data has two pieces: the N by r matrix of the multivariate longitudinal data, Y^* and the N by p matrix of the predictors which includes the design matrices for both the fixed and random effects, X_i^* and Z_i^*. N is the total number of observations, thus each observation is a row in both matrices. This is an advantage when there is wide variation in the timing of observations. The algorithm requires a *prior* distribution for the variance parameters. The prior is specified as a list of four components: a, Binv, c, and Dinv. For an uninformative prior a=r, c=$r * q$, Binv is a r x r identity matrix and Dinv is a rq x rq identity matrix where q is the number of random effects. The following code generates the first two imputed datasets for a single longitudinal variable (FACT_T2):

```
R> # Create Matrix of Predictors (X and Z)
R> Intcpt = matrix(1,ncol=1,nrow=length(Lung$PatID))      # Intercept
R> TxMONTHS=Lung$ExpTx*Lung$MONTHS                        # Interaction
R> pred=cbind(Intcpt,Lung$MONTHS,TxMONTHS,Lung$cycles,
   + Lung$PD_LT6,Lung$ln_surv)
R> xcol=c(1,2,3,4,5,6)                                    # X columns
R> zcol=c(1,2)                                            # Z columns

R> # Single Longitudinal Variable
R> y=Lung$FACT_T2                                         # longitudinal variable
R> I2=cbind(c(1,0),c(0,1))                                # 2x2 identity matrix
R> prior <- list(a=1,Binv=1,c=2,Dinv=I2)                 # hyperparameters
```

```
R> results1=pan(y,Lung$PatID,pred,xcol,zcol,prior,seed=13579,iter=1000)
R> Lung$Y1=results1$y
R> results2=pan(y,Lung$PatID,pred,xcol,zcol,prior,seed=77777,iter=1000)
R> Lung$Y2=results2$y
```

This is repeated for each of the M imputations.

The pan function also allows multiple longitudinal variables. The following example simultaneously imputes values of the Funtional Well-being, Physical Well-being, and Additional Concerns subscales of the FACT-L:

```
R> # Multiple Longitudinal Variables
R> y=cbind(Lung$FUNC_WB2,Lung$PHYS_WB2,Lung$ADD_CRN2)
R> I3=cbind(c(1,0,0),c(0,1,0),c(0,0,1))        # 3x3 identity matrix
R> I6=I2 %x% I3                                # 6x6 identity matrix
R> prior <- list(a=3,Binv=I3,c=6,Dinv=I6)
R> results1=pan(y,Lung$PatID,pred,xcol,zcol,prior,seed=13579,iter=1000)
R> Y1=results1$y
R> results2=pan(y,Lung$PatID,pred,xcol,zcol,prior,seed=77777,iter=1000)
R> Y2=results2$y
```

This is repeated for each of the M imputations.

With both of these examples, the pan function for some seeds sometime took much longer to execute. Checking the results using the str function indicated that there was a problem with the convergance though no error message was generated. A new seed was used when this occurred.

9.7   Analysis of the M Datasets

After the M datasets are generated, they are individually analyzed as previously described in Step 3 (Section 9.2). This will yield M sets of parameter estimates, $\hat{\beta}^{(m)}$, and their variance, $Var(\hat{\beta}^{(m)})$. Linear combinations of the parameters $(\hat{\theta}^{(m)} = C\hat{\beta}^{(m)})$, which will be used to test specific hypotheses (for example, $H_0 : \hat{\theta}^{(m)} = 0$) and the corresponding variance, $(U_\theta^{(m)} = Var(\hat{\theta}^{(m)}))$, will also be estimated. The following procedures are used to combine the information from the M analyses (Step 4 of the general procedure in Section 9.2).

9.7.1   Univariate Estimates and Statistics

Estimates

The combined parameter estimates $(\bar{\beta}$ and $\bar{\theta})$ are obtained by simply averaging the M within-imputation estimates $(\hat{\beta}^{(m)}$ and $\hat{\theta}^{(m)})$.

$$\bar{\beta} = \frac{1}{M} \sum_{m=1}^{M} \hat{\beta}^{(m)} \tag{9.14}$$

$$\bar{\theta} = \frac{1}{M} \sum_{m=1}^{M} \hat{\theta}^{(m)} \tag{9.15}$$

Variance of Estimates

The total variance of the parameter estimates incorporates both the average within imputation variance of the estimates ($\bar{U}_\beta$ and $\bar{U}_\theta$) and the between imputation variability of the M estimates (B_β and B_θ). The total variance (V) is computed by the sum of the within-imputation component ($\bar{U}$) and the between-imputation component (B) weighted by a correction for a finite number of imputations ($1 + M^{-1}$).

$$\bar{U}_\beta = \sum_{m=1}^{M} Var(\hat{\beta}^{(m)})/M \tag{9.16}$$

$$B_\beta = \frac{1}{M-1} \sum_{m=1}^{M} (\hat{\beta}^{(m)} - \bar{\beta})^2 \tag{9.17}$$

$$V_\beta = \bar{U}_\beta + (1 + \frac{1}{M})B_\beta \tag{9.18}$$

The procedure is identical for both β and θ. Finally, the standard errors are simply the square root of the variances.

Other Useful Information

There are other useful statistics that can be computed from the data. The first is the between to within variance ratio, r_β, which is relative increase in variance due to non-response. The second is the fraction of missing information about β (or θ), γ_β (γ_θ). The fraction of information about the parameters that is missing due to non-response (γ) for each parameter can be estimated from the ratio of the between imputation variance to the total variance.

$$r_\beta = (1 + M^{-1})B_\beta/U_\beta \tag{9.19}$$

$$\nu_{m\beta} = (M-1)(1 + r_\beta^{-1})^2 \tag{9.20}$$

$$\gamma_\beta = (r + 2/\nu_{m\beta} + 3)/(r + 1) \tag{9.21}$$

Both statistics are helpful diagnostics for assessing how the missing data contribute to the uncertainty about β (or θ). As the amount of missing data increases, γ increases. In contrast, as the amount of information about the missing data in the covariates of the imputation model increases, γ decreases.

Tests of $\hat{\beta} = \beta_0$ or $\hat{\theta} = \theta_0$

For tests with a single degree of freedom (θ is a scalar), confidence interval estimates and significance levels can be obtained using a t distribution with ν degrees of freedom [Rubin and Schenker, 1986, Rubin, 1987].

$$t_\beta = (\bar{\beta} - \beta_0)/V_\beta^{1/2} \sim t_{\nu_\beta} \tag{9.22}$$

This approximation assumes the dataset is large enough that if there were no missing values, the degrees of freedom for standard errors and denominators of F statistics are effectively infinity. Barnard and Rubin [1999] suggest an adjustment for the degrees of freedom for small sample cases. However, in most cases, if the dataset is large enough to use multiple imputation techniques then this adjustment will not be necessary.

$$\nu^*_{m\beta} = \left[\frac{1}{\nu_{m\beta}} + \frac{1}{\nu_{obs}} \right]^{-1} \tag{9.23}$$

$$\nu_{obs} = (1 - \nu_{m\beta})\nu_O(\nu_O + 1)/(\nu_O + 3) \tag{9.24}$$

9.7.2   Multivariate Tests

For tests with multiple degrees of freedom (θ is a $k \times 1$ vector), significance levels can be obtained using the multivariate analog [Rubin and Schenker, 1991]. The statistic

$$F = (\bar{\theta} - \theta_0)'U_\theta^{-1}(\bar{\theta} - \theta_0)/[(1 + r_\theta)k] \tag{9.25}$$

has an approximate F distribution with ν_1 and ν_2 degrees of freedom. $\nu_1 = k$ and $r_\theta = (1 + \frac{1}{M})trace(B_\theta U_\theta^{-1})/k$.

$$\nu_2 = 4 + [k(M - 1) - 4](1 + a/r)^2,$$
$$a = 1 - 2/[k(M - 1)] \quad \text{if } k(M - 1) > 4 \text{ or}$$
$$\nu_2 = (k + 1)(M - 1)(1 + r)^2/2 \quad \text{if } k(M - 1) \le 4.$$

As before, this approximation assumes the dataset is large enough that if there were no missing values, the degrees of freedom for standard errors and denominators of F statistics are effectively infinity. While adjustment of the degrees of freedom for small sample cases can be made, if the dataset is large enough to use multiple imputation techniques then this adjustment will not be necessary.

9.7.3   Analysis of M Datasets in SAS

In the following example, the imputed dataset has been transformed from a dataset with a single record per subject for each of the M imputations to a dataset with a record for each of the four assessments for each subject (`work.MCMC4`). PROC MIXED is then used to generate estimates of the primary and secondary parameters for each of the M imputed datasets.

```
proc mixed data=work.mcmc4;
  BY _IMPUTATION_;
  CLASS Trtment PatID;
  Model Fact_T2=Trtment Trtment*Weeks/noint solution;
  random intercept weeks/subject=PatID type=UN;
```

```
estimate 'Control Wk17' Trtment 1 0 Trtment*Weeks 17 0;
estimate 'Expmntl Wk17' Trtment 0 1 Trtment*Weeks 0 17;
estimate 'Slope Diff' Trtment*Weeks -1 1;
ods output SolutionF=MIXBeta Estimates=MIXTheta;
run;
```

The M imputations are identified by the variable `_IMPUTATION_`. For the model `FACT_T2=Trtment Trtment*Weeks`, the primary parameters ($\hat{\beta}$) are the means at baseline and the slopes in each treatment group. These are stored in a table labeled `SolutionF` and exported to a SAS dataset using the `ODS` statement above. Secondary parameters ($\hat{\beta}$) are generated by the `ESTIMATE` statement and also exported to a SAS dataset. In the above example, these are the estimates at 17 weeks in each treatment group and the differences in the slopes. The resulting `WORK.MIXBeta` and `WORK.MIXTheta` datasets will contain M sets of parameter estimates.

The M sets primary parameter estimates can be combined and analyzed using SAS `Proc MIanalyze`. This procedure will generate the pooled estimates of $\hat{\beta}$ and its standard error, 95% confidence limits and tests of $\beta = 0$.

```
Proc MIanalyze parms=MIXBeta;
  class Trtment;
  modeleffects Trtment Trtment*Weeks;
  run;
```

While there is an option to test linear combinations of the βs within `Proc MIanalyze`, it excludes models that use a class statement or interaction terms in the model statement (e.g. `Trtment*Weeks`). I recommend construction of secondary parameters ($\theta = C\beta$) within `Proc Mixed`, modifying the dataset containing the M estimates of θ and using `Proc MIanalyze` again to generate pooled estimates of $\hat{\theta}$ and its standard error, 95% confidence limits and tests of $\theta = 0$.

```
*** Linear Contrasts ***;
data work.MIXTheta2;
  set work.MIXTheta;
  Effect='Theta';
  rename label=Theta;
proc MIanalyze parms=MIXTheta2;
  class Theta;
  modeleffects Theta;
  run;
```

9.7.4 Analysis of M Datasets in SPSS

The `SPLIT FILE` and `SET` commands ensure that the subsequent analyses are performed separately for each imputed dataset and that the results are pooled. These commands are then followed by any analysis command such as `MIXED`.

```
SPLIT FILE BY Imputation_.
```

```
SET MIOUTPUT[OBSERVED IMPUTED POOLED Diagnostics].
MIXED FACT_T2 BY ExpTx WITH Months
  /FIXED=ExpTx*Months|SSTYPE(3)
  /PRINT G R SOLUTION TESTCOV
  /RANDOM=Intercept Months|SUBJECT(PatID) COVTYPE(UN)
  /TEST ='Difference in Slopes' ExpTx*Months -1 1.
```

The estimates, standard errors and associated test statistics of the fixed effects and covariance parameters are reported for the pooled analysis. In SPSS version 17.0.2 the estimates associated with the TEST option are not pooled and the analyst will need to perform these calculations by hand using the formulas presented at the beginning of this section.

9.7.5   Analysis of M Datasets in R

In R the procedure would be to analyze each dataset then combine the estimates and standard errors. Use of the lme function was described in Chapter 4.

```
R> M1=lme(fixed=Y1~TrtGrp:MONTHS,data=Lung,random=~1+MONTHS|PatID)
R> M2=lme(fixed=Y2~TrtGrp:MONTHS,data=Lung,random=~1+MONTHS|PatID)
R> M3=lme(fixed=Y3~TrtGrp:MONTHS,data=Lung,random=~1+MONTHS|PatID)
R> M4=lme(fixed=Y4~TrtGrp:MONTHS,data=Lung,random=~1+MONTHS|PatID)
R> M5=lme(fixed=Y5~TrtGrp:MONTHS,data=Lung,random=~1+MONTHS|PatID)

R> est.beta=rbind(M1$coef$fix,M2$coef$fix,M3$coef$fix,M4$coef$fix,
  + M5$coef$fix)
R> est.beta

R> se.beta=sqrt(rbind(diag(M1$varFix),diag(M2$varFix),diag(M3$varFix),
  + diag(M4$varFix),diag(M5$varFix)))
R> se.beta
```

The function mi.inference from the cat package generates the pooled estimates. Linear contrasts of the primary parameters can also be generated (see Chapter 4) and pooled in the same manner.

```
library(cat)
pooled1=mi.inference(est.beta[,1],se.beta[,1]) # Beta1
pooled2=mi.inference(est.beta[,2],se.beta[,2]) # Beta2
pooled3=mi.inference(est.beta[,3],se.beta[,3]) # Beta3
pooled=cbind(pooled1,pooled2,pooled3)          # Join results
dimnames(pooled)[[2]]=dimnames(se.beta)[[2]]   # Add column headings
pooled                                         # Print
```

The results appear as follows:

```
         (Intercept) TrtGrp0:MONTHS TrtGrp1:MONTHS
est       65.12152    -1.245133      -1.165042
std.err   0.7416646    0.4564894      0.1815791
```

```
df       55.10646    5.988199      25.97456
signif   0           0.03436219    8.527995e-07
lower    63.63525    -2.362656     -1.538301
upper    66.60778    -0.1276094    -0.7917826
r        0.3687742   4.473475      0.6458855
fminf    0.2945656   0.8579539     0.4343629
```

`df`, `r` and `fminf` correspond to $\nu_{m\beta}$, r_β, and γ_β as defined above.

9.8   Miscellaneous Issues

9.8.1   Sensitivity Analyses

Many of the articles describing multiple imputation incorporate sensitivity analyses as part of the presentation. These sensitivity analyses include both comparisons of multiple imputation with simple methods [Crawford et al., 1995, Lavori et al., 1995, Cook, 1997] and explorations of the effects of assumptions that have been made in the process of imputing the missing observations [Heitjan and Landis, 1994, Little and Yau, 1996, vanBuuren et al., 1999]. There are several outcomes of these sensitivity analyses. The analyses may demonstrate that the estimates and inference are insensitive to the results. Or, if the results do depend on the model used for imputation, precise statements can be made about the conditions under which the conclusions are valid.

While these sensitivity analyses generally focus on the primary hypotheses of the study, other components can also facilitate interpretation of the results. One such component of these analyses is the examination of distributions of the imputed values. In the lung cancer trials with auxiliary information about other clinical outcomes, we note that the distribution of the imputed values are shifted to lower values than the observed values (Figures 9.1-9.4). A second component of these exploratory analyses are plots of the data and the imputed values as a function of the time of dropout. Figure 9.5 illustrates a comparison of the MCMC method with and without auxiliary information. Without the auxiliary information the scores remain roughly constant after dropout. In contrast, with the auxiliary information, the scores continue to decline. As previously mentioned, there are no analytic methods that can be used to infer which approach is correct, but given the progressive nature of lung cancer the latter would be more credible clinically. These examples are only a few of many possible ways that one could explore the sensitivity of results to the imputation procedure.

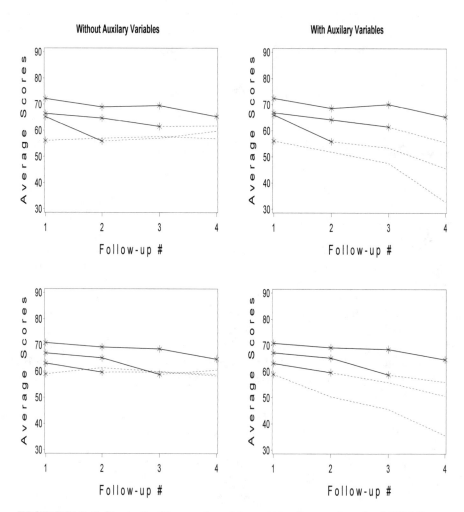

FIGURE 9.5 Study 3: Observed and imputed values using the MCMC procedure with and without auxiliary variables (complete or partial response, early progressive disease, number of cycles of therapy and log(time to death)) for the Control (upper) and Experimental (lower) arms by time of last assessment. Observed data is indicated by solid line and ⋆. Imputed data is indicated by the dashed line.

9.8.2 Imputation after Death

Whether or not one should impute values for observations that would have occurred after death is a controversial topic. I am not going to attempt to resolve the existential question about rating the quality of life after death. I would like to point out the statistical implications of not using imputed values after death in the analyses. All analyses result in either explicit or implicit imputation of the missing values. The analyst should be aware of any implicit imputation that occurs. Generally, in most analyses that do not explicitly impute missing values (Chapters 3, 4, and 7), we assume that the data are MAR and HRQoL in the patient who has died is similar to HRQoL in the survivors (conditional on the observed scores). As discussed in Chapter 7, values used in the E-step of the EM algorithm are imputed using the BLUPs. The resulting estimates will be similar to those obtained using MCMC without auxiliary information (Figure 9.5). Ultimately, the final decision will rest on the intent of the analysis. For example, consider the lung cancer trial. If the goal of the analysis is to compare two treatments using intent-to-treat (ITT) principles, explicit imputation (or use of one of the models in the subsequent chapters) would result in more rapid declines in the average scores for a treatment that was associated with more or earlier deaths. On the other hand, if the goal was to estimate scores within groups of surviving patients, explicit imputation of scores after death would not be warranted.

9.8.3 Imputation versus Analytic Models

If the multiple imputation models only use the same data that is used in the analytic models (the observed response data and baseline covariates), the resulting estimates are almost identical to those obtained using maximum likelihood methods with the same information. Without auxiliary information, multiple imputation is the hard way to analyze data where missingness is MAR. MI procedures will only provide a benefit when either complete data is required for analysis or the analyst has additional information (auxiliary data) that is related to HRQoL both when the response is observed and missing.

9.8.4 Implications for Design

If multiple imputation is proposed as an analysis strategy for a clinical trial, a number of factors should be considered. As mentioned above, these procedures all require large datasets. Initially, multiple imputation was developed for large surveys. Application of multiple imputation to smaller clinical trials should be proposed cautiously. How large is necessary will depend on how much auxiliary information is available and the expected proportion of missing data.

Anticipating the use of multiple imputation, it is wise to ensure the collection of auxiliary information. When, as a result of careful planning of a study, there is adequate documentation of the reasons for missing data along with information that will link these reasons to changes in HRQoL, it is possible to develop a good imputation model. For example, a possible strategy is to use surrogate assessments of HRQoL or related measures obtained from the health care providers or caregivers. These measures can be obtained both concurrently with the patients' assessment of HRQoL and also when the patients' assessments are missing. Although there has been considerable documentation of the discrepancies between the patients' self-evaluation of HRQoL and that of others, these assessments may be stronger predictors than other measures. This strategy is particularly useful in settings where subjects are expected to be unable to provide their own assessment of HRQoL over the course of the study (e.g. patients with brain tumors or Alzheimer's disease).

9.9   Summary

- MI provides a flexible way of handling missing data from multiple unrelated causes or when the mechanism changes over time. For example, separate models can be used for early and late dropout.

- MI will only provide a benefit when the analyst has additional information (data) that is related to HRQoL both when the response is observed and missing.

- MI will be difficult to implement in studies with mistimed observations and where the sample size is small.

- Sequential univariate regression and predictive mean matching will be useful when the missing data patterns are predominately monotone and the variables explaining dropout are very different over time.

- Markov chain monte carlo (MCMC) methods will be useful when the missing data pattern is not strictly monotone and the same set of variables can be used to explain dropout over time.

- Approximate Bayesian bootstrap (ABB) is not recommended for longitudinal studies as it ignores the correlation of observations over time.

10

Pattern Mixture and Other Mixture Models

10.1 Introduction

Mixture models that have been proposed for studies with missing data. These were briefly introduced in Chapter 7 (see Section 7.4.2). The most well known are *pattern mixture models*. The strength of these models is that the portion of the model specifying the missing data mechanism ($f[\mathbf{M}]$) does not depend on the missing values (Y^{mis}). Thus, for these mixture models, we only need to know the proportion of subjects in each strata and we do not need to specify how missingness depends on Y_i^{mis}. This is balanced by other assumptions that are described throughout this chapter. In pattern mixture models, the strata are defined by the pattern of missing assessments. Other strategies are used for the other mixture models. In concept the procedure is simple, but as I will illustrate in this chapter there are two major challenges. The first is to estimate <u>all</u> of the model parameters within each strata. The second is to justify the assumption that estimates within each strata are unbiased. There are special cases where mixture models are useful, but there are also numerous situations where justifying the assumptions will be difficult.

10.1.1 General Approach

The basic concept is the true distribution of the measures of HRQoL for the entire group of patients is a mixture of the distributions from each of the P groups of patients [Little, 1993, 1994, 1995]. The distribution of the responses, Y_i, may differ across the P strata with different parameters, $\beta^{\{p\}}$, and variance, $\Sigma^{\{p\}}$.

$$Y_i | M^{\{p\}} \sim N\left(X_i \beta^{\{p\}}, \Sigma_i^{\{p\}}\right), \quad p = 1, \ldots, P. \tag{10.1}$$

For example, let us assume that the change in HRQoL among subjects in each strata could be described using a stratum specific intercept ($\beta_0^{\{p\}}$) and slope ($\beta_1^{\{p\}}$). This would allow patients in one strata (e.g. those who drop out earlier) to have lower HRQoL scores initially and to decline more rapidly over time. The same patients may also have more or less variability in their scores (different variance) than patients in other strata, thus the variance may also differ across strata. The quantities of interest are the marginal values of the parameters averaged over the strata

$$\hat{\beta} = \sum_{}^{P} \hat{\pi}^{\{p\}} \hat{\beta}^{\{p\}} \tag{10.2}$$

where $\pi^{\{p\}}$ is the proportion of subjects observed with the pth stratum.

10.1.2   Illustration

Pauler et al. [2003] illustrate the use of a mixture model in a trial of patients with advanced stage colorectal cancer. The patients were to complete the SF-36 questionnaire at baseline, 6 weeks, 11 weeks and 21 weeks post randomization. While the authors describe the model as a pattern-mixture model, they did not form the strata based on the patterns of observed data but on a combination of survival and completion of the last assessment. Specifically, they proposed two strategies for their sensitivity analysis. In the first, they defined two strata for each treatment group based on whether the patient survived to the end of the study (21 weeks). In the second, they split the patients who survived 21 weeks based on whether they completed the last assessment. They assumed that the trajectory within each strata was linear and that the covariance structure is the same across all strata. Thus two untestable assumptions were made: missing data are ignorable within each strata and that linear extrapolation is reasonable for strata with no assessments after 11 weeks. The first assumption implies that within the group of patients who did not survive 21 weeks, there are no systematic differences between those who die early versus later, and within those who survived, there are no differences between those who drop out early versus later within a stratum.

Lung Cancer Trial (Study 3)

To illustrate we apply the strategy proposed by Pauler et al. [2003] to the lung cancer trial. Table 10.1 summarizes the proportions in each strata for using the two definitions (A and B). The last mixture model (Definition C) is an adaptation of a pattern mixture model and will be discussed later in this chapter.

The first step in our analysis is to check the assumption that a linear model is appropriate within each strata. Figure 10.1 displays (upper plots) a piecewise linear model with knots at 6, 12 and 26 weeks estimated within each strata using definition B. While the estimated curve for patients in strata 3 appears to be roughly linear, there are bends in the curves in the other two strata. If we examine the number of subjects who have observed data, we note that the number of observations in strata 1 and 2 (the lower two rows) drop rapidly over time with almost no observations available at the final follow-up. The questions are whether this is enough evidence to reject the notion of applying a model that assumes linearity within strata, how influential will the small number of later assessments be on the estimate of the slope and if extrapolation of the slope is reasonable. Unfortunately there are no formal tests to answer these questions and the analyst will have to rely on clinical opinions and intuition.

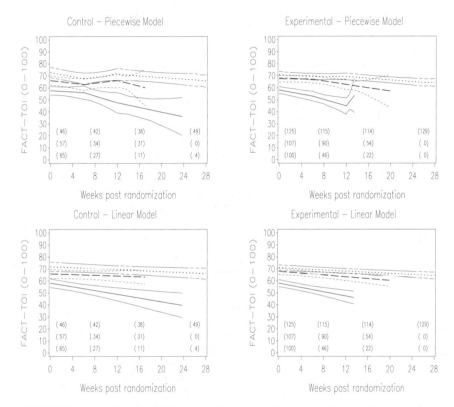

FIGURE 10.1 Study 3: Estimated trajectories and 95% confidence intervals by strata (see Table 10.1) using a piecewise linear model (upper plots) and a linear model (lower plots) for patients on control (right plots) or experimental (left plots) arms. Curves and number of observations are displayed for strata B1 ——— (lower row), B2 – – (middle row) and B3 - - - (upper row).

For the purposes of illustration, let us assume that we accept the model and assumptions as reasonable. Figure 10.1 displays in the lower plots the estimated linear trajectories. The estimates from strata B1, formed from individuals who died in the first 26 weeks, are noticeably different from those of the other two strata. If we combine the estimates using the proportions displayed in Table 10.1 with estimates obtained within each of the strata, we

TABLE 10.1 Study 3: Proportion of lung cancer subjects in each strata using definitions proposed by Pauler et al. [2003] and by time of last assessment.

			Control		Experimental	
Definition		Description	N	(%)	N	(%)
A	1	Died within 26 weeks	67	(38.3)	107	(30.6)
	2	Alive at 26 weeks	108	(61.7)	243	(69.4)
B	1	Died within 26 weeks	67	(38.3)	107	(30.6)
	2	Alive, incomplete data	59	(33.7)	114	(32.6)
	3	Alive, complete data	49	(28.0)	129	(36.9)
C	1	Baseline only or no assessments	48	(27.4)	75	(21.4)
	2	Last assessment near 6 weeks	34	(19.4)	71	(20.3)
	3	Last assessment near 12 weeks	39	(22.3)	71	(20.3)
	4	Last assessment near 26 weeks	54	(30.9)	133	(38.0)

note that the decline over 26 weeks within treatment groups is dramatically (2 to 3 times) greater when estimated using either definition A or B for the proposed mixture models (Table 10.2) than when estimated using a simple mixed effect model without stratification (first row). The differences between groups is much smaller across the different analyses; all tests of treatment differences would be non-significant. The greater sensitivity to dropout of the within group estimates of change than the between group comparisons is very typical of studies where all treatment arms have similar reasons for and proportion of missing data.

TABLE 10.2 Study 3: Results of a sensitivity analysis of the lung cancer trial using three mixture models.

	Change over 26 weeks					
----------------------------	Control		Experimental		Difference	
Mixture Model	Est	(S.E.)[*]	Est	(S.E.)[*]	Est	(S.E.)[*]
Reference (single strata)	-4.2	(2.02)	-5.5	(1.32)	-1.25	(2.4)
Definition A	-10.4	(2.69)	-11.4	(2.00)	-1.05	(3.35)
Definition B	-10.6	(3.01)	-12.7	(2.22)	-2.12	(3.74)
Definition C	-21.4	(6.02)	-11.3	(3.42)	10.2	(6.93)

[*] Standard Errors are estimated assuming the proportions of subjects in each strata are known/fixed quantities. Corrected S.E.s will be slightly larger.

As a final comment, implementing the mixture models proposed by Pauler et al. in the lung cancer trial (Study 3) was relatively straightforward and the assumptions appeared reasonable. But this will not be the case for all studies. For example, in the renal cell carcinoma trial (Study 4), the trajectories in strata defined by the time of dropout (see Figure 6.4) are definitely nonlinear. New stratification strategies may also be required in other clinical settings in which death is not a common event or the proposed schema results in strata that are too small to obtain stable estimates. In general, the challenge will be to specify both a stratification schema in which the missing data are likely to be ignorable within each strata and any necessary restrictions that would allow one to estimate all the parameters in the model. This may be especially difficult if one needs to specify the analysis plan in detail without prior experience with the same measure and population or before observing the data.

10.2 Pattern Mixture Models

In pattern mixture models, the strata are defined by different missing data patterns ($R_i \in M^{\{p\}}$). As with the general mixture model, we need to know the proportion of subjects within each strata but we do not need to specify how missingness depends on Y_i^{mis}. This advantage is balanced by 1) the large number of potential patterns of missing data and 2) the difficulties of estimating all parameters in the model or identifying appropriate restrictions. The first difficulty is the large number of missing data patterns that occur where there may only be a few subjects with some patterns. In a study with J assessments over time, there are theoretically 2^J possible patterns. Thus, with only four assessments, there are 16 possible patterns.

The second difficulty is that ($X_i \beta^{\{p\}}$) is *underidentified* (can not be directly estimated) for most of the patterns the model. This means that all the parameters cannot be estimated in each pattern unless additional assumptions are made. The remainder of this chapter focuses on the various restrictions and assumptions required to estimate parameters in these underidentified models. Section 10.3 describes strategies for growth curve models. Section 10.4 describes the identifying restrictions for repeated measures data for two special cases: bivariate data (Section 10.4.1) and monotone dropout (Section 10.4.2).

10.2.1 Specifying Patterns

As mentioned before, in a study with J planned assessments, there are theoretically 2^J possible patterns. Some studies will by design restrict this number, generally by dropping subjects from the study when they miss a follow-up.* When there are a large number of possible patterns, many stratum will have a small number of subjects. The usual strategy is to simplify the problem by

---

*This type of design is not a good policy as it can result in additional selection bias. Attempts to assess the patient response should continue even when the previous assessment is missing unless the patient has requested to have no further assessments.

combining the subjects in the smaller stratum with another stratum. When we do this, we are making one of two possible assumptions. Either the data that are missing within the combined strata are ignorable or the proportion is so small that it will have a minimal effect on the estimates of parameters within that strata.

One of the most typical methods of combining strata is to pool groups by the timing of the last assessment. Hogan et al. [2004a] go one step further in a study with dropout at each of the 12 planned assessments. Their strategy was to first fit a mixed model with interactions between all of the covariate parameters and indicators of the dropout times. They then plotted the estimates of the covariate effects versus the dropout times. From these plots, they attempted to identify by visual inspection, natural groupings where the parameters were roughly constant. They acknowledge that the procedure is subjective, and the sensitivity to different groupings should be examined.

Lung Cancer Trial

The existence of a large number of patterns is clearly illustrated in the lung cancer trial. Fifteen of the 16 possible patterns were observed (see Table 6.3). Ten of the 15 patterns have less than 5% of the observations. Most of these patterns will have fewer than 10 subjects in either of the treatment groups, generating very unstable estimates. If we adopt the strategy of defining the patterns by the time of dropout, we have five possible patterns (one without any data). If the intermittent missing values are the result of administrative problems, then we can safely assume the missing data are ignorable. However, if the missing values occurred because the patient was feeling badly, perhaps because of acute toxicity, we will need to demonstrate that the proportions of patients with intermittent missing data are small or likely to have minimal impact on estimates.

10.3   Restrictions for Growth Curve Models

In longitudinal studies in which growth curve models are used, the approach is to fit growth curve models to the data in each pattern. Polynomial models can be fit within each of the P patterns where there are sufficient observations over time to estimate the parameters. It is necessary to make additional restrictions to estimate all the parameters; generally this involves extrapolating past the point of dropout [Hogan and Laird, 1997a, Curren, 2000].

$$Y_{ij}^{\{p\}} = \beta^{\{p\}} X_{ij}^{\{p\}} + \epsilon_{ij}^{\{p\}}. \tag{10.3}$$

The fixed effects and the covariance parameters may differ across the patterns. The pooled parameter estimates are

$$\hat{\beta} = \sum_{}^{P} \hat{\pi}^{\{p\}} \hat{\beta}^{\{p\}}. \tag{10.4}$$

10.3.1 Linear Trajectories over Time

In a limited number of studies, it is reasonable to believe that the change in HRQoL is linear over time (t):

$$Y_{hij}^{\{p\}} = \beta_0^{\{p\}} + \beta_1^{\{p\}} t_{hij}^{\{p\}} + \epsilon_{hij}^{\{p\}}. \tag{10.5}$$

But even with this simple model, we can immediately see the challenges. The two fixed-effect parameters (intercept and slope) can be estimated only in the patterns with at least two observations per subject. Thus we need to impose an additional restriction to estimate the parameters for patterns with less than two observations. Consider the patterns observed in the lung cancer trial after collapsing the 15 observed patterns by time of dropout (Table 10.1, Definition C). None of the parameters are estimable in the patients with no data and the slope is not estimable in the pattern with only the baseline assessment without additional assumptions.

There are a number of approaches that one can take which may or may not be reasonable in different settings. One strategy is to collapse patterns until there is sufficient follow-up to estimate both the intercept and slope within each strata. In this example, we would combine those with only the baseline assessment (Stratum C1) with those who dropped out after the second assessment (Stratum C2).

$$\hat{\beta}_0^{\{1\}} = \hat{\beta}_0^{\{2\}} \text{ and } \hat{\beta}_1^{\{1\}} = \hat{\beta}_1^{\{2\}}. \tag{10.6}$$

This solves the problem only if the resulting parameters are an unbiased representation of the subjects in the pooled patterns. There are no formal tests to assure this, but examining the estimates prior to pooling and understanding the reasons for dropout will inform the decision. Another possible restriction is to allow different intercepts ($\hat{\beta}_0^{\{1\}} \neq \hat{\beta}_0^{\{2\}}$) and to assume that the slope for subjects with only the baseline assessment (Stratum C1) is the same as the slope for subjects with two assessments (Stratum C2):

$$\hat{\beta}_1^{\{1\}} = \hat{\beta}_1^{\{2\}}. \tag{10.7}$$

The plots in the upper half of Figure 10.2 illustrates this for the lung cancer trial.

An alternative approach is to place parametric assumptions on the parameters using the time of dropout as a covariate [Curren, 2000, Michiels et al., 1999]. For example, one might assume that there was an interaction between the time of dropout $(d^{\{p\}})$ and the intercept and slope in each pattern. With both linear and quadratic terms for the time of dropout the model might appear as:

$$Y_{ij}^{\{p\}} = \underbrace{\beta_0^{\{p\}} + \beta_1^{\{p\}} d^{\{p\}} + \beta_2^{\{p\}} d^{\{p\}2}}_{Intercept}$$
$$+ \underbrace{\beta_3^{\{p\}} t_{ij} + \beta_4^{\{p\}} t_{ij} d^{\{p\}} + \beta_5^{\{p\}} t_{ij} d^{\{p\}2}}_{Slope} + \epsilon_{ij}^{\{p\}} \qquad (10.8)$$

Pattern-specific estimates using this approach are illustrated in the plot in the lower half of Figure 10.2. This restriction is equivalent to the conditional linear model that will be described in the next chapter (see Section 11.3).

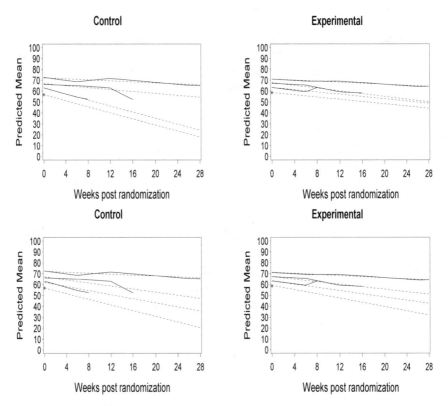

FIGURE 10.2 Study 3: Extrapolation of linear trends in patterns defined by the time of the last observation. Solid lines are based on MLE of available data using a piecewise linear regression model. Dashed lines in upper plots are based on restrictions identified in equation 10.7. Dashed lines in the lower plots are based on restrictions identified in equation 10.8.

It is not possible to statistically determine which models are correct, as we are missing the necessary data to test the assumption. Examination of all plots suggest that both approaches reasonably approximate the observed data. This is indicated by the close approximation of the curves to estimates of change obtained using a piecewise linear regression model. Not surprisingly, the major difference between the two methods of extrapolation occurs for subjects who have only a baseline observation (Stratum C1).

10.3.2 Estimation of the Parameters

There are two approaches to obtain the pooled parameter (or marginal) estimates, $\hat{\beta}$. The first uses the weighted average model described in equation 10.3. Parameters are first estimated within each strata, $\hat{\beta}^{\{p\}}$, and then combined by weighting by the proportion of subjects within each strata as described in equation 10.4. This approach is conceptually straightforward but somewhat cumbersome to implement.

The second approach [Fitzmaurice et al., 2001] involves reparameterizing the model using centered indicator variables as follows:

$$Y_{ij} = \beta X_{ij} + \sum_{p=1}^{P-1} \alpha_p W_{ip} + \epsilon_{ij} \tag{10.9}$$

where W_{ip} is a known function of the P dropout times or strata. In this model, we wish to estimate the parameters, β. The terms αW_{ip} model the pattern specific deviations from βX. If we restrict the expected value of W_{ip} to be zero, the expected value of Y_{ij} is βX_{ij} and estimates of $\hat{\beta}$ will come directly from the model. Typically W_{ip} will be constructed from centered indicator variables for the time of dropout or the strata.

To illustrate the equivalence of the two models, consider a very simple example with a single group and two strata with one and two-thirds of the subjects respectively. Both models will assume that change is linear over time. If D_{i1} is an indicator of belonging to the first strata, then the average of D_{i1} across all subjects, $\bar{D}_1 = 1/3$. The centered indicator variable $W_{i1} = D_{i1} - \bar{D}_1 = 1 - 1/3$ for subjects in the first strata and $0 - 1/3$ for subjects not in the first strata. Table 10.3 illustrates the equivalence of the two strategies.

To illustrate the procedure for multiple dropout times, consider the lung cancer trial where dropout is defined by the time of the last assessment (Definition C, Table 10.1). D_i would be a vector of indicator variables where $D_{ik} = 1$ if the last assessment occurred at the kth assessment and $D_{ik} = 0$ otherwise. So for an individual who dropped out after the third assessment, $D_i = (0, 0, 1, 0)$. Because the elements of D_i always sum to one, we must drop one of the indicator variables. It does not matter which, so for illustration we drop the last indicator. We then center the indicator variables: $W_i = D_i - \bar{D}_i$ where $\bar{D}_i$ is the average of D_i or the proportions in each dropout group. Thus for an individual in the experimental arm who dropped out after the third

TABLE 10.3 Study 3: Equivalence of two estimation strategies for mixture models: weighted average (equation 10.3) and centered indicator (equation 10.9).

Strata	$\hat{\pi}$	Weighted Average	W_{i1}	Centered Indicator
1	1/3	$\beta_0^{\{1\}} + \beta_1^{\{1\}}t$	2/3	$\beta_0 + \beta_1 t + \frac{2}{3}(\alpha_{01} + \alpha_{11})$
2	2/3	$\beta_0^{\{2\}} + \beta_1^{\{2\}}t$	-1/3	$\beta_0 + \beta_1 t - \frac{1}{3}(\alpha_{01} + \alpha_{11})$
β_0		$\frac{1}{3}\beta_0^{\{1\}} + \frac{2}{3}\beta_0^{\{2\}} = \beta_0$		$\frac{1}{3}(\beta_0 + \frac{2}{3}\alpha_{01}) + \frac{2}{3}(\beta_0 - \frac{1}{3}\alpha_{01}) = \beta_0$
β_1		$\frac{1}{3}\beta_1^{\{1\}} + \frac{2}{3}\beta_1^{\{2\}} = \beta_1$		$\frac{1}{3}(\beta_1 + \frac{2}{3}\alpha_{11}) + \frac{2}{3}(\beta_1 - \frac{1}{3}\alpha_{11}) = \beta_1$

assessment $W_i = (0, 0, 1) - (.214, .203, .203) = (-.214, -.203, .797)$. W_i could have alternative forms, such as functions of the actual times of dropout.

An important caution: If all the parameters in the model described in equation 10.3 can not be estimated, the second model described equation 10.9 will be less than full rank. In this case, while estimates of the βs are generated, they can not be interpreted as the average across all the strata.

Lung Cancer Trial

The reparameterization using centered indicator variables can be useful when imposing restrictions on the model. Consider the two sets of restrictions for the pattern mixture models that are proposed for the lung cancer trial. The first set of restrictions (Model 1) is described by equation 10.7. We can reparameterize it as follows:

$$Y_{ij} = \beta_0 + \alpha_{02}W_{i2} + \alpha_{03}W_{i3} + \alpha_{04}W_{i4} +$$
$$\beta_1 t_{ij} + \alpha_{13}t_{ij}W_{i3} + \alpha_{14}t_{ij}W_{i4} + \epsilon_{ij} \qquad (10.10)$$

where $W_{ik}, k = 2, 3, 4$ are centered indicators of dropout after the 2nd, 3rd and 4th assessments. Note that we did not include the term $\alpha_{12}t_{ij}W_{i2}$, which would allow the slopes to be different in the 1st and 2nd strata. Omitting the term imposes the restriction that the slopes are equal in those two patterns (equation 10.7).

We can also implement the second restriction described by equation 10.8 as follows:

$$Y_{ij} = \beta_0 + \alpha_{01}W_{1i} + \alpha_{02}W_{2i} +$$
$$\beta_1 t_{ij} + \alpha_{11}t_{ij}W_{1i} + \alpha_{12}t_{ij}W_{2i}\epsilon_{ij} \qquad (10.11)$$

where $W_{1i} = T_i^D - \bar{T}_i^D$ and $W_{2i} = T_i^{2D} - \bar{T}_i^{2D}$ are the centered time of dropout (T_i^D) and time of dropout squared.

10.3.3 Nonlinear Trajectories over Time

Renal Cell Carcinoma Trial

Implementation of pattern mixture models becomes considerably more difficult when the trajectories are nonlinear. In the renal cell carcinoma study (Table 10.4), slightly over half the patients survived to 52 weeks (Definition A) and there are six strata defined by the timing of the last assessment (Definition C). The trajectories of the observed data within those strata are displayed in Figure 10.3. The challenges become immediately obvious. First, the trajectories are dramatically nonlinear, particularly during the early phase of the study when scores drop over the first 8 weeks and then start to recover. Second, there is considerably more variation among subjects as a function of the timing of the last assessment than is captured by Definition A. Finally, to estimate the marginal (pooled) estimates of the parameters, we must extrapolate the curves in most of the strata.

TABLE 10.4 Study 4: Proportion of renal cell carcinoma subjects in each strata using definitions proposed by Pauler et al. [2003] and by time of last assessment.

			Control		Experimental	
Definition		Description	N	(%)	N	(%)
A	1	Died within 52 weeks	41	(41.0)	47	(47.0)
	2	Alive at 52 weeks	59	(59.0)	53	(53.0)
B	1	Died within 52 weeks	41	(41.0)	47	(47.0)
	2	Alive at 52 weeks, incomplete data	57	(57.0)	47	(47.0)
	3	Alive at 52 weeks, complete data	2	(2.0)	8	(8.0)
C	1	Baseline only or no assessments	5	(5.0)	14	(14.0)
	2	Last assessment near 2 weeks	9	(9.0)	11	(11.0)
	3	Last assessment near 8 weeks	32	(32.0)	24	(24.8)
	4	Last assessment near 17 weeks	21	(21.0)	14	(14.0)
	5	Last assessment near 34 weeks	25	(25.0)	13	(13.0)
	6	Last assessment near 52 weeks	8	(8.0)	24	(24.0)

One of the strengths of the pattern mixture approach is that it is easy to display the trajectories that result from a particular set of restrictions and assess whether the extrapolations are clinically reasonable. For the purposes of illustration (not because it is necessarily recommended), we combine the six strata into three strata, combining C1 with C2, C3 with C4, and C5 with C6. Figure 10.4 illustrates three of many possible sets of restrictions. In the upper plots, the estimate at the end of the period with data is extended. In the middle plots, the slopes observed in the last observed segment of time are extended. In the lower plots, we assume that the changes in slopes would follow that of the nearest neighbor. Thus, we would use the change in slope

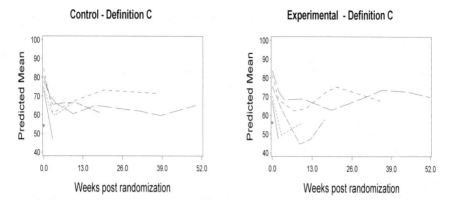

FIGURE 10.3 Trial 4: Estimated trajectories in the renal cell carcinoma trial with strata defined by the last assessment (Definition C) using a piecewise-linear model.

after 17 weeks from strata C5/6 to extrapolate the curve for those in strata C3/4. It is immediately obvious that there is considerable variation in the extrapolated estimates, with some trajectories dropping below the lower limit of the scale. Perhaps some scenarios could be eliminated as clinically unrealistic, such as the assumption that scores would be maintained over time in patients who drop out primarily due to disease progression. In summary, this example illustrates the difficulty of identifying a set (or sets) of restriction(s) that are clinically reasonable, especially if this is required prior to examining the data.

10.3.4   Implementation in SAS

Average of Stratum Specific Estimates

To illustrate the procedure for the weighted sum of stratum specific estimates (equation 10.3), I will consider the mixture using definition B (Table 10.1) for the lung cancer trial. In the following illustration, we will need the proportion of subjects in each strata. In this illustration, I will also be estimating the 26 week change, so it will be helpful to have the values of those proportions multiplied by 26. The following SQL code creates global macro variables that we will use later.

```
*** Calculate proportion of subjects in each strata ***;
proc sql;
   *** Calculate Proportions within Strata (Definition B) ***;
   *** Multiply Proportions times 26 for 26 week change ***;
   select count(PatID)/&Grp0,count(PatID)/&Grp0*26 into :IntOB1,:WkOB1
      from work.lung1
      where Exp=0 and StrataB=1;
```

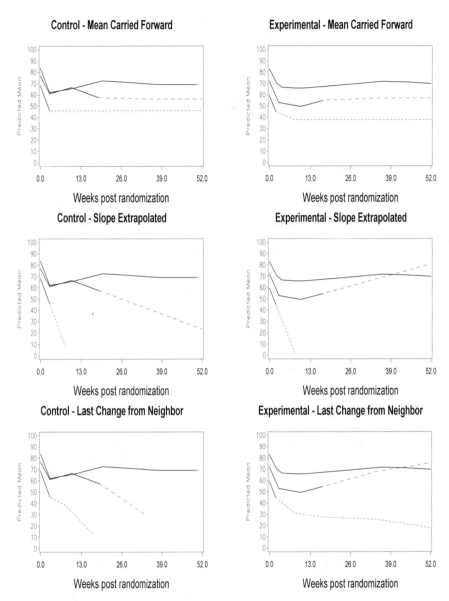

FIGURE 10.4 Study 4: Estimated trajectories for strata defined as C1/2, C3/4 and C5/6 for the control (left) and experimental (right) treatment arms. In the upper plots, estimates are extrapolated by extending the mean estimates forward in time. In the middle plots, the slope for the last observed segment is extended. In the lower plots, the change in slope from the nearest neighbor is used. Bold solid lines represent the trajectories based on observed data; dashed lines indicate the extrapolated trajectories.

```
   select count(PatID)/&Grp0,count(PatID)/&Grp0*26 into :IntOB2,:WkOB2
      from work.lung1
      where Exp=0 and StrataB=2;
   select count(PatID)/&Grp0,count(PatID)/&Grp0*26 into :IntOB3,:WkOB3
      from work.lung1
      where Exp=0 and StrataB=3;
   select count(PatID)/&Grp1,count(PatID)/&Grp1*26 into :Int1B1,:Wk1B1
      from work.lung1
      where Exp=1 and StrataB=1;
   select count(PatID)/&Grp1,count(PatID)/&Grp1*26 into :Int1B2,:Wk1B2
      from work.lung1
      where Exp=1 and StrataB=2;
   select count(PatID)/&Grp1,count(PatID)/&Grp1*26 into :Int1B3,:Wk1B3
      from work.lung1
      where Exp=1 and StrataB=3;
   quit;
*%put _global_; * Checks Macro variables *;
```

In this example, we assume that the trajectory is linear in each strata and estimate an intercept and slope for each stratum and treatment combination. The resulting model produces 12 estimates, six for the intercept terms (StrataB*Exp) and six for the slope terms (StrataB*Exp*Weeks). The pooled estimates are then generated using the macro variables (e.g. &IntOB1, &IntOB2, &IntOB3, etc.) in the ESTIMATE statements.

```
proc mixed data=work.lung3 noclprint order=internal;
 class PatID Exp StrataB;
 model FACT_T2=StrataB*Exp StrataB*Exp*Weeks/noint solution;
 random Intercept Weeks/subject=PatID type=UN gcorr;
 Estimate 'Cntl Week=0' StrataB*Exp &IntOB1 &IntOB2 &IntOB3 0 0 0;
 Estimate 'Exp  Week=0' StrataB*Exp 0 0 0 &Int1B1 &Int1B2 &Int1B3;
 Estimate 'Cntl Week=26' StrataB*Exp &IntOB1 &IntOB2 &IntOB3 0 0 0
                         StrataB*Exp*Weeks &WkOB1 &WkOB2 &WkOB3 0 0 0;
 Estimate 'Exp Week=26'  StrataB*Exp 0 0 0 &Int1B1 &Int1B2 &Int1B3
                         StrataB*Exp*Weeks 0 0 0 &Wk1B1 &Wk1B2 &Wk1B3;
 Estimate 'Cntl Change' StrataB*Exp*Weeks &WkOB1 &WkOB2 &WkOB3 0 0 0;
 Estimate 'Exp  Change' StrataB*Exp*Weeks 0 0 0 &Wk1B1 &Wk1B2 &Wk1B3;
 Estimate 'Diff Change' StrataB*Exp*Weeks -&WkOB1 -&WkOB2 -&WkOB3
                                           &Wk1B1  &Wk1B2  &Wk1B3;
 run;
```

We have assumed that the proportions are known (fixed) quantities when they are in fact unknown quantities that we have estimated. Thus, the resulting standard errors of the pooled estimates will underestimate the actual standard errors (see Section 10.5). The use of the macro variables will facilitate implementation of any bootstrapping procedures to obtain acurate estimates of the standard errors (or using the same code as the study matures).

Centered Indicator Variables

The following procedure implements the reparametered model using centered indicator variables described in Section 10.3.2 (equation 10.9). Two indicator variables (StrataB1, StrataB2) were previously defined (StrataB1 = (StrataB eq 1); StrataB2 = (StrataB eq 2);). Centered indicator variables, D1B and D2B, are then created using the following SQL procedure:

```
*** Center the Dropout Indicators within Exp Group ***;
proc sql;
  create table work.centered as
  select PatID,
    (StrataB1 - mean(StrataB1)) as D1B,
    (StrataB2 - mean(StrataB2)) as D2B,
  from work.lung1A
  group by Exp order by PatID;
quit;
data work.lung3A;
  merge work.lung3 work.centered;
  by PatID;
  run;
```

The parameter estimates are then obtained as follows:

```
proc mixed data=work.lung3A noclprint order=internal;
  title2 'Strata B definition';
  class PatID Exp;
  model FACT_T2=Exp Exp*Weeks Exp*D1b Exp*Weeks*D1b
        Exp*D2b Exp*Weeks*D2b
     /noint solution;
  random Intercept Weeks/subject=PatID type=UN gcorr;
  Estimate 'Ctnl Week=0'    Exp 1 0;
  Estimate 'Exp  Week=0'    Exp 0 1;
  Estimate 'Cntl Week=26'   Exp 1 0 Exp*Weeks 26 0;
  Estimate 'Exp  Week=26'   Exp 0 1 Exp*Weeks 0 26;
  Estimate 'Cntl Change'    Exp*Weeks 26  0;
  Estimate 'Exp  Change'    Exp*Weeks 0 26;
  Estimate 'Diff Change'    Exp*Weeks  -26 26;
  run;
```

Note that because the variables that define the strata are centered, the parameters associated with the terms Exp and Exp*Weeks are the same as those obtained in the previous section.

10.3.5   Implementation in R

I will again use the mixture using definition B (Table 10.1) for the lung cancer trial to illustrate the weighted sum and centered indicator approaches using R. The first steps are required in both approaches.

```
# Find maximum FUNO where FACT_T2 is not missing
Last_FU<-tapply(Lung$FUNO[!is.na(Lung$FACT_T2)],
                Lung$PatID[!is.na(Lung$FACT_T2)],max,na.rm=T)
Last_FU<-data.frame(Last_FU=Last_FU,PatID=names(Last_FU))
Lung<-merge(Lung,Last_FU,by="PatID",all.x=TRUE)
Lung$Last_FU[is.na(Lung$Last_FU)]=0 # Missing eq 0


# Define strata (1=Died, 2=Alive incomplete, 3=Alive complete)
Lung$Strata=2
Lung$Strata[Lung$Last_FU==4]=3
Lung$Strata[Lung$SURV_DUR<365.25/2]=1


# Factor Variables for Treatment and Strata
Lung$StrataF=factor(Lung$Strata)
Lung$ExpF=factor(Lung$Exp)
```

Average of Stratum Specific Estimates

The procedure for the weighted sum of stratum specific estimates (equation 10.3) follows. We again assume that the trajectory is linear in each strata and estimate an intercept and slope for each stratum and treatment combination. The resulting model produces 12 estimates, six for the intercept terms (StrataF*ExpF) and six for the slope terms (StrataF*ExpF*Weeks).

```
#-----------------------------------------------------------------------
# Linear Mixed Effects Model with 3 Strata
#-----------------------------------------------------------------------
StratModel=lme(fixed=FACT_T2~0+StrataF:ExpF+StrataF:ExpF:WEEKS,
               data=Lung,random=~1+WEEKS|PatID,na.action = na.exclude)
print(StratModel)      # Summary of results
summary(StratModel)    # Details of results
```

We will then need the proportion of subjects in each strata to construct the pooled estimates.

```
# Calculate proportions (Note equal # obs per subject)
Freqs=table(Lung$Exp,Lung$Strata)
Props=prop.table(Freqs,1)
print(Props,digits=3)
Prop1=Props[1,]
Prop2=Props[2,]
```

```
# Construct C matrix to generate Theta=C*Beta
null=c(0,0,0)
C1=cbind(Prop1,null,null,null);          dim(C1)=c(1,12)
C2=cbind(null,Prop2,null,null);          dim(C2)=c(1,12)
C3=cbind(Prop1,null,Prop1*26,null);      dim(C3)=c(1,12)
C4=cbind(null,Prop2,null,Prop2*26);      dim(C4)=c(1,12)
C5=cbind(null,null,Prop1*26,null);       dim(C5)=c(1,12)
C6=cbind(null,null,null,Prop2*26);       dim(C6)=c(1,12)
```

```
C7=cbind(null,null,Prop1*26*-1,Prop2*26); dim(C7)=c(1,12)
CStrat=rbind(C1,C2,C3,C4,C5,C6,C7)
rownames(CStrat)=c("T0 Cntl","T0 Exp","Wk26 Cntl","Wk26 Exp",
                   "Chg Cntl","Chg Exp","Diff")

# Obtain estimates, etc for Theta=C*Beta
StratResults=estCbeta(CStrat,StratModel$coef$fix,StratModel$varFix)
print(StratResults,digits=3)
```

The function `estCBeta` can be found in Appendix R. Note we have assumed that the proportions are known (fixed) quantities and the resulting standard errors of the pooled estimates will underestimate the actual standard errors (see Section 10.5).

Centered Indicator Variables

Begin to implement the second estimation procedure described in Section 10.3.2 by generating the centered indicator variables (M1, M2). When the number of records is not equal to 4 records per subject the following code will need to be altered slightly. We then fit the model described in equation 10.9.

```
# Centered Indicators (M1 and M2): Note 4 records per subject
Lung$Strata_1=0
Lung$Strata_1[Lung$Strata==1]=1
Mean_S1<-tapply(Lung$Strata_1[Lung$FUNO==1],
                Lung$Exp[Lung$FUNO==1],mean,na.rm=T)
Mean_S1<-data.frame(Mean_S1=Mean_S1,Exp=names(Mean_S1))
Lung<-merge(Lung,Mean_S1,by="Exp")
Lung$M1=Lung$Strata_1-Lung$Mean_S1
Lung$Strata_2=0
Lung$Strata_2[Lung$Strata==2]=1
Mean_S2<-tapply(Lung$Strata_2[Lung$FUNO==1],
                Lung$Exp[Lung$FUNO==1],mean,na.rm=T)
Mean_S2<-data.frame(Mean_S2=Mean_S2,Exp=names(Mean_S2))
Lung<-merge(Lung,Mean_S2,by="Exp")
Lung$M2=Lung$Strata_2-Lung$Mean_S2

CentModel=lme(fixed=FACT_T2~0 + ExpF+ExpF:WEEKS+
              ExpF:M1+ExpF:WEEKS:M1 + ExpF:M2+ExpF:WEEKS:M2,
              data=Lung,random=~1+WEEKS|PatID,na.action = na.exclude)
summary(CentModel)   # Details listing of results
```

The linear combinations and associated test statistics of the parameter estimates are then obtained as follows:

```
# Construct C matrix to generate Theta=C*Beta
null=c(0,0,0,0)
C1=c(1, 0, 0, 0);   C1=cbind(C1,null,null);  dim(C1)=c(1,12)
C2=c(0, 1, 0, 0);   C2=cbind(C2,null,null);  dim(C2)=c(1,12)
C3=c(1, 0, 26, 0);  C3=cbind(C3,null,null);  dim(C3)=c(1,12)
```

```
C4=c(0, 1, 0, 26);    C4=cbind(C4,null,null);  dim(C4)=c(1,12)
C5=c(0, 0, 26, 0);    C5=cbind(C5,null,null);  dim(C5)=c(1,12)
C6=c(0, 0, 0, 26);    C6=cbind(C6,null,null);  dim(C6)=c(1,12)
C7=c(0, 0, -26, 26);  C7=cbind(C7,null,null);  dim(C7)=c(1,12)
CCent=rbind(C1,C2,C3,C4,C5,C6,C7)
rownames(CCent)=c("T0 Cntl","T0 Exp","Wk26 Cntl","Wk26 Exp",
                  "Chg Cntl","Chg Exp","Diff")

# Obtain estimates, etc for Theta=C*Beta
CentResults=estCbeta(CCent,CentModel$coef$fix,CentModel$varFix)
print(CentResults,digits=3)
```

10.4 Restrictions for Repeated Measures Models

Alternative strategies exist for repeated measures models to "identify" the unknown parameters of a repeated model. For example, if we were using a cell means model in the lung cancer trial we would need to estimate a mean at each time in each pattern $(\hat{\mu}_1^{\{p\}}, \hat{\mu}_2^{\{p\}}, \hat{\mu}_3^{\{p\}}, \hat{\mu}_4^{\{p\}})$ and the 10 covariance parameters $(\hat{\sigma}_{11}^{\{p\}}, \hat{\sigma}_{12}^{\{p\}}, \ldots, \hat{\sigma}_{44}^{\{p\}})$. Without making additional assumptions, we could obtain all 14 parameters only in strata with all four assessments. In the following section, we describe possible strategies for two special cases of the pattern mixture models: bivariate data (Section 10.4.1) and monotone dropout (Section 10.4.2).

10.4.1 Bivariate Data (Two Repeated Measures)

The simplest case for longitudinal studies consists of two repeated measures, typically a pre and post-intervention measure. There are four possible patterns of missing data (Table 10.5). The first pattern, in which all responses are observed, contains the *complete cases*. The second and third patterns have one observation each. In the fourth pattern, none of the responses is observed. In trials where the pre-intervention measure is required, only the first two patterns will exist.

In each of the four patterns, there are five possible parameters to be estimated: two means $(\hat{\mu}_1^{\{p\}}, \hat{\mu}_2^{\{p\}})$ and three parameters for the covariance $(\hat{\sigma}_{11}^{\{p\}}, \hat{\sigma}_{12}^{\{p\}}, \hat{\sigma}_{22}^{\{p\}})$. We can estimate 9 of the 20 total parameters from the data: all five parameters from pattern 1 and two each from patterns 2 and 3. Thus the model is underidentified and some type of restriction (assumption) is required to estimate the remaining parameters.

TABLE 10.5 All possible missing data patterns for two repeated measures and the estimable parameters.

Pattern	R	Y_1	Y_2	Means		Covariance		
1	(1,1)	$Y_1^{\{1\}}$	$Y_2^{\{1\}}$	$\hat{\mu}_1^{\{1\}}$	$\hat{\mu}_2^{\{1\}}$	$\hat{\sigma}_{11}^{\{1\}}$	$\hat{\sigma}_{12}^{\{1\}}$	$\hat{\sigma}_{22}^{\{1\}}$
2	(1,0)	$Y_1^{\{2\}}$	Missing	$\hat{\mu}_1^{\{2\}}$	?	$\hat{\sigma}_{11}^{\{2\}}$	?	?
3	(0,1)	Missing	$Y_2^{\{3\}}$	?	$\hat{\mu}_2^{\{3\}}$	?	?	$\hat{\sigma}_{22}^{\{3\}}$
4	(0,0)	Missing	Missing	?	?	?	?	?

Complete-Case Missing Variable (CCMV) Restriction

One possible set of restrictions is based on the complete cases [Little, 1993]. For the bivariate case shown in Table 10.5, the restrictions are:

$$\theta_{[2\cdot1]}^{\{2\}} = \theta_{[2\cdot1]}^{\{1\}}, \quad \theta_{[1\cdot2]}^{\{3\}} = \theta_{[1\cdot2]}^{\{1\}}, \quad \text{and} \quad \theta^{\{4\}} = \theta^{\{1\}} \tag{10.12}$$

where $\theta_{[2\cdot1]}^{\{1\}}$ denotes the parameters from the regression of Y_2 on Y_1 (or the conditional distribution of Y_2 given Y_1) using the complete cases in pattern 1.

Consider an example where we have only the first two patterns. All subjects were observed initially, but some are missing at the second assessment. We estimate $\mu_1^{\{1\}}, \mu_2^{\{1\}}$, and $\mu_1^{\{2\}}$ directly from the data. We then apply this complete-case missing variable restriction to estimate $\mu_2^{\{2\}}$ using the regression of Y_2 on Y_1:

$$Y_{i2}^{\{1\}} = \beta_{0[2\cdot1]}^{\{1\}} + \beta_{1[2\cdot1]}^{\{1\}} Y_{i1}^{\{1\}} + e_i \tag{10.13}$$

$$Y_{i2}^{\{2\}} = \beta_{0[2\cdot1]}^{\{2\}} + \beta_{1[2\cdot1]}^{\{2\}} Y_{i1}^{\{2\}} + e_i \tag{10.14}$$

Since we cannot estimate the parameters in the second equation due to missing data, we assume the same relationship holds in pattern 2 as in pattern 1.

$$\beta_{0[2\cdot1]}^{\{2\}} = \beta_{0[2\cdot1]}^{\{1\}}, \quad \beta_{1[2\cdot1]}^{\{2\}} = \beta_{1[2\cdot1]}^{\{1\}} \tag{10.15}$$

The estimated mean for the second assessment in pattern 2 is:

$$\begin{aligned} \hat{\mu}_2^{\{2\}} &= \hat{\beta}_{0[2\cdot1]}^{\{1\}} + \hat{\beta}_{1[2\cdot1]}^{\{1\}} \bar{Y}_1^{\{2\}} \\ &= \bar{Y}_2^{\{1\}} - \frac{\hat{\sigma}_{12}^{\{1\}}}{\hat{\sigma}_{11}^{\{1\}}} \left(\bar{Y}_1^{\{1\}} - \bar{Y}_1^{\{2\}} \right). \end{aligned} \tag{10.16}$$

Combining the estimates for the two patterns, the overall estimates of the two means are

$$\hat{\mu}_1 = \hat{\pi}^{\{1\}} \hat{\mu}_1^{\{1\}} + \hat{\pi}^{\{2\}} \hat{\mu}_1^{\{2\}} = \hat{\pi}^{\{1\}} \bar{Y}_1^{\{1\}} + \hat{\pi}^{\{2\}} \bar{Y}_1^{\{2\}} = \bar{Y}_1 \tag{10.17}$$

$$\hat{\mu}_2 = \hat{\pi}^{\{1\}} \hat{\mu}_2^{\{1\}} + \hat{\pi}^{\{2\}} \hat{\mu}_2^{\{2\}} = \bar{Y}_2^{\{1\}} + \frac{\hat{\sigma}_{12}^{\{1\}}}{\hat{\sigma}_{11}^{\{1\}}} \left(\hat{\mu}_1 - \bar{Y}_1^{\{1\}} \right) \tag{10.18}$$

Procedures for estimating the covariance parameters are outlined in detail by Little [1993, 1994].

Note that for this special case, these estimates are the same as those obtained using MLE with all available data. The restrictions are equivalent to assuming that the missingness of Y_2 depends only on Y_1. Recall that this is exactly the definition of MAR. Thus, this restriction is helpful when trying to understand pattern mixture models, but is not of much practical use when we believe that the data are MNAR.

Brown's Protective[†] Restrictions

A second set of restrictions was proposed by Brown [1990] for monotone dropout where patterns 1 and 2 are observed. The assumption is that the missingness of Y_2 depends on Y_2. This is the MNAR assumption. For the bivariate case, the restriction is: $\theta^{\{2\}}_{[1\cdot2]} = \theta^{\{1\}}_{[1\cdot2]}$. (Note that this is the mirror image of the complete-case restriction).

Consider the bivariate example where we have only the first two patterns. This time, we will regress Y_1 on Y_2.

$$Y^{\{1\}}_{i1} = \beta^{\{1\}}_{0[1\cdot2]} + \beta^{\{1\}}_{1[1\cdot2]} Y^{\{1\}}_{i2} + e_i \tag{10.19}$$

$$Y^{\{2\}}_{i1} = \beta^{\{1\}}_{0[1\cdot2]} + \beta^{\{1\}}_{1[1\cdot2]} Y^{\{2\}}_{i2} + e_i \tag{10.20}$$

The assumption is that the same relationship holds in both patterns:

$$\beta^{\{2\}}_{0[1\cdot2]} = \beta^{\{1\}}_{0[1\cdot2]} \qquad \beta^{\{2\}}_{1[1\cdot2]} = \beta^{\{1\}}_{1[1\cdot2]} \tag{10.21}$$

To estimate $\mu^{\{2\}}_2$, we assume

$$\bar{Y}^{\{2\}}_1 = \beta^{\{1\}}_{0[1\cdot2]} + \beta^{\{1\}}_{1[1\cdot2]} \hat{\mu}^{\{2\}}_2 \tag{10.22}$$

and then solve for $\hat{\mu}^{\{2\}}_2$:

$$\begin{aligned}
\hat{\mu}^{\{2\}}_2 &= (\bar{Y}^{\{2\}}_1 - \hat{\beta}^{\{1\}}_{0[1\cdot2]})/\hat{\beta}^{\{1\}}_{1[1\cdot2]} \\
&= \bar{Y}^{\{1\}}_2 - \frac{\hat{\sigma}^{\{1\}}_{22}}{\hat{\sigma}^{\{1\}}_{12}} \left(\bar{Y}^{\{1\}}_1 - \bar{Y}^{\{2\}}_1 \right).
\end{aligned} \tag{10.23}$$

Combining the estimates for the two patterns, the overall estimates of the two means are:

$$\hat{\mu}_1 = \hat{\pi}^{\{1\}} \hat{\mu}^{\{1\}}_1 + \hat{\pi}^{\{2\}} \hat{\mu}^{\{2\}}_1 = \hat{\pi}^{\{1\}} \bar{Y}^{\{1\}}_1 + \hat{\pi}^{\{2\}} \bar{Y}^{\{2\}}_1 = \bar{Y}_1 \tag{10.24}$$

$$\hat{\mu}_2 = \hat{\pi}^{\{1\}} \hat{\mu}^{\{1\}}_2 + \hat{\pi}^{\{2\}} \hat{\mu}^{\{2\}}_2 = \bar{Y}^{\{1\}}_2 + \frac{\hat{\sigma}^{\{1\}}_{22}}{\hat{\sigma}^{\{1\}}_{12}} \left(\hat{\mu}_1 - \bar{Y}^{\{1\}}_1 \right) \tag{10.25}$$

[†]This term was used in the orginal article to indicate protecting against nonrandomly missing data.

Sensitivity Analyses with Intermediate Restrictions

Although the two approaches use the complete cases to define the restrictions, the first approach assumes that dropout is completely dependent on the initial measure of the outcome, Y_1, and the second approach assumes that dropout is completely dependent on the final measure of the outcome, Y_2. Reality is likely to be somewhere in between. Little [1994] proposed a mixture of these two approaches in which missingness depends on $Y_1 + \lambda Y_2$.

$$\hat{\mu}_2 = \bar{Y}_2^{\{1\}} + b^{(\lambda)}\left(\hat{\mu}_1 - \bar{Y}_1^{\{1\}}\right), \quad b^{(\lambda)} = \frac{\lambda\hat{\sigma}_{22}^{\{1\}} + \hat{\sigma}_{12}^{\{1\}}}{\lambda\hat{\sigma}_{12}^{\{1\}} + \hat{\sigma}_{11}^{\{1\}}}. \tag{10.26}$$

where $\hat{\sigma}_{11}^{\{1\}}, \hat{\sigma}_{12}^{\{1\}}, \hat{\sigma}_{22}^{\{1\}}$ are the parameters of the covariance of Y_1 and Y_2 estimated from the complete cases in pattern 1.

If $\lambda = 0$, this is equivalent to the complete-case missing value restriction.

$$b^{(\lambda)} = \frac{\lambda\hat{\sigma}_{22}^{\{1\}} + \hat{\sigma}_{12}^{\{1\}}}{\lambda\hat{\sigma}_{12}^{\{1\}} + \hat{\sigma}_{11}^{\{1\}}} = \frac{\hat{\sigma}_{12}^{\{1\}}}{\hat{\sigma}_{11}^{\{1\}}}. \tag{10.27}$$

As $\lambda \to \infty$, by L'Hôpital's rule, we have

$$\lim_{\lambda\to\infty} b^{(\lambda)} = \lim_{\lambda\to\infty} \frac{\lambda\hat{\sigma}_{22}^{\{1\}} + \hat{\sigma}_{12}^{\{1\}}}{\lambda\hat{\sigma}_{12}^{\{1\}} + \hat{\sigma}_{11}^{\{1\}}} = \frac{\hat{\sigma}_{22}^{\{1\}}}{\hat{\sigma}_{21}^{\{1\}}}. \tag{10.28}$$

This is equivalent to Brown's protective restriction.

Unfortunately, we are unable to estimate λ. We can use a range of values of λ to perform a sensitivity analysis. Sensitivity to λ will decrease as the correlation between Y_1 and Y_2 increases; when the variance of Y is constant over time ($\sigma_{11}^{\{1\}} \approx \sigma_{22}^{\{1\}}$) and the correlation approaches 1, then $b^{(\lambda)}$ will be approximately 1 regardless of the value of λ.

Large-Sample Inferences for μ_2

The large-sample variance of $\hat{\mu}_2$ is derived using Taylor series approximations [Little, 1994]:

$$\begin{aligned}
var(\hat{\mu}_2) = {} & \frac{\hat{\sigma}_{22}}{N} + (\mu_1 - \bar{Y}_1^{\{1\}})^2 V_b \\
& + \frac{n_2}{n_1 N}\left[\hat{\sigma}_{22}^{\{1\}} - 2b^{(\lambda)}\hat{\sigma}_{12}^{\{1\}} + b^{(\lambda)2}\hat{\sigma}_{11}^{\{1\}}\right]
\end{aligned} \tag{10.29}$$

$$\hat{\sigma}_{11} = \frac{1}{N}\sum(Y_{i1} - \hat{\mu}_1)^2$$

$$\hat{\sigma}_{22} = \hat{\sigma}_{22}^{\{1\}} + b^{(\lambda)2}\left(\hat{\sigma}_{11} - \hat{\sigma}_{11}^{\{1\}}\right)$$

$$V_b = var\left(b^{(\lambda)}\right) = \frac{(\hat{\sigma}_{11}^{\{1\}}\hat{\sigma}_{22}^{\{1\}} - \hat{\sigma}_{12}^{\{1\}2})(\lambda^2\hat{\sigma}_{22}^{\{1\}} + 2\lambda\hat{\sigma}_{12}^{\{1\}} + \hat{\sigma}_{11}^{\{1\}})^2}{n_1(\lambda\hat{\sigma}_{12}^{\{1\}} + \hat{\sigma}_{11}^{\{1\}})^4}$$

While it is also possible to derive estimates of the standard errors of other functions of the estimate, such as the change between the two time points, bootstrap procedures to estimate standard errors may be more practical when there are multiple estimators.

Lung Cancer Trial

To illustrate, consider the initial and 12-week assessments in the lung cancer trial using only subjects who had a baseline assessment. Application of the sensitivity analysis proposed by Little is illustrated in Table 10.6. The two special cases, the CCMV ($\lambda = 0$) and Brown's protective ($\lambda = \infty$) restrictions, are included. The estimates of the 12-week means ($\hat{\mu}_{h2}$) and of the change over time ($\hat{\mu}_{h2} - \hat{\mu}_{h1}$) are very sensitive to the value of λ, with the estimated change increasing in magnitude as the missingness is assumed to depend more heavily on the missing 12 week values. The differences between the two treatments is less sensitive to the value and all differences are non-significant. Thus one would feel much more confident making inferences about treatment differences at 12 weeks than one would making inferences about the presence or absence of change over time within each group. However, with approximately 50% of the 12 week data missing, all conclusions about the differences should be made cautiously. It is also not surprising that the estimated variance of the parameters increases as the dependence shifts from the observed data (Y_{i1}) to the missing data (Y_{i2}).

TABLE 10.6 Study 3: Sensitivity analysis. Estimated means for baseline and 12-week FACT-Lung TOI scores including means estimated under the CCMV ($\lambda = 0$) and Brown's protective restriction ($\lambda = \infty$). Example limited to subjects with a baseline assessment. Standard errors were obtained using bootstrap procedure.

	Control			Experimental			Difference	
λ	$\hat{\mu}_{11}$	$\hat{\mu}_{12}$	$\hat{\mu}_{1\Delta}$	$\hat{\mu}_{21}$	$\hat{\mu}_{22}$	$\hat{\mu}_{2\Delta}$	$\hat{\mu}_{22}$-$\hat{\mu}_{12}$	(S.E.)
0	64.8	63.4	-1.4	65.9	63.7	-2.2	-0.86	(2.47)
1	64.8	59.4	-5.5	65.9	61.0	-4.9	0.53	(2.85)
2	64.8	57.0	-7.8	65.9	59.4	-6.5	1.34	(3.56)
4	64.8	54.3	-10.5	65.9	57.8	-8.1	2.38	(5.48)
∞	64.8	48.3	-16.6	65.9	48.3	-11.9	4.67	(39.6)

μ_{hk} is the mean at the kth assessment for the hth treatment group. $\mu_{h\Delta}$ is the change between the initial and 12-week assessments for the hth treatment group.

Extensions of Bivariate Case

Little and Wang [1996] extend the bivariate case for normal measures to a more general case for multivariate measures with covariates. However, their extension is still limited to cases where there are only two patterns of missing data, one of which consists of complete cases. For the non-ignorable missing data, the multivariate analog of the restriction is used $(\Theta_{[1.2]}^{\{2\}} = \Theta_{[1.2]}^{\{1\}})$. The model is *just* identified when the number of missing observations exactly equals the number of non-missing observations in the second pattern. Explicit expressions can be derived for the maximum likelihood estimates. The model is *overidentified* when the number of non-missing observations exceeds the number of missing observations. Additional restrictions are required if the number of missing observations is greater than the number of non-missing observations.

Extensions of the Sensitivity Analysis

Small-sample Bayesian inference is described by Little [1994] for the bivariate case described in Section 10.4.1. Daniels and Hogan [2000] describe an extension of the sensitivity analysis to a more general missing data pattern. They illustrate the extension with a study that has three repeated measures and monotone dropout. The sensitivity analysis is no longer a function of a single parameter, λ, but of multiple parameters. The attraction of their approach is that by reparameterizing the restriction, the unknown parameters are theoretically interpretable as the between pattern differences in means and variances, though communication of this to clinical investigators may be challenging.

10.4.2 Monotone Dropout

In this section I extend the concepts to longitudinal studies with monotone dropout. Three sets of restrictions have been proposed for monotone missing data patterns: an extension of Little's CCMV restrictions, available case missing value (ACMV) restrictions and neighboring case missing value (NCMV) restrictions.

Lung Cancer Trial

In the lung cancer trial, patients with one of the four patterns of data conforming exactly to a monotone dropout pattern account for 85% of the patients. In practice one is reluctant to omit 15% of the subjects from the analysis. However, for the purpose of illustration, we will use only the patients with a monotone dropout pattern. Note that each pattern has approximately one-fourth of the patients, so that no pattern contain fewer than 25 subjects (Table 10.7).

TABLE 10.7 Study 3: Patients with monotone dropout patterns by treatment.

	Assessment				Control		Experimental	
Pattern	1	2	3	4	N	%	N	%
1	X	X	X	X	36	24.8 %	103	34.2 %
2	X	X	X		30	20.7 %	64	21.3 %
3	X	X			25	17.2 %	61	20.3 %
4	X				54	37.2 %	73	24.2 %

Complete Case Missing Value (CCMV) Restriction

In the CCMV restriction, the data from the subjects in pattern 1 are used to impute the means for the missing observations in the remaining patterns:

$$\theta^{\{2\}}_{[4\cdot123]} = \theta^{\{1\}}_{[4\cdot123]} \tag{10.30}$$

$$\theta^{\{3\}}_{[34\cdot12]} = \theta^{\{1\}}_{[34\cdot12]} \tag{10.31}$$

$$\theta^{\{4\}}_{[234\cdot1]} = \theta^{\{1\}}_{[234\cdot1]} \tag{10.32}$$

This restriction is only feasible when the number of cases in pattern 1 is sufficient to estimate these parameters reliably. The predicted values are likely to be between those obtained in a complete case analysis and MLE of all available data.

Available Case Missing Value (ACMV) Restriction

In the ACMV restriction, available data from subjects in all the patterns are used to impute the means for the missing observations in the remaining patterns. The restrictions for the patterns in Table 10.7 are:

$$\theta^{\{2\}}_{[4\cdot123]} = \theta^{\{1\}}_{[4\cdot123]} \tag{10.33}$$

$$\theta^{\{3\}}_{[4\cdot123]} = \theta^{\{1\}}_{[4\cdot123]}, \quad \theta^{\{3\}}_{[3\cdot12]} = \theta^{\{1,2\}}_{[3\cdot12]} \tag{10.34}$$

$$\theta^{\{4\}}_{[4\cdot123]} = \theta^{\{1\}}_{[4\cdot123]}, \quad \theta^{\{4\}}_{[3\cdot12]} = \theta^{\{1,2\}}_{[3\cdot12]}, \quad \theta^{\{4\}}_{[2\cdot1]} = \theta^{\{1,2,3\}}_{[2\cdot1]} \tag{10.35}$$

This restriction is a bit more feasible than the CCMV restriction as more observations are used to estimate some of these parameters. It is important to note that the results using this restriction will be the same as MLE of all available data [Curren, 2000]. While this restriction is important when trying to understand methods, MLE of all available data is much easier to implement.

FIGURE 10.5 Study 3: Observed and imputed means for control (left) and experimental (right) arms under CCMV (upper), ACMV (middle), and NCMV (lower) restrictions displayed by pattern of dropout. Observed means indicated by solid line. Imputed means indicated by dashed lines.

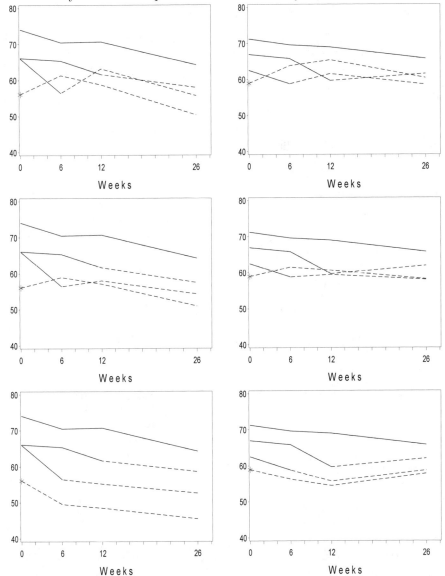

Neighboring Case Missing Value (NCMV) Restriction

In the NCMV restriction, available data from subjects in the neighboring pattern are used to impute the means for the missing observations.

$$\theta^{\{2\}}_{[4\cdot123]} = \theta^{\{1\}}_{[4\cdot123]} \tag{10.36}$$

$$\theta^{\{3\}}_{[4\cdot123]} = \theta^{\{1\}}_{[4\cdot123]}, \; \theta^{\{3\}}_{[3\cdot12]} = \theta^{\{2\}}_{[3\cdot12]} \tag{10.37}$$

$$\theta^{\{4\}}_{[4\cdot123]} = \theta^{\{1\}}_{[4\cdot123]}, \; \theta^{\{4\}}_{[3\cdot12]} = \theta^{\{2\}}_{[3\cdot12]}, \; \theta^{\{4\}}_{[2\cdot1]} = \theta^{\{3\}}_{[2\cdot1]} \tag{10.38}$$

Of the three restrictions, this is the one that might be the most useful. However, as will be demonstrated in the following example, the assumption that the missing values are random conditional on the nearest neighbor may be hard to justify for the later assessments as the neighboring cases are the subjects with complete data. Specifically, there is an assumption that relationship between assessments is similar in those who have complete data and those who drop out early in the trial.

Implementation

With four assessments, these restrictions result in six equations that must be solved for the unknown means and variance parameters. Although this is burdensome, solving the equations for the unknown parameters is straightforward. Deriving the appropriate variance for the pooled estimates is very complex. Curren [2000] suggest an analytic technique using multiple imputation (see Section 9.6) to avoid this problem.

The procedure for the NCMV restriction is as follows:

1. Impute M sets of missing values at T2 using cases in patterns 3 and 4.

2. Add cases in pattern 2 to results of previous step.

3. Impute M sets of missing values at T3 using cases in patterns 2, 3 and 4.

4. Add cases in pattern 1 to results of previous step.

5. Impute M sets of missing values at T4 using cases in patterns 1, 2, 3 and 4.

6. Analyze each set of imputed data and combine estimates as previously described in Chapter 9 for multiple imputation.

Comparison of CCMV, ACMV and NCMV Estimates

The resulting estimates for the NSCLC patients are displayed by strata in Figure 10.5 and pooled across strata in Figure 10.6. Note that the imputed values (Figure 10.5 upper plots) under the CCMV restriction tend to increase initially after the last observed FACT-Lung TOI score, especially for patients who had only the initial assessments. This illustrates the consequences of the implicit assumption with the CCMV restriction. Obviously, in the setting of the lung cancer trial, we do not believe that the HRQoL of the individuals who drop out early is likely to be similar to that of individuals who have all four assessments. The imputed values (middle plot) under the ACMV restriction no longer tend to increase, but rather tend to remain at the same level as the last observed FACT-Lung TOI measure. This is a slight improvement over the CCMV, but still seems to overestimate the HRQoL of patients who drop out. The imputed values (lower plots) under the NCMV restriction tend to fall initially over time, especially for subjects who dropped out early, but tend to increase by the last assessment. This would seem to be the most appropriate of the three restrictions, but it may still overestimate the HRQoL of subjects who drop out of the study especially at the last assessment.

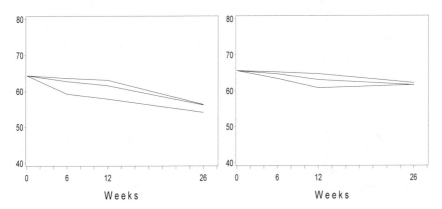

FIGURE 10.6 Study 3: Estimated means for the control (left) and experimental arms (right) under CCMV, ACMV and NCMV restrictions for patients with monotone dropout patterns. Curves from highest to lowest correspond to CCMV, ACMV and NCMV.

10.5   Standard Errors for Mixture Models

In the previous sections we have been assuming that the proportions in each strata are known fixed quantities, $\pi^{\{p\}}$. They are actually unknown and estimates derived from a random sample obtained for a particular trial, $\hat{\pi}^{\{p\}}$. The estimated variance (and standard errors) assuming they are known values will be smaller than the true variance, potentially inflating the Type I errors associated with any tests of hypotheses.

$$Var[\hat{\pi}^{\{p\}} \hat{\beta}^{\{p\}}] > Var[\pi^{\{p\}} \hat{\beta}^{\{p\}}] \tag{10.39}$$

Two approaches can be taken to obtain more precise estimates. The first strategy is based on a Taylor series approximation (also referred to as the *Delta Method*). In the simplest form, the product of an estimated proportion, $\hat{\pi}^{\{p\}}$, and a parameter estimate, $\hat{\beta}^{\{p\}}$, the variance of the product is:

$$Var[\hat{\pi}\hat{\beta}] \approx \hat{\pi}^2 Var[\hat{\beta}] + \hat{\beta}^2 Var[\hat{\pi}] \tag{10.40}$$

The second term in this equation, $\hat{\beta}^2 Var[\hat{\pi}]$, is ignored when we assume $\hat{\pi}$ is known. The delta method will be described in Section 10.5.1. The second approach is to use a bootstrap procedure and described in Section 10.5.2.

10.5.1 Delta Method

To describe the estimation of the variance of the pooled parameter estimates we need to introduce some matrix notation [Curren, 2000]. In this notation, equation 10.4 for the pooled parameter estimates is:

$$\hat{\beta}_k = \sum^P \hat{\pi}^{\{p\}} \hat{\beta}^{\{p\}} = (\hat{\pi}^P)' A_k \hat{\beta}^P \tag{10.41}$$

$\hat{\pi}^P$ and $\hat{\beta}^P$ are the stacked vectors of the r estimates of $\pi^{\{p\}}$ and the c estimates of $\beta^{\{p\}}$ from all P patterns. A_k is a $r \times c$ matrix of known constants (usually 0s and 1s) derived from the partial derivatives of equation 10.4 with respect to π^P and β^P that causes the appropriate estimates to be multiplied:

$$A_k = \left[\frac{\partial^2 \sum^P \hat{\pi}^{\{p\}} \hat{\beta}^{\{p\}}}{\partial \pi^{\{p\}} \partial \beta^{\{p\}}} \right] \tag{10.42}$$

When the proportions are known (and not estimated), the variance of $\hat{\beta}_k$ is solely a function of the variance of the parameter estimates:

$$Var[\hat{\beta}_k] = (\hat{\pi}^P)' A_k Var[\hat{\beta}^P] A_k' \hat{\pi}^P. \tag{10.43}$$

Using the delta method (Taylor series approximation) to approximate the variance of the pooled estimates:

$$Var[\hat{\beta}_k] = (\hat{\pi}^P)' A_k Var[\hat{\beta}^P] A_k' \hat{\pi}^P + \hat{\beta}^{P'} A_k' Var[\hat{\pi}^P] A_k \hat{\beta}^P \tag{10.44}$$

where $Var[\hat{\pi}_h^P] = [diag(\hat{\pi}_h^P) - \hat{\pi}_h^P (\hat{\pi}_h^P)']/N_h$ and

$$Var[\hat{\pi}^P] = \begin{bmatrix} Var[\hat{\pi}_1^P] & & \\ & \ddots & \\ & & Var[\hat{\pi}_H^P] \end{bmatrix}$$

for the H independent groups (treatment arms).

Consider the first approach for the linear patterns where the slopes of the third and fourth patterns are constrained to be equal, $\beta_{h1}^{\{4\}} = \beta_{h1}^{\{3\}}$.

$$
\begin{aligned}
\beta_{h1} &= \pi_h^{\{1\}} \beta_{h1}^{\{1\}} + \pi_h^{\{2\}} \beta_{h1}^{\{2\}} + \pi_h^{\{3\}} \beta_{h1}^{\{3\}} + \pi_h^{\{4\}} \beta_{h1}^{\{4\}} \\
&= \pi_h^{\{1\}} \beta_{h1}^{\{1\}} + \pi_h^{\{2\}} \beta_{h1}^{\{2\}} + \pi_h^{\{3\}} \beta_{h1}^{\{3\}} + \pi_h^{\{4\}} \beta_{h1}^{\{3\}} \quad (10.45)
\end{aligned}
$$

If $\beta^{\{p\}} = [\beta_{h0}^{\{1\}}, \beta_{h1}^{\{1\}}, \dots, \beta_{h0}^{\{4\}}, \beta_{h1}^{\{4\}}]$, the first derivative with respect to β_{h1} is

$$
\frac{\partial \beta_{h1}}{\partial \beta^{\{p\}}} =
\begin{bmatrix}
\frac{\partial \beta_{h1}}{\partial \hat{\beta}_{h0}^{\{1\}}} \\
\vdots \\
\frac{\partial \beta_{h1}}{\partial \hat{\beta}_{h1}^{\{4\}}}
\end{bmatrix}
= \left(0, \ \pi_h^{\{1\}}, \ 0, \ \pi_h^{\{2\}}, \ 0, \ \pi_h^{\{3\}} + \pi_h^{\{4\}}, \ 0, \ 0 \right).
$$

The columns that correspond to the intercept parameters are all zero as these parameters are not used in the estimate of the slope. Then if $\pi^{\{p\}} = [\pi_h^{\{1\}}, \pi_h^{\{2\}}, \pi_h^{\{3\}}, \pi_h^{\{4\}}]$, the second derivative with respect to π is:

$$
\begin{aligned}
\frac{\partial^2 \beta_{h1}}{\partial \pi^{\{p\}} \partial \beta^{\{p\}}} &=
\begin{bmatrix}
\left(0, \pi_h^{\{1\}}, 0, \pi_h^{\{2\}}, 0, \pi_h^{\{3\}} + \pi_h^{\{4\}}, 0, 0 \right) / \partial \pi_h^{\{1\}} \\
\left(0, \pi_h^{\{1\}}, 0, \pi_h^{\{2\}}, 0, \pi_h^{\{3\}} + \pi_h^{\{4\}}, 0, 0 \right) / \partial \pi_h^{\{2\}} \\
\left(0, \pi_h^{\{1\}}, 0, \pi_h^{\{2\}}, 0, \pi_h^{\{3\}} + \pi_h^{\{4\}}, 0, 0 \right) / \partial \pi_h^{\{3\}} \\
\left(0, \pi_h^{\{1\}}, 0, \pi_h^{\{2\}}, 0, \pi_h^{\{3\}} + \pi_h^{\{4\}}, 0, 0 \right) / \partial \pi_h^{\{4\}}
\end{bmatrix} \\
&=
\begin{bmatrix}
0 & 1 & 0 & 0 & 0 & 0 & 0 & 0 \\
0 & 0 & 0 & 1 & 0 & 0 & 0 & 0 \\
0 & 0 & 0 & 0 & 0 & 1 & 0 & 0 \\
0 & 0 & 0 & 0 & 0 & 1 & 0 & 0
\end{bmatrix}.
\end{aligned}
$$

This is more work than one needs to do to derive the pooled estimates for a single estimate, but it provides a general framework with wide applications.

This approximation is appropriate for large and moderate sized samples. In very large samples, $Var(\hat{\pi}_h^{\{p\}})$ is very small and for all practical purposes ignorable. Implementation is facilitated by software that allows matrix manipulation (e.g. **SAS** Proc IML or R).

10.5.2 Bootstrap Methods

When the estimation of the variance of parameter estimates is intractable or even moderately challenging, sample sizes are small or the confidence intervals are asymmetric, bootstrap procedures are useful. There are many variations of these procedures that can become increasingly complex for correlated observations. I have chosen to present the most straightforward and general of these options. The procedure will be to randomly sample with replacement the subjects. In most cases, we will do this within each treatment group. As a word of caution, many statistical analysis packages contain procedures/functions that perform a bootstrap procedure, however, most are designed for setting where all observations are independent. In most clinical trials we are working with correlated longitudinal observations and need to sample patients rather than observations.

The basic procedure assumes that there are two sets of data, one with only a single observation containing subject level data and the second with multiple observations containing the longitudinal data. The procedure is as follows:

1. Sample with replacement N subjects from the first set of data, where N is the number of subjects. Combine data from the strata and generate a unique identifier for each of the N subjects in the bootstrap sample.

2. Merge the bootstrap sample with the longitudinal data.

3. Analyze the bootstrap sample as appropriate and save the estimates of interest.

4. Repeat these three steps 1000 times.

5. Calculate the standard deviation of the estimates of interest. This is the standard error.

SAS macros that facilitate these steps are included in Appendix S.

10.6   Summary

- Mixture models have the advantage that a model for the dropout mechanism does not need to be specified.

- This advantage is balanced by either

   - the need to specify a set of restrictions to estimate all of the parameters or

   - create strata where all parameters are estimable and missing values are assumed to be ignorable within each strata.

- The validity of the restrictions can not be tested and the results may be sensitive to the choice of restrictions.

- It is, however, easy to display the underlying assumptions by plotting the trajectories for each pattern.

11

Random Effects Dependent Dropout

11.1 Introduction

In this chapter I present three models that all assume that there is random variation among subjects that is related to the time of dropout. The models incorporate the actual time of dropout or another outcome that is related to dropout. In some trials, it is reasonable to believe that the rate of change over time (slope) in HRQoL is associated with the length of time a subject remains on the study. This is typical of patients with rapidly progressing disease where more rapid decline in HRQoL is associated with earlier termination of the outcome measurement.

The first model is the *conditional linear model* (CLM) proposed by Wu and Bailey [1989] (see Section 11.2). Each individual's rate of change in HRQoL is assumed to depend on covariates and the time to dropout where the time to dropout is known. While this model is rarely used in practice, it forms the basis for this class of models. The second model is a *varying coefficient model* (VCM) proposed by Hogan et al. [2004b] that expands this idea to include variation in the intercept and uses a semi-parametric method to model the relationship of the outcome to the time of dropout. The third model is the *joint model with shared parameters* proposed by Schluchter [1992] and DeGruttola and Tu [1994]. This model relaxes the assumption that the time to dropout is observed in all subjects (allowing censoring) but assumes a parametric distribution for the time to dropout. All of these models are appropriate to settings where simple growth curve models describe the changes in the outcome and there is variation in the rates of change among the individual subjects (Table 11.1). Further distinctions between these models are discussed in more detail later in the chapter.

Random Effects

In all three models, a practical requirement is non-zero variation in the random effects, d_i. If the variance of the random effects is close to zero ($Var(d_i) \approx 0$), it is difficult, if not impossible, to estimate the association between the random effects and the time to dropout. Prior to embarking on analyses using the joint model, it is wise to check the estimates of variance in the simpler mixed-effects model that you intend to use in the joint model. In SAS, the COVTEST

TABLE 11.1 General requirements of the conditional linear model (CLM), varying-coefficient model (VCM) and joint shared parameter model (Joint).

Model Characteristic	CLM	VCM	Joint
Repeated measures	No	No	No
Growth curve model	Linear[1]	Yes	Yes
Random effects	Slope only[2]	Intercept + Slope	Flexible
Baseline missing	Not allowed	Allowed	Allowed
Mistimed observations	Allowed	Allowed	Allowed
Monotone dropout	Yes	Yes	Yes
Intermittent pattern	Yes if MAR	Yes if MAR	Yes if MAR
Censoring of T^D	No	No	Yes

[1]Higher order polynomials possible but challenging.
[2]Random intercept is unrelated to dropout.

option in the MIXED procedure statement generates these estimates and an approximation of their standard errors. In R, the model can be fit with and without each random effect and then compared using the anova function.

Consider a simple example, using the lung cancer trial (Study 3), in which the fixed effects include an intercept and slope term for two treatment groups and two corresponding random effects. The estimated variance of the random effects for all subscales of the FACT-Lung are summarized in Table 11.2. The results suggest that there is minimal variation in the individual slopes for social and physical well-being subscale and possibly for the emotional well-being subscale and attempting to model variation in the slopes would be futile.

TABLE 11.2 Study 3: Estimates of variance of random effects for subscales of the FACT-Lung in the lung cancer study. p-value reported for test of the hypothesis that $\widehat{Var}(d_i) = 0$.

	Intercept			Slope		
Subscale	$\widehat{Var}(d_{1i})$	(s.e.)	p	$\widehat{Var}(d_{2i})$	(s.e.)	p
Functional Well-being	257	(28)	<0.001	4.84	(1.99)	0.008
Lung CA specific issues	154	(16)	<0.001	2.55	(1.06)	0.008
Emotional Well-being	202	(19)	<0.001	1.31	(0.91)	0.08
Physical Well-being	166	(25)	<0.001	0.93	(1.70)	0.29
Social Well-being	112	(13)	<0.001	No estimate*		
FACT-Lung TOI	142	(15)	<0.001	1.95	(0.98)	0.023

* Variance too close to 0 to estimate.

Alternatives to Dropout

In some setting, dropout may occur for various reasons only some of which would be related to the subject's trajectory. In general we are looking for a characteristic such that conditional on the observed HRQOL outcome and that characteristic, the missing data are ignorable. Alternatives for time to dropout might include time to death or disease progression in the cancer trials or changes in the frequency of migraines in the migraine prevention trial.

11.2 Conditional Linear Model

Wu and Bailey [1989] proposed a *conditional linear model* for studies where the primary interest focuses on estimating and comparing the average rate of change of an outcome over time (slope). The basis of their models is the assumption that the slope depends on covariates, the baseline value of the outcome and the time of dropout, T_i^D. Consider a model where each individual's HRQoL can be described by a linear function of time,

$$Y_i = X_i\beta_i + e_i, \quad X_i' = \begin{bmatrix} 1 & 1 & \cdots & 1 \\ t_{i1} & t_{i2} & \cdots & t_{in_i} \end{bmatrix}, \quad \beta_i = \begin{bmatrix} \beta_{i1} & \beta_{i2} \end{bmatrix} \qquad (11.1)$$

with random variation of the intercept, β_{i1}, and rate of change (slope), β_{i2}.*

$$\beta_i \sim N(\beta_h, \mathcal{G}) \quad \beta_h' = [\beta_{h1} \; \beta_{h2}] \qquad (11.2)$$
$$e_i \sim N(0, \sigma^2 \mathbf{I}) \qquad (11.3)$$

Each individual's slope may depend on M covariates (V_{mi}), the initial value of the outcome (Y_{i1}), as well as a polynomial function of the time of dropout (T_i^D). The form of the relationship is allowed to vary across the h treatment groups. The expected slope for the ith individual is

$$E[\beta_{i2}|T_i^D, V_{mi}, Y_{i1}] = \sum_{l=0}^{L} \gamma_{hl}(T_i^D)^l + \sum_{m=1}^{M} \gamma_{h(L+m)}V_{mi} + \gamma_{h(L+M+1)}Y_{i1} \quad (11.4)$$

where $\gamma_{h0}, \ldots, \gamma_{h(L+M+1)}$ are the coefficients for the hth group and L is the degree of the polynomial. The intercept for the ith individual, β_{i1}, is not dependent on covariates or the time of dropout, thus, the expected intercept is

$$E[\beta_{i1}] = \beta_{h1}. \qquad (11.5)$$

---

*Note that the model is equivalent to a mixed-effects model, $X_i\beta_i = X_i\beta + Z_i d_i$ when $X_i = Z_i$ and $\beta_i = \beta + d_i$. $\mathcal{G} = Var[\beta_i]$ (see chapter 4).

Substituting equations 11.4 and 11.5 into equation 11.1

$$Y_{ij} = E[\beta_{i1}] + E[\beta_{i2}]t_{ij} + \epsilon_{ij}$$

$$= \beta_{h1} + \left(\sum_{l=0}^{L} \gamma_{hl}(T_i^D)^l + \right.$$

$$\left. \sum_{m=1}^{M} \gamma_{h(L+m)} V_{mi} + \gamma_{h(L+M+1)} Y_{i1} \right) t_{ij} + \epsilon_{ij} \qquad (11.6)$$

The mean slope in the hth group is the expected value of the individual slopes of the subjects in the hth group ($i \in h$):

$$\beta_{h2} = E_{i \in h} \left[\beta_{i2} | T_i^D, V_{mi}, Y_{i1} \right]. \qquad (11.7)$$

One of the estimates proposed by Wu and Bailey is referred to as the *Linear Minimum Variance Unbiased Estimator* (LMVUB):

$$\hat{\beta}_{h2} = \sum_{l=0}^{L} \hat{\gamma}_{hl}(\bar{T}_h^D)^l + \sum_{m=1}^{M} \hat{\gamma}_{h(L+m)} \bar{V}_{hm} + \hat{\gamma}_{h(L+M+1)} \bar{Y}_{h1} \qquad (11.8)$$

where $\bar{T}_h^D$ is the mean dropout time in the hth group, $\bar{V}_{hm}$ is the mean of the mth covariate in the hth group and $\bar{Y}_{h1}$ is the mean of the baseline measure in the hth group. In a randomized trial, pre-randomization characteristics are theoretically the same in all treatment groups. To avoid introducing differences that are the result of random differences in these baseline characteristics, $\bar{V}_{hm}$ and $\bar{Y}_{h1}$ are estimated using all randomized subjects ($\bar{V}_m$ and $\bar{Y}_1$). Centering the values of T_i^D, V_{mi}, and Y_{i1} so that $\bar{T}_h^D = 0$, $\bar{V}_m = 0$, and $\bar{Y}_1 = 0$ facilitates the analysis as the estimates of the slopes are now the conditional estimates.

11.2.1   Assumptions

There are several practical consequences and assumptions of this model:

1. Trajectories over time are assumed to be roughly linear.

2. There is enough variation in the rate of change among subjects to allow modeling of the variation.

3. All subjects must have a baseline measurement and complete data for the selected covariates (V) or they will be excluded.

4. The time of dropout is known for all subjects or subjects with an assessment at the last follow-up behave as if they dropped out immediately after that point in time.

It is theoretically possible to extend this model to non-linear trajectories (e.g. polynomial or piecewise linear growth curves); the models are very complex and parameters are difficult to estimate unless the size of the sample is very large. In small studies there may be more parameters than observations. Even in moderate studies, there will be insufficient information to obtain precise estimate of the parameters.

The second condition is that there is random variation in the slopes among subjects $(Var[\beta_{i2}] >> 0)$.

Censoring of the time to dropout is also a limitation. In the example that I have presented, we used the time to the last assessment as a surrogate for the time to dropout for the purposes of illustration of the method, but in practice it may not be valid assumption. In the next section, we will see that the relationship between dropout and the slope may only exist prior to the last assessment (true dropouts).

11.2.2 Testing MAR versus MNAR under the Assumptions of Conditional Linear Model

Given the assumptions of this model, the missing data are non-ignorable when the terms involving functions of the time of dropout, T_i^D, remain in the model. Thus, testing the hypothesis $\gamma_{hl} = 0$ versus $\gamma_{hl} \neq 0, l = 1, \ldots, L$ is a test of the MAR assumption against MNAR. If it is rejected, there is evidence that missingness is non-ignorable. However, if the test is not rejected one can only conclude that the missingness is ignorable only if this particular model is correct. Unfortunately, we cannot test or prove that the model is correctly specified. Thus, failing to reject the hypothesis can not be considered proof that the data are MAR.

11.2.3 Lung Cancer Trial (Study 3)

Previous examination of the Lung Cancer data suggests that the change in the FACT-Lung TOI scores over time is approximately linear. Assuming that the endpoint of interest is comparison of the slopes of patients on the control and experimental arms, one might proceed as follows:

Step 1: Estimate the intercept and slope for each treatment group in a simple mixed-effects model.

$$\text{Model 1: } Y_{ij} = \beta_{hi1} + \gamma_{h0}t_{ij} + \epsilon_{ij} \tag{11.9}$$

where $\epsilon_i = Z_i d_i + e_i$ with a random intercept and slope. Note that this example is restricted to the subset of subjects who have complete baseline assessments for this analysis so that the various models are comparable.

At this point, check the variance of the random slope effects, $\text{Var}(d_{2i})$. If this value is small (i.e. not significantly different from zero), seriously reconsider using a conditional linear model as an analysis strategy. In this example, the variance of the slopes is significant, but only moderately different from zero (Table 11.3).

TABLE 11.3 Study 3: Summary of slope estimates and standard errors estimated using a Conditional Linear Model. $\text{Var}(d_{2i})$ is the variance of the random effects associated with the slope. Model 1 is the reference, 2 adds baseline covariates, 3 adds baseline outcome, 4 and 5 add linear and quadradic models for time of last assessment.

Model	$\text{Var}(d_{2i})$ Est (s.e.)	Control Est (s.e.)	Experimntl Est (s.e.)	Difference Est (s.e.)	-2logL	χ_2^2
1	1.89 (0.98)	-0.82 (0.34)	-0.94 (0.22)	0.12 (0.41)	10395.1	
2	1.85 (0.97)	-0.88 (0.34)	-0.96 (0.22)	0.08 (0.41)	10386.7	8.4
3	0.49 (0.80)	-0.92 (0.35)	-0.90 (0.22)	-0.02 (0.41)	10380.2	4.5
4	0.71 (0.82)	-2.07 (0.69)	-2.17 (0.42)	0.11 (0.80)	10364.0	16.2
5	0.57 (0.85)	-4.10 (1.14)	-2.95 (0.61)	-1.14 (1.30)	10356.2	7.8

Step 2: Identify baseline covariates that might predict change and test the significance of their interaction with time in a mixed-effects model

$$\text{Model 2:} \quad Y_{ij} = \beta_{hi1} + \gamma_{h0}t_{ij} + \underbrace{\sum_{m=1}^{M} \gamma_{hm}V_{mi}t_{ij}}_{\text{Addition to Model 1}} + \epsilon_{ij} \qquad (11.10)$$

Symptoms of metastatic disease (SX_MET) was the strongest predictor of the slope among the available demographic[†] and disease measures prior to treatment.[‡] Note that the three way interaction of treatment, time and SX_MET_C is added to the model, where SX_MET_C is centered (SX_MET - the average value of SX_MET). Addition of symptoms of metastatic disease prior to treatment explained a significant proportion of the variability of the outcome ($\chi_2^2 = 8.14, p = 0.02$), but did not affect the estimates of the slopes in the two treatment groups (Table 11.3).

Step 3: Add the baseline measure of the outcome variable to the model and test for an interaction with time.

$$\text{Model 3:} \quad Y_{ij} = \beta_{hi1} + \gamma_{h0}t_{ij} \sum_{m=1}^{M} \gamma_{hm}V_{mi}t_{ij} +$$

[†]Age and gender.

[‡]Stage of disease, ECOG performance status, > 5% weight loss in last 6 months, primary disease symptoms, metastatic disease symptoms, systemic disease symptoms.

$$+ \quad \underbrace{\gamma_{h(M+1)} Y_{i1} t_{ij}}_{\text{Addition to Model 2}} \quad + \; \epsilon_{ij} \qquad (11.11)$$

The three way interaction term of treatment, time and the centered BASELINE value is added to the model. Again, centering simplifies the analysis because $\bar{Y}_h 1 = 0$. Addition of the baseline value of the outcome did not explain much additional variability ($\chi_2^2 = 4.5, p = 0.11$) and did not affect the estimates of the slopes in the two treatment groups (Table 11.3). It should not be surprising that the estimates do not change, since the baseline values are already part of observed data.

Step 4: Finally, the interaction of time of dropout with the slope is added to the model.

$$\text{Models 4 \& 5: } Y_{ij} = \; \beta_{hi1} \; + \; \gamma_{h0} t_{ij} \; + \; \underbrace{\sum_{l=1}^{L} \gamma_{hl} (T_i^D)^l t_{ij}}_{\text{Addition to Model 3}} \qquad (11.12)$$

$$+ \sum_{m=1}^{M} \gamma_{h(L+m)} V_{mi} t_{ij} + \gamma_{h(L+M+1)} Y_{i1} t_{ij} + \epsilon_{ij}$$

There are several possibilities at this point for defining T_i^D, including the planned time of the last assessment and the observed time of the last assessment. In the following illustration, T_i^D was defined as the observed time in months from randomization to the last HRQoL assessment centered around the average time in the trial for each treatment group (LAST_MO). Other possibilities are the time to disease progression, termination of therapy, or death. In the Lung Cancer example, a linear (Model 4: $L = 1$) and quadratic (Model 5: $L = 2$) model for the time of dropout were tested. The quadratic model provided the best fit. Addition of the time of dropout also explained a significant proportion of the variability of the slope (Model 3 vs. 4: $\chi_2^2 = 16.2, p < 0.001$; Model 4 vs. 5: $\chi_2^2 = 7.8, p = 0.02$). In contrast with the previous models, there was a dramatic effect on the estimates of the slopes with a doubling of the estimated rate of decline in both treatment groups when the linear interaction was added and a tripling of the rates when the quadratic interaction was added (Table 11.3). The differences in the estimates of the slope between Models 4 and 5 suggest that the estimates of change within each group can be very sensitive to the form of $\sum_{l=1}^{L} \gamma_{hl} (T_i^D)^l t_{ij}$. (In the next section (Section 11.3), an alternative model that creates a semi-parametric model for this relationship addresses this concern.)

Of practical note, variation in the slopes may exist in Model 1 but disappear as more variation of the slopes is explained. As the variance approaches zero, problems with convergence of the algorithm can develop and the second random effect may need to be dropped from the model. In the Lung Cancer example, the addition of baseline as an interaction explained approximately 70% of the variability of the slopes (Table 11.3).

Examination of the coefficients of Model 5 (Table 11.4) suggests that the HRQoL measure decreases roughly 1 point per month faster in subjects with symptoms of metastatic disease than in those without symptoms prior to randomization (-1.15 and -0.75 in the two groups). It also predicts a decline of the same magnitude in a subject who scored 16-17 points lower at baseline than another subject (10/0.62 and 10/0.57). The rate of decline is slower in those who stay on therapy longer; initially the slope will increase 2-3 points per month for each additional month of follow-up (positive linear terms). However, the benefit will diminish with time (negative quadratic terms).

TABLE 11.4 Study 3: Summary of coefficients from the Conditional Linear Model 5.

	Control		Experimental	
Effect	Estimate	(S.E.)	Estimate	(S.E.)
Intercept	65.2	(1.19)	66.30	(0.84)
Slope	-4.10	(1.14)	-2.95	(0.62)
Slope*Metastatic Disease[a]	-1.15	(0.63)	-0.75	(0.40)
Slope*Baseline[b]	-0.57	(0.23)	-0.62	(0.14)
Slope*Time of Dropout(linear)[c]	3.16	(1.24)	1.91	(0.81)
Slope*Time of Dropout(quadratic)[c]	-0.29	(0.13)	-0.15	(0.09)

[a] 0=No, 1=Yes   [b] Score/10   [c] Last HRQoL assessment (months)

All covariates are centered.

Table 11.5 contrasts the results of the conditional linear model with the two pattern mixture models described in the previous chapter. The estimates of change are between those estimated under the MAR assumptions and the pattern mixture models.

TABLE 11.5 Study 3: Comparison of estimates of change in FACT-Lung TOI per month from selected models where change over time is assumed to be linear.

Method	Control	Experimental	Difference
Ignorable (MLE)	-0.75 (0.32)	-0.91 (0.21)	-0.16 (0.39)
Pattern Mixture 1	-3.63 (0.96)	-2.06 (0.53)	1.57 (1.10)
Pattern Mixture 2	-5.03 (1.75)	-2.21 (0.85)	2.82 (1.94)
Conditional Linear Model 4	-2.07 (0.69)	-2.17 (0.42)	-0.11 (0.80)
Conditional Linear Model 5	-4.10 (1.14)	-2.95 (0.61)	1.11 (1.30)
VCM Time to last Assessment	-3.27 (0.92)	-2.12 (0.44)	1.15 (1.02)
VCM ln(Time to Death)	-2.70 (0.67)	-2.71 (0.48)	-0.01 (0.82)

Implementation in SAS

The SAS statements for Model 1 are:

```
PROC MIXED DATA=work.analysis METHOD=ML COVTEST;
  CLASS Trtment PatID;
  MODEL FACT_T2=Trtment Trtment*MONTHS/NOINT SOLUTION;
  RANDOM INTERCEPT MONTHS/SUBJECT=PatID TYPE=UN;
  ESTIMATE 'DIFF - SLOPE' Trtment*MONTHS -1 1;
  RUN;
```

In Model 2, all the statements remain the same except for the addition of the term `Trtment*MONTHS*SX_MET_C` to the `MODEL` statement:

```
MODEL FACT_T2=Trtment Trtment*MONTHS Trtment*MONTHS*SX_MET_C
              /NOINT SOLUTION;
```

In Model 3 we add `Trtment*BASELINE*MONTHS` to the `MODEL` statement:

```
MODEL FACT_T2=Trtment Trtment*MONTHS Trtment*MONTHS*SX_MET_C
              Trtment*MONTHS*BASELINE /NOINT SOLUTION;
```

In Model 4 we add terms for the interaction of a linear function of dropout `Trtment*MONTHS*LstFu_C`. Finally, a quadratic term, `Trtment*MONTHS*LstFU_C2`, is added to Model 5:

```
MODEL FACT_T2=Trtment ExpTx*months*Sx_Met_C ExpTx*months*Baseline
        ExpTx*months*LstFU_C ExpTx*months*LstFU_C2
              /NOINT SOLUTION;
```

Note that in Models 2-5, the covariates (`SX_MET_C`, `BASELINE`, etc.) are centered so that their expected value is 0. Thus, the parameters associated with `Trtment*MONTHS` are the parameters of interest, $E[\beta_{i2}|V_i = \bar{V}$, etc.].

Implementation in SPSS

The first steps are to center the covariates (See Appendix P).

The statements to fit the models 1 and 5 are:
Model 1:

```
/* Model 1 */
MIXED FACT_T2 BY ExpTx WITH Months
  /FIXED=ExpTx ExpTx*Months|NOINT SSTYPE(3)
  /PRINT G R SOLUTION
  /RANDOM=Intercept Months|SUBJECT(PatID) COVTYPE(UN)
  /TEST 'Difference in Slopes' ExpTx*Months -1 1 .
```

Model 5:

```
MIXED FACT_T2 BY ExpTx WITH Months Sx_Met_C Baseline LstFU_C LstFU_C2
  /FIXED=ExpTx ExpTx*Months ExpTx*Months*Sx_Met_C  ExpTx*Months*Baseline
        ExpTx*Months*LstFU_C ExpTx*Months*LstFU_C2|NOINT SSTYPE(3)
  /PRINT G R SOLUTION
  /RANDOM=Intercept Months|SUBJECT(PatID) COVTYPE(UN)
  /TEST 'Difference in Slopes' ExpTx*Months -1 1 .
```

Implementation in R

The first steps are to create a factor variable for the treatment groups, TrtGrp, and to center the other explanatory variables (See Appendix R).

The statements to fit the models 1 and 5 are:
Model 1:

```
Model1=lme(fixed=FACT_T2~0+TrtGrp+TrtGrp:MONTHS,data=Lung,
    random=~1+MONTHS|PatID, na.action = na.exclude,method="ML")
```

Model 5:

```
Model5=update(Model4,fixed=FACT_T2~0 + TrtGrp+ TrtGrp:MONTHS +
    TrtGrp:MONTHS:Sx_Met_C + TrtGrp:MONTHS:Baseline+
    TrtGrp:MONTHS:Last_FU_c + TrtGrp:MONTHS:Last_FU_c2)
```

The anova function can be used to compare the models:

```
anova(Model1,Model2,Model3,Model4,Model5)
```

11.2.4   Estimation of the Standard Errors

Computations of the standard errors in the above examples assume that the means of the covariates, baseline scores, and time to dropout are fixed and known. Because they are estimates, the standard errors will underestimate the true variance of the slopes. Wu and Bailey [1989] provide corrected estimates of the variance for a special case. Bootstrapping is a useful tool to handle all models especially with small or moderately sized samples. Table 11.6 illustrates the increase in the standard errors of estimates for the lung cancer trial example.

TABLE 11.6 Study 3: Comparison of naive and bootstrap estimates of the variance for Model 5. Naive estimate assumes that means of covariates, baseline and time to dropout are fixed and have no variance.

Method	Control	Experimental	Difference
Naive	-4.10 (1.14)	-2.95 (0.61)	-1.14 (1.30)
Bootstrap	-4.10 (1.16)	-2.94 (0.73)	-1.16 (1.32)

Random-Coefficient versus Pattern Mixture Models

The conditional linear model has been described as a *random-coefficient pattern mixture model* [Little, 1995] and a *random-effects mixture model* [Hogan and Laird, 1997b]. Each subject has a unique pattern defined by the dropout time, covariates and the baseline measure. If we omit the covariates and baseline measure and if the time of dropout has a limited number of fixed values, the model is equivalent to a pattern mixture model with constraints placed on the slopes (see Section 10.3.1, equation 10.7).

11.3 Varying Coefficient Models

Hogan et al. [2004b] proposed a *varying coefficient random effects model* as an extension of the conditional linear model described in the previous section. The regression coefficients (intercept and slope) depend on dropout time through semi-parametric functions that are estimated using smoothing functions when the dropout time is continuous. They define the basic model as:

$$Y_i | T_i^D = X_i \beta(T_i^D) + Z_i d_i + e_i \tag{11.13}$$

The model reduces to the standard mixed effects model when the functions $\beta_j(T_i^D)$ are constant and do not depend on T_i^D. If the functions associated with the intercepts $(\beta_1(T_i^D))$ are independet of T_i^D and with the slopes $(\beta_2(T_i^D))$ are simple polynomial functions of T_i^D, then the model reduces to the conditional linear model described in the previous section.

To estimate the semi-parametric functions $\beta_j(T_i^D)$ using a smoothing spline, the β_js (dropping (T_i^D) for simplicity) are rewritten as

$$\beta_j = U\gamma_j + Ba_j, \tag{11.14}$$

where $U = (1, T^0)$, T^0 is a vector of the r distinct values of T_i^D, γ_j the corresponding fixed effect parameters, B is an $rxr - 2$ design matrix for the smoothing function and a_j are the corresponding random effects. For theoretical details see Hogan et al. [2004b]. The β_j parameters can be estimated using a parametric mixed effects model

$$Y = \sum_j (X_j U)\gamma_j + \sum_j (X_j B)a_j + Zd + e \tag{11.15}$$

While this equation appears complicated, it is relatively straightforward. The term $\sum_j (X_j U)\gamma_j$ is equivalent to $E[\beta_{i1}] + E[\beta_{i2}]t_{[ij]}$ in the conditional linear model (equation 11.6). For a model that is expected to be linear in the fixed effects, $\sum_j (X_j U)\gamma_j$ includes a term for the intercept and slope as well as interactions with the time to dropout T_i^D. Interpretation is facilitated by centering T_i^D as the parameters for the intercept and slope are estimated at the expected value (average) of T_i^D. Zd are the usual random intercept and slope. $\sum_j (X_j B)a_j$ is divided into two components, one corresponding to the intercept and the other the slope. If we have r dropout times then each of these design matrices defined by B has $r - 2$ columns.

Implementation in SAS

The algorithm for calculating $X_j B$ is in Appendix C. The SAS macro can be found on the website. Because of computational requirements, the model is generally fit separately for each treatment group. Implementation of this in SAS appears as follows for a group with 80 distinct dropout times; zint1–zint78 and zslp1–zslp78 are the two components of $X_j B$:

```
proc mixed data=Zdata1 covtest;
   class patid;
   where trtment eq 0; * Fit model for control group *;
   model Fact_t2=Weeks Last_weeks_C Weeks*Last_weeks_C/s;
   random intercept weeks /subject=patid type=un;
   random zint1-zint78/type=toep(1) s;
   random zslp1-zslp78/type=toep(1) s;
run;
```

indexSAS procedures, MIXED

If problems occur with the algorithm, a number of suggestions are as follows: If $Var(d_i)$ is not positive definite, substitute type=FA0(2) for type=UN in the first set of random effects. If the message continues and one of the two components labeled Variance in the listing of covariance parameters has no value, it can be interpreted that there is no systematic time varying deviation from a simple linear relationship between intercepts/slopes and the time to dropout. If the procedure runs on forever, there are a couple of potential solutions. If there are a large number of distinct dropout times, you might consider reducing the number of distinct dropout times. For example, if dropout times are recorded in days, convert them to weeks (rounding weeks to integer values). Other options include limiting the number of iterations (maxiter=200) or reducing the convergence criteria (convh=1e-4).

11.3.1   Assumptions

Two of the assumptions imposed by the conditional linear model have been relaxed;

1. Trajectories over time are not required to be linear.

2. Subject specific intercepts may be related dropout times.

The following remain:

2. There is enough variation in the intercept and slope among subjects to allow modeling of the variation.

3. The time of dropout is known for all subjects or if the time of the last assessment is used, subjects behave similarly regardless of whether they would have continued to have assessments or would have dropped out before the next assessment if the follow-up had been extended.

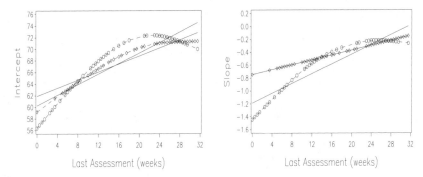

FIGURE 11.1 Study 3: Association of intercept and slope with the time to last assessment estimated with a varying coefficient model (VCM): Cubic smoothing spline estimators of $\beta_j = U\gamma_j + Ba_j$ for the intercept (left) and slope (right). $U\gamma_j(T_i^D)$ is indicated by the solid lines without symbols. $U\gamma_j(T_i^D) + Ba_j(T_i^D)$ is indicated by the dashed lines overlayed with symbols. The control group is indicated by a circle ($\circ$) and the experimental group by a diamond ($\diamond$).

11.3.2 Application

Continuing the example of the lung cancer trial (Study 3), let us further examine the assumption that the slope (and the intercept) are linear functions of the dropout time. Again we will use the time of the last assessment as a surrogate for the time of dropout. In Figure 11.1, two components of the varying coefficient model are plotted for each treatment group. The first is the relationship of the fixed effect estimates of the intercept and slope as a function of the dropout time ($\sum_j (X_j U)\gamma_j$). These are represented by the solid lines in Figure 11.1. Both the intercept and slope increase with increasing time to the last assessment. The second is the estimated semiparametric function $\sum_j (X_j U)\gamma_j + \sum_j (X_j B)a_j$ of the time to dropout. These are represented by dashed lines overlayed by the symbols. Several patterns arise. First, the assumption that the intercept is a linear function of the time of the last assessment appears not to hold and there is a plateau that occurs around 18 weeks. This is not surprising as the fourth assessment (planned at 26 weeks) is a mixture of subjects who would drop out after that assessment and subjects who would continue if further assessments had been planned. The slope for the control group follows a similar pattern but the slopes for the experimental group seem to follow the linear trajectory.

Variables other than time to dropout can also be used in this model. Figure 11.2 illustrates the relationship of the intercept and slope with the log time to death. The lines defined by $U\gamma_j(T_i^D)$ and $U\gamma_j(T_i^D) + Ba_j(T_i^D)$ almost overlay indicating that the log transformation is appropriate. It also

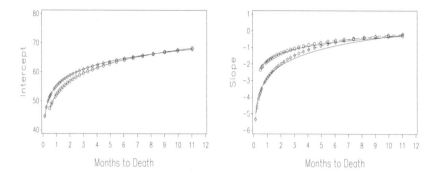

FIGURE 11.2 Study 3: Association of intercept and slope with the log time to death estimated with a varying coefficient model (VCM): Cubic smoothing spline estimators of $\beta_j = U\gamma_j + Ba_j$ for the intercept (left) and slope (right). $U\gamma_j(T_i^D)$ is indicated by the solid lines without symbols. $U\gamma_j(T_i^D)+Ba_j(T_i^D)$ is indicated by the dashed lines overlayed with symbols. The control group is indicated by a circle (○) and the experimental group by a diamond (◇).

makes sense that deaths that are farther out in time, especially those past the duration of the trial would have increasingly less impact on the outcome. Note that this study had almost complete follow-up to death, so that the issue of censoring was not relevant.

11.3.3   General Application

This is still an experimental procedure. However, it may be very useful as a tool for exploring the relationship between individual trajectories and time to dropout. A number of research questions still remain. The most obvious is whether the deviations from the simpler relationships (e.g. linear in dropout time) are significant. One option to answer this question is in the framework of sensitivity analyses. Do the results change when the assumption of a linear relationship is relaxed? A second option requires more research; specifically, can one use a test that the variation associated with a_J is negligible ($H_0 : var(a_h) = 0$) to differentiate an ignorable versus important nonlinear relationship?

11.4 Joint Models with Shared Parameters

In the two previous sections, we have assumed that the time to dropout (or another event) is observed for all subjects. The joint models for the outcome and dropout relaxes this assumption. But, to do this, we must assume a parametric distribution for the time to dropout and its relationship to the random effects. In the examples presented here, I illustrate this approach with normal or log normal models. There are many other parametric and semi-parametric distributions that can be considered and are appearing in the statistical literature (see Section 11.4.8).

To begin, consider the same basic mixed-effects model described by equations 11.1-11.3 where changes in HRQoL are described by a simple two-stage mixed-effects model. Each individual's HRQoL is described by a linear function of time, with random variation among subjects of the intercept, β_{i1}, and the linear rate of change (slope), β_{i2}. The time of an event associated with the discontinuation of HRQoL measurement (T_i^D) is incorporated into the model by allowing some function of the time to dropout ($f(T_i^D)$) to be correlated (σ_{bt}) with the random effects of the longitudinal model for HRQoL [Schluchter, 1992, Schluchter et al., 2001, 2002, DeGruttola and Tu, 1994, Ribaudo et al., 2000, Touloumi et al., 1999].

$$\begin{bmatrix} \beta_i \\ f(T_i^D) \end{bmatrix} \sim N \left(\begin{bmatrix} \beta \\ \mu_T \end{bmatrix}, \begin{bmatrix} \mathcal{G} & \sigma_{bt} \\ (\sigma_{bt})' & \tau^2 \end{bmatrix} \right). \tag{11.16}$$

T_i^D does not have to be the time to dropout, but can be the time to any event associated with dropout that is related to the outcome. This is helpful when some of the dropout is unrelated to the outcome. For example, if the events associated with the outcome were termination of therapy due to toxicity or lack of efficacy, then individuals who drop out for unrelated reasons could be censored and would not be treated as if they experienced a negative outcome.

One implication of this model is that the expected changes in HRQoL are a function of the dropout time. More formally, the conditional expectation of the individual trajectories are a function of the dropout time.

$$E[\beta_i | T_i^D] = \beta + \sigma_{bt} \tau^{-2} (f(T_i^D) - \mu_t) \tag{11.17}$$

This is illustrated in Figure 11.3. Note that the patients with earlier dropout start with lower scores and decline more rapidly than subjects who remain longer. In the example, both the intercepts (β_{i1}) and the slopes (β_{i2}) are positively correlated with longer survival ($\sigma_{bt} > 0$). Substituting estimates for the parameters derived from the lung cancer trial (Study 3) into equation 11.17, the expected intercept for a subject surviving to T_i^D is

$$E[\beta_{i1} | T_i^D] = 65.3 + 8.381 * 1.721^{-1} (ln(T_i^D) + 0.088)$$
$$= 65.7 + 4.870 * ln(T_i^D).$$

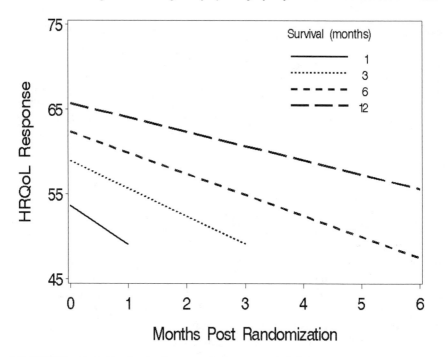

FIGURE 11.3 Study 3: Expected change in FACT-Lung TOI among lung cancer patients given death occurred at 1, 3, 6 and 12 months.

The predicted baseline scores are 59.0 and 65.7 for subjects surviving 3 months ($ln(0.25$ years$) = -1.386$) and 12 months ($ln(1.00$ years$) = 0.00$) respectively. The predicted change over time is

$$E[\beta_{i2}|T_i^D] = -1.78 + 1.974 * 1.721^{-1}(ln(T_i^D) + 0.088)$$
$$= -1.77 + 1.147 * ln(T_i^D).$$

Thus, the predicted decline is greater (3.4 points per month) for a patient who survives 3 months than for a patient surviving 12 months (1.8 points per month).

The second implication of the joint model is that we can express the expected time of dropout as a function of the initial HRQoL scores as well as the rate of change over time. This is of interest when the focus of the investigation is on the time to the event and the HRQOL measures improve the prediction of the time to that event. More formally, the conditional distribution of the dropout times is a function of the random effects.

$$E[f(T_i^D)|\beta_i] = \mu_t + \sigma_{bt}' \mathcal{G}^{-1}(\beta_i - \beta) \tag{11.18}$$

11.4.1 Joint versus Conditional Linear Model

The *joint model* differs from the *conditional linear model* in several respects. The first two allow the model to be more general, whereas the third is potentially more restrictive.

1. The joint model allows both the intercept and slope to be related to the time of dropout.

2. The algorithms [Schluchter, 1992, DeGruttola and Tu, 1994] allow censoring of T_i^D. This allows us to differentiate a subject who completes the 6-month evaluation, but dies shortly thereafter (e.g. $T_i^D = 8$ months) from a subject who remains alive (e.g. $T_i^D > 8$ months). This frees the analyst from assigning an arbitrary dropout time to subjects who complete the study.

3. There is an added restriction that the relationships are linear functions of $f(T_i^D)$.

$$
\begin{aligned}
E[\beta_i | T_i^D] &= \beta + \sigma_{bt}\tau^{-2}(f(T_i^D) - \mu_t) \\
&= \underbrace{\beta - \sigma_{bt}\tau^{-2}\mu_t}_{\gamma_{h0}} + \underbrace{\sigma_{bt}\tau^{-2}}_{\gamma_{h1}} f(T_i^D)
\end{aligned}
\tag{11.19}
$$

11.4.2 Testing MAR versus MNAR under the Assumptions of the Joint Model

Under this model, the missing data are non-ignorable if the random effects (particularly the slope) are correlated with the time of dropout ($\sigma_{bt} \neq 0$). For example, if patients with more rapid rates of decline in their HRQoL scores failed earlier (and thus were more likely to be missing subsequent assessments), the random effect corresponding to the rate of change is positively correlated with the failure time. Again, it should be emphasized that the lack of significant correlation implies the missing data are ignorable *only if the model for dropout is correct*. If dropout was the result of a sudden change in the outcome rather than a gradual change (as measured by slopes), then the dropout model is misspecified and would not necessarily identify the non-ignorable process.

11.4.3 Alternative Parameterizations

Two equivalent parameterizations have been proposed for this model [Schluchter, 1992, DeGruttola and Tu, 1994, Touloumi et al., 1999]. Both use the same general mixed-effects model for the HRQoL outcome:

$$
Y_i = X_i\beta + Z_id_i + e_i.
\tag{11.20}
$$

They differ in the manner in which *time* is related to the random effects for the HRQoL outcome. In the first alternative, the model for time to the event is

$$f(T_i) = \mu_T + r_i. \tag{11.21}$$

The two models are joined by allowing the random effects (d_i) to covary with the residual errors of the time model (r_i) and thus with time to the event itself.

$$\begin{bmatrix} d_i \\ r_i \end{bmatrix} \sim N\left(\begin{bmatrix} 0 \\ 0 \end{bmatrix}, \mathcal{G}\sigma_{bt}\tau^2 \right). \tag{11.22}$$

$$\begin{bmatrix} Y_i \\ f(T_i) \end{bmatrix} \sim N\left(\begin{bmatrix} X_i\beta \\ \mu_T \end{bmatrix}, \begin{bmatrix} Z_i\mathcal{G}Z_i' + \sigma^2 I & Z_i\sigma_{bt} \\ \sigma_{bt}Z_i' & \tau_a^2 \end{bmatrix} \right). \tag{11.23}$$

In the second alternative, the random effects (d_i) are included in the time to event model:

$$f(T_i) = \mu_T + \lambda d_i + t_i. \tag{11.24}$$

$$\begin{bmatrix} Y_i \\ f(T_i) \end{bmatrix} \sim N\left(\begin{bmatrix} X_i\beta \\ \mu_T \end{bmatrix}, \begin{bmatrix} Z_i\mathcal{G}Z_i' + \sigma^2 I & Z_i\mathcal{G}\lambda' \\ \lambda\mathcal{G}Z_i' & \lambda\mathcal{G}\lambda' + \tau_b^2 \end{bmatrix} \right). \tag{11.25}$$

The two models are equivalent as the parameters of one can be written as a function of the other: $\sigma_{bt} = \lambda\mathcal{G}$ and $\tau_a^2 = \lambda\mathcal{G}\lambda' + \tau_b^2$. Both alternatives have specific uses. The first alternative may be more intuitive when the focus is on the HRQoL outcome and corresponds to displays such as Figure 11.3. The second alternative allows us to use one of the SAS procedures to obtain maximum likelihood (ML) estimates of the parameters.

11.4.4   Implementation

Choice of $f(T_i^D)$

In the lung cancer trial, the protocol specified that HRQoL was to be collected until the final follow-up, regardless of disease progression or discontinuation of treatment. Thus, theoretically death is the event that censored the measurement of HRQoL. In practice, it is difficult to follow patients after disease progression for various reasons. So in addition to time to death, one might consider time to the last HRQoL measurement as a candidate for the joint model. Finally there is the possibility that the rate of change in HRQoL depends on other clinical events, such as time to disease progression. The choice in other trials will depend on the disease, treatment, study design and likely relationship of the individual trajectories to the event.

Two considerations will influence the choice of the transformation $f(T_i^D)$: the first is the distribution of T_i and the second is the relationship of T_i^D and d_i. Examples in the literature have used both untransformed and log transformed values of time. We can assess the fit by comparing the empirical distribution (Kaplan-Meier estimates) with distributions estimated assuming normal and lognormal distributions as displayed in Figures 11.4 and 11.5. Visual examination of the times of the last HRQoL measurement (Figure 11.4) suggested that the distribution is roughly normal while time to death (Figure 11.5) more closely fits a log normal distribution.

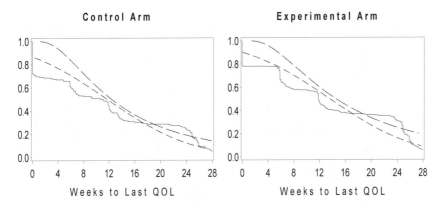

FIGURE 11.4 Study 3: Time to last QOL assessment. Empirical estimates (Kaplan Meier) are indicated by the solid line. Predicted curves assuming normal and log normal are indicated by the short and long dashed lines respectively.

As previously mentioned, the second consideration is the relationship of $\mathcal{T}_i^D$ and d_i. If we utilize the untransformed times ($f(\mathcal{T}_i^D) = \mathcal{T}_i^D$), we are assuming that the change in slopes has the same proportional relationship with time regardless of whether $\mathcal{T}_i^D$ occurs early or later in the trial. In contrast, if we utilize the log transformed times ($f(\mathcal{T}_i^D) = log(\mathcal{T}_i^D)$), we are assuming that the change in slopes has a diminishing relationship over time, with early dropout having a stronger effect than later dropout. This is consistent with the results that we observed for the VCM in the previous section.

11.4.5   Implementation in SAS

Initial Estimates

The algorithms for maximization of the likelihood function of the joint model require initial estimates of the parameters. *Good* starting estimates speed up the convergence of the program, and for some algorithms avoid non-positive definite covariance matrices. Using multiple starting values avoids finding local maximums.

One possible starting point assumes that there is no correlation between the random effects and time: $\lambda_1 = \lambda_2 = 0$. The following procedure is suggested:

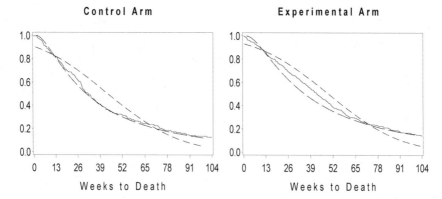

FIGURE 11.5 Study 3: Proportion surviving. Empirical estimates (Kaplan Meier) are indicated by the solid line. Predicted curves assuming normal and log normal are indicated by the short and long dashed lines respectively.

1. Fit a mixed-effects model for the HRQoL data alone (`SAS Proc MIXED` or R `lme`). In `SAS`, obtain the Cholesky decomposition of $\mathcal{G}$ ($\mathcal{G} = LL'$) by adding GC to the options of the `RANDOM` statement. (This is the default in R). We will use this to ensure that the estimates of $\mathcal{G}$ remain positive definite. For a $2x2$ symmetric matrix the Cholesky decomposition is:

$$\begin{bmatrix} \mathcal{G}_{11} & \mathcal{G}_{12} \\ \mathcal{G}_{21} & \mathcal{G}_{22} \end{bmatrix} = \begin{bmatrix} L_{11} & 0 \\ L_{21} & L_{22} \end{bmatrix} \begin{bmatrix} L_{11} & 0 \\ L_{21} & L_{22} \end{bmatrix}'$$

$$= \begin{bmatrix} L_{11}^2 & L_{11} * L_{21} \\ L_{11} * L_{21} & L_{21}^2 + L_{22}^2 \end{bmatrix}$$

   Use the results as initial estimates for β, D and σ^2.

2. Estimate the distribution of $f(T_i^D)$. To estimate μ_T and τ^2 when a natural log transformation is used and T_i^D is censored for some subjects. In `SAS`:

   ```
   PROC LIFEREG data=work.TIMETOEVENT;
     MODEL Surv_Dur*Surv_Cen(1)= / DISTRIBUTION=LNORMAL;
     RUN;
   ```

   When the times (T^D) are assumed to be normally distributed, the estimates can be obtained using `DISTRIBUTION=NORMAL`. Note that the `SCALE` parameter equal $\sqrt{\hat{\tau}^2}$. In R, the `survreg` function can be used.

A second alternative includes initial estimates of λ_1 and λ_2. This strategy estimates d_i and incorporates them into the estimation of $f(T_i^D)$. The strategy is as follows:

1. The first step is to fit a mixed-effects model for the HRQoL data alone and obtain the empirical best linear unbiased predictors (EBLUPs) of the random effects, $\hat{d}_i$:

$$\hat{d}_i = \hat{G}Z_i'(Z_i\hat{G}Z_i' + \sigma^2 I)^{-1}(Y_i - X_i\hat{\beta}) \qquad (11.26)$$

These estimates can be generated by adding the `Solution` option to the `RANDOM` statement in `Proc MIXED` and saving the results:

```
proc mixed data=work.lung3;
   title 'Longitudinal model for FACT_T2';
   class PatID Trtment;
   model FACT_T2=Months*Trtment/Solution;
   random intercept months/subject=PatID type=UN GC Solution;
   ods output SolutionR=work.SolutionR; * Output EBLUPS *;
   run;
```

The EBLUPs are merged with the time to event data. In `SAS`, the data set is then transposed to create one record per subject and merged with the dataset containing the time variable its censoring indicator.

```
*** Transpose Estimates ***;
proc transpose data=work.solutionR Prefix=D out=Random;
   by Patid;
   var Estimate;
   run;
*** Merge with Original Data ***;
data work.TIMETOEVENT2;
   merge work.TIMETOEVENT work.Random;
   by PatID;
   run;
```

2. The parameters of the time to event model are then estimated with the estimates of d_i as covariates:

```
proc lifereg data=work.timetoevent2;
   model Surv_Dur*Surv_cen(1)= D1 D2/dist=lognormal;
   run;
```

Maximization of Likelihood

There are numerous ways to maximize the likelihood function for the joint model. Schluchter [1992], Schluchter et al. [2001] describes an EM algorithm and provides a link to a program that implements it in `SAS`. Guo and Carlin [2004] present a Bayesian version implemented in `WinBUGS`. Vonesh et al. [2006] uses the `SAS NLMIXED` procedure that uses numerical integration to maximize an approximation to the likelihood integrated over the random effects assuming Weibull and piecewise exponential distributions for the time to event.

Li et al. [2007] propose a poissonization of the Cox model. In this section, implementation in SAS NLMIXED procedure assuming a normal or lognormal distribution is illustrated as follows:

The intimal estimates are specified in the PARMS statement.

```
proc nlmixed data=work.lung3(where=(FACT_T2 ne .));
   title3 'Joint Longitudinal and Time to Event';

   *** Initial Estimates ***;
   PARMS b0=65.86 b1=-1.19 b2=-0.59
         L11=12.61 L21=-0.277 L22=0.822 s2w=116.7
         mu0=3.57 tau2b=1.2 lambda1=0 lambda2=0;
```

The BOUNDS statement constrains σ_w^2 and τ_b^2 to be positive and the Cholesky decomposition constrains $\mathcal{G}$ to be positive definite.

```
   * Variance constrained to be Positive *;
   bounds s2w>0, tau2b>0;
   D11=L11*L11; D12=L11*L21; D22=L21*L21 + L22*L22;
```

We then specify the log of the likelihood for $Y_{it}|d_i$ recalling that assuming a normal distribution:

$$
\begin{aligned}
log(f[Y_{it}|d_i]) &= log\left(\frac{1}{\sqrt{2\pi\sigma^2}}e^{-\frac{1}{2}(Y_{it}-(X_{it}\beta+Z_{it}d_i))^2/\sigma^2}\right) \quad (11.27)\\
&= -\frac{1}{2}\left(log(2\pi) + log(\sigma^2) + \frac{(Y_{it}-(X_{it}\beta+Z_{it}d_i))^2}{\sigma^2}\right)
\end{aligned}
$$

```
   *** Mixed effect Model for longitudinal outcome***;
   IF Trtment eq 0 then Pred=b0 +b1*Months +d1 +d2*months;
   IF Trtment eq 1 then Pred=b0 +b2*Months +d1 +d2*months;
   ll_Y= -(log(2*3.14159) + log(s2w) + (FACT_T2-Pred)**2/s2w)/2;
```

Next we specify the log likelihood for $g(T_i^D)|d_i$ when some of the times are censored. If we define $\delta_i = 0$ when the time is observed, $\delta_i = 1$ when right censored and $\delta_i = -1$ when left censored, and let T_i be the observed or censored value of $g(T_i^D)$, then the general form of the log likelihood assuming a normal distribution is:

$$
\begin{aligned}
log(f[g(T_i^D)|d_i]) &= -\frac{1}{2}\left(log(2\pi) + log(\tau_b^2) + z_i^2\right) \quad &(\delta_i = 0) \quad &(11.28)\\
&= log\left[1 - \Phi(z_i)\right] \quad &(\delta_i = 1) \quad &(11.29)\\
&= log\left[\Phi(z_i)\right] \quad &(\delta_i = -1) \quad &(11.30)\\
z_i &= \frac{T_i-(\mu_T+\lambda d_i)}{\tau_b}
\end{aligned}
$$

where $\Phi(\cdot)$ is the cumulative probability function of the standard normal distribution.

```
*** Time to Event ***;
if FUNO eq 1 then do; * First Obs *;
    Pred_T=mu0 + lambda1*d1 +lambda2*d2;
    *** Residual of Measure of Dropout Variable ***;
    Z_T=(log(Surv_Dur)-Pred_T)/sqrt(tau2b);
    *** Left censored ***;
    *if Censor eq -1 then ll_t=log(probnorm(Z_T));
    *** Uncensored ***;
    if Surv_Cen eq 0 then ll_T=-(log(2*3.14159)+log(tau2b)+Z_T**2)/2;
    *** Right censored ***;
    if Surv_Cen eq 1 then ll_T=log(1-probnorm(Z_T));
end;
else ll_T=0;
```

The joint log likelihood is specified, adding the two components and specifying the distribution of the random effects as multivariate normal.

```
*** Joint Log Likelihood ***;
model FACT_T2 ~ general(ll_Y+ll_T);
random d1 d2 ~ normal([0,0],[D11,D12,D22]) sub=patid;
```

Finally, we can request both linear and non-linear function of the parameters. In this example, we first contrast the estimated slopes for the two groups, $H_0 : \beta_2 - \beta_1 = 0$. We can also estimate the correlation of the random effects with the time to death or dropout:

```
*** Estimates and Contrasts ***;
estimate 'Diff in Slopes' b2-b1 ;
estimate 'Rho1T' (lambda1*D11+Lambda2*D12)/(sqrt(D11)*
        sqrt(lambda1**2*D11+2*lambda1*lambda2*D12+lambda2**2*D22+tau2b));
estimate 'Rho2T' (lambda1*D12+Lambda2*D22)/(sqrt(D22)*
        sqrt(lambda1**2*D11+2*lambda1*lambda2*D12+lambda2**2*D22+Tau2b));
run;
```

Results

Tables 11.7 and 11.8 summarizes the results from a number of joint models for the lung cancer study and compares the estimates to the corresponding mixed-effects model. The results support the hypothesis that the random effects of the longitudinal model are associated with the time to the events. The associations were stronger for the time to death than for the last assessments. The events were moderately correlated with the intercept (ρ is in the range of 0.40-0.44). The correlation with the slopes ranged from ($\rho = .46$) for last HRQoL assessment to ($\rho = 0.75$) for log time to death. The strong correlation ($\rho > 0.7$) of change with time to death fit with the observation that deterioration in physical and functional well-being accelerate in the months prior to death.

Estimates of the intercept are insensitive to the choice of model. This is not unexpected as there is minimal missing data at baseline. In contrast, the rate

TABLE 11.7 Study 3: Joint Model for FACT-Lung TOI and various measures of the time to dropout $(\mathcal{T}^D)$. Estimates of λs and correlation between time $(\mathcal{T}^D)$ and random effects(β_i) .

	Intercept			Slope		
Dropout Event	$\hat{\lambda}_1$ (s.e)	p-value	Corr	$\hat{\lambda}_2$ (s.e)	p-value	Corr
ln(Survival)	0.04 (0.01)	<0.01	0.44	0.59 (0.15)	<0.01	0.75
Last assessment	0.35 (0.09)	<0.01	0.40	4.63 (2.47)	0.061	0.46

of decline within each group roughly doubles when the outcome is modeled jointly with either time to death or last assessment. Given the extensive missing data and the patterns observed in Figure 6.1, this is also expected. The between group differences exhibit less variation among the models; the span of estimates being roughly half the standard error. This is typical of studies where treatment arms have roughly similar rates and reasons for dropout.

TABLE 11.8 Study 3: Joint Model for FACT-Lung TOI and various measures of the time to dropout $(\mathcal{T}^D)$. Parameter estimates of intercept (β_0), slopes for control group (β_1) and experimental group (β_2) and the difference in slopes $(\beta_2 - \beta_1)$.

	Estimates (s.e.)			
Dropout Event	$\hat{\beta}_0$	$\hat{\beta}_1$	$\hat{\beta}_2$	$\hat{\beta}_2 - \hat{\beta}_1$
None (MLE)	65.9 (0.66)	-1.18 (0.29)	-0.58 (0.19)	0.60 (0.31)
ln(Survival)	65.7 (0.66)	-1.85 (0.30)	-1.43 (0.24)	0.47 (0.31)
Last assessment	66.1 (0.66)	-2.15 (0.39)	-1.53 (0.31)	0.62 (0.32)

11.4.6 Implementation in R

The `jointModel` function in R uses a slightly different approach for the survival portion of the joint model. Instead of incorporating the random effects into the survival model, they incorporate $W_i(t)$ the value of the longitudinal outcome at time point t for the ith subject; evaluating $\mathbf{X}_i\beta + Z_i d_i$ at t. The default survival function is a Weibull accelerated failure time model where r_i follows an extreme value distribution:

$$log(\mathcal{T}_i^D) = \mu_T + \alpha W_i(t) + \sigma_t r_i \tag{11.31}$$

The function also allows the time to event portion to be modeled as a time-dependent proportional hazards model [Wulfsohn and Tsiatis, 1997] or an additive log cummulative hazard model [Rizopoulos et al., 2009].

Fit the longitudinal part of the model creating the object LME (see Appendix R for required libraries).

```
R> Lung3$trtgrp=factor(Lung3$ExpTrt)        # Factor version
R> comp=Lung3[!is.na(Lung3$FACT_T2),]       # Select non=missing
R> LME=lme(fixed=FACT_T2~MONTHS:trtgrp,random=~MONTHS|PatID,data=comp)
```

Create a dataset that has one record for each subject with at least one measurement for the survival part of the model. Then run Weibull model creating the object `Surv`.

```
R> Surv=unique(comp[,c("PatID", "SURV_DUR", "Death","trtgrp")])
R> Surv$Surv_wks = Surv$SURV_DUR/7
R> Surv2 = survreg(Surv(Surv_wks,Death)~1,data=Surv,x=TRUE)

R> Joint=jointModel(lmeObject=LME,survObject=Surv2,timeVar="MONTHS")
R> summary(Joint)
```

With this code, the algorithm encountered a non-PD estimate of D, the covariance of the random effects. Restricting the algorithms to EM `control = list(only.EM=TRUE)` allowed the procedure to finish although there was still a warning message about the Hessian. Partial results appear as:

```
Coefficients:
Longitudinal Process
                Value Std.Err   z-value p-value
(Intercept)    67.0653  0.5854 114.5730 <0.0001
MONTHS:TrtGrp0 -1.6903  0.1014 -16.6633 <0.0001
MONTHS:TrtGrp1 -1.6772  0.0947 -17.7072 <0.0001

Event Process
                Value Std.Err  z-value p-value
(Intercept)    3.5126  0.0555 63.3451 <0.0001
Assoct        -0.0140  0.0008 -16.5566 <0.0001
log(scale)    -0.9734  0.0485 -20.0543 <0.0001
```

The parameter for the association of the two models, α, is indicated as `Assoct` and is highly significant. Note that while the estimates of the slope parameters, β, of the longitudinal model are similar to those obtained previously, their standard errors are much smaller. As an interesting side note, when only a single between-subject random effect was included (`random ~1`) the results were similar (with no problems with the Hessian).

11.4.7 Multiple Causes of Dropout

One model that accommodates multiple causes of dropout was proposed by Jaros [2008]. The model extends the model presented in Section 11.4.3 to two competing causes of dropout. This model assumes that both reasons for dropout can not be observed and once the individual has dropped out for one reason, they are censored with respect to the second reason.

This model can be adapted to the osteoarthritis trial (Study 6) in which participants discontinued treatment early due to inadequte pain relief requiring rescue medication and due to side effects during treatment (see Section 1.8). Figure 11.6 illustrates the differences in the trajectories for these patients. Visual inspection suggests that individual variation in change (but probably not initial scores) will be associated with the reason for (and time to) dropout.

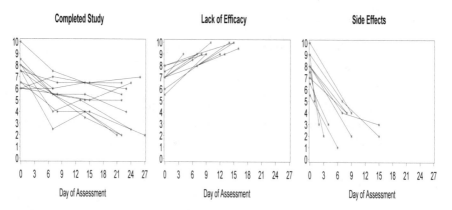

FIGURE 11.6 Study 6: Pain intensity scores of randomly selected subjects who completed study, dropped out due to lack of efficacy or side effects.

Again the first step is to develop working models for the longitudinal and time to event processes. In the longitudinal model for pain intensity, a piecewise linear model for the fixed effects includes an intital slope (`Time`) and a change in slope at 7 days (`Time7=max(Time-7,0)`). The random effects have a similar structure as the migraine prevention trial that was described in Section 4.6.2. Unlike the lung cancer trial where patients continue to decline throughout the period of observation, a model for the random effects with indicators for baseline (i.e. initial pain intensity) and change from baseline to follow-up (i.e. response) fits the observed data. The correlation between the baseline and follow-up assessments is weak and the correlation among the follow-up assessments is strikingly strong (Table 11.9).

For most patients, dropout occurs after the first assessment if it occurs at all and there is no suggestion of an association of time with trajectories of the pain scores. This suggests considering an alternative model for dropout. For example, one might consider T_i^D to be an indicator variable for dropout and $g(T_i^D)$ to be the logistic function. The conditional likelihood is:

$$log(f[g(T_i^D)|d_i]) = T_i^D(\mu_t + \lambda d_i) - log(1 + e^{(\mu_t + \lambda d_i)}) \qquad (11.32)$$

The following code could be used with `DO_LackEff` and `DO_SideEff` as in-

TABLE 11.9 Study 6: Estimated covariance and correlation of the four assessments using a model with two random effects: baseline (i.e. initial pain intensity) and change from baseline to follow-up (i.e. response).

Covariance				Correlation			
1.07	0.11	0.11	0.11	1.00	0.04	0.04	0.04
0.11	6.40	5.47	5.47	0.04	1.00	0.85	0.85
0.11	5.47	6.40	5.47	0.04	0.85	1.00	0.85
0.11	5.47	5.47	6.40	0.04	0.85	0.85	1.00

dicator variables for dropout due the two reasons and `ExpTx` an indicator of the experimental arm:

```
*** Binomial Models for Dropout ***;
*** Lack of Efficacy ***;
if First eq 1 then do; * First Obs *;
    EffModel=mu0a+mu1a*ExpTx+lambda1a*d1+lambda2a*d2;
    ll_LackEff =DO_LackEff*(EffModel) -log(1+exp(EffModel));
end;
else ll_LackEff=0;

*** Side Effects ***;
if First eq 1 then do; * First Obs *;
    SEModel=mu0b+mu1b*ExpTx+lambda1b*d1+lambda2b*d2;
    ll_SideEff =DO_SideEff*(SEModel) -log(1+exp(SEModel));
end;
else ll_SideEff=0;
```

The results from the longitudinal portion of the model are very similar to those obtained when modeled separately. This is not unexpected given the strong correlation among the follow-up assessments. The first follow-up assessment has much of the information about the subsequent assessments thus dropout after the first follow-up is likely to be MAR. The results are sensitive to variations in the models, such as dropping the `mu1a*ExpTx` or `mu1b*ExpTx` terms. There is still much to be learned about the performance of these models.

11.4.8 Other Model Extensions

There have been numerous extensions to the joint or shared parameter models. The following examples do not represent a comprehensive review of the literature, but are presented to illustrate the richness of this class of models. Vonesh et al. [2006] extended the model by relaxing the assumptions of normality allowing distributions of the random effects from the quadratic exponential family and event-time models from accelerated failure-time models (e.g., Weibull, exponential extreme values and piece-wise exponential). Numerous investigators have joined proportional hazard models with the longitudinal models. Thiebaut et al. [2005], Chi and Ibrahim [2006], and Elashoff et al. [2007] consider multiple longitudinal outcomes. Chi and Ibrahim [2006] and Elashoff et al. [2007] have also proposed models for multiple reasons for dropout. For example, in the migraine prevention trial (Study 2) and the osteoarthrtis trial (Study 6) subjects may terminate treatment because of side effects or lack of efficacy. Both the timing and the HRQoL trajectories are likely to be different for these two reasons. Law et al. [2002], Yu et al. [2004] and Chi and Ibrahim [2006] consider the possibility that some subjects would not eventually experience the dropout event and could stay on the intervention indefinitely.

11.5   Summary

- There is a rich class of models that relate the individual trajectories (generally through random effects) to the time to dropout or other clinically relevant events.

- All models are based on strong assumptions.

- These assumptions cannot be formally tested. Defense of the assumptions must be made on a clinical basis rather than statistically.

- Lack of evidence of non-ignorable missing data for any particular model does not prove the missing data are ignorable.

- Estimates are not robust to model misspecification, thus more than one model should be considered (a sensitivity analysis).

- The random effect dependent dropout models can be very useful as part of a sensitivity analysis when non-ignorable dropout is suspected.

12

Selection Models

12.1 Introduction

In this chapter we examine a final model for non-ignorable missing data. As with the models presented in the previous two chapters,

1. All models for non-ignorable data require the analyst to make strong assumptions.

2. These assumptions cannot be formally tested. Defense of the assumptions must be made on a clinical basis rather than a statistical basis.

3. Lack of evidence of non-ignorable missing data for any particular model does not prove the missing data are ignorable.

4. Estimates are not robust to model misspecification.

The term *selection model* was originally used to classify models with a univariate response, y_i, where the probability of being *selected* into a sample depended on the response. The same idea is extended to longitudinal studies. As previously described, the joint distribution of the outcome, Y_i and the missing data mechanism, M_i is factored into two parts.

$$f(Y_i, M_i | \Theta, \Psi) = f(Y_i | \Theta) f(M_i | Y_i^{obs}, Y_i^{mis}, \Psi) \tag{12.1}$$

The model for the outcome, $f(Y_i | \Theta)$, does <u>not</u> depend on the missing data mechanism. The model for the missing data mechanism, $f(M_i | Y_i^{obs}, Y_i^{mis}, \Psi)$, may depend on the observed and missing outcome data. Θ and Ψ are the parameters of the two models. We can expand this definition to differentiate among selection models. Specifically, in *outcome-dependent* [Hogan and Laird, 1997b] selection models the mechanism depends directly on the elements of $\mathbf{Y}$ and in *random-effects* [Hogan and Laird, 1997b] or *random-coefficient* [Little, 1995] selection models missingness depends on $\mathbf{Y}$ through the subject-specific random effects, β_i or d_i.

$$\text{Outcome-dependent selection } f(M_i | Y_i^{obs}, Y_i^{mis}) \tag{12.2}$$
$$\text{Random effects dependent selection } \quad f(M_i | \beta_i) \tag{12.3}$$

An example of a outcome-dependent selection model is the model proposed by [Diggle and Kenward, 1994] that is described in the next section (Section 12.2). The joint or shared parameter models described in the previous chapter can be written as a random-effects dependent selection model (see Section 11.4).

The model for $f(Y_i)$ of the outcome dependent selection model is straightforward, typically either a repeated measures or growth curve model described in Chapters 3 or 4. The challenge is defining the model for the missing data mechanism $f(M_i)$, specifically the portion of the model that depends on the unobserved data, Y_i^{mis} or the random effects d_i. In particular, for the outcome dependent selection model, this requires a strong <u>untestable</u> assumption about the distribution of the outcome measure, Y_i. Typically the assumption is that the outcome has a normal distribution. While many of the previously described methods appear relatively insensitive (robust) to deviations from this assumption, the selection models have been shown to be particularly sensitive. In the example that will be presented in Section 12.2, I will illustrate the sensitivity in the context of a HRQoL outcome.

12.2   Outcome Selection Model for Monotone Dropout

Diggle and Kenward [1994] proposed a selection model for monotone missing data in the context of a repeated measures design. This model is appropriate to settings where there are equally spaced repeated measures and the missing data patterns are strictly monotone, thus $M_i = D_i^T$. The *response model* is the same multivariate linear regression model that we have used throughout, $f(Y_i|\Theta)$. For the *dropout model* they assume a logistic regression, $f(R_i|Y_i,\Gamma)$ which may depend on covariates, $\mathcal{X}_i$, previous observations, y_{ij-1} or the unobserved measurement at the time of dropout, y_{ij}. The conditional probability of dropout at time t_j given the history through the previous assessment at t_{j-1} is denoted by

$$P_j = Pr(T_i^D = t_j|Y_{i1},\ldots,Y_{ij-1}). \tag{12.4}$$

The logistic linear model for the dropout process takes the form

$$logit[P_j] = \gamma_0 \, \mathcal{X}_i + \gamma_1 \, y_{ij} + \gamma_2 \, y_{ij-1} \cdots . \tag{12.5}$$

Diggle and Kenward defined the dropout process in terms that correspond to MCAR, MAR and MNAR. *Completely random dropout* (CRD) corresponds to MCAR where dropout is completely independent of measurement, $\gamma_1 = \gamma_2 = 0$. *Random dropout* (RD) corresponds to MAR where dropout depends on only observed measurements (prior to dropout), $\gamma_1 = 0$ and $\gamma_2 \neq 0$. *Informative dropout* (ID) corresponds to MNAR where dropout depends on unobserved measures. If $\gamma_1 \neq 0$ then dropout depends on the previously observed

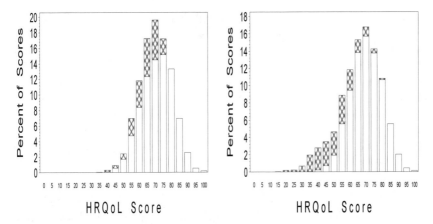

FIGURE 12.1 Contrasting two distributions with 20% missing observations. Missing scores are indicated by the hatched pattern and observed scores are indicated by the empty portion. In figure A (left) the complete (observed and missing) data have a normal distribution. In figure B (right) the observed scores have a normal distribution but the distribution of the complete data is skewed.

response (y_{ij-1}) and if $\gamma_1 \neq 0$ then dropout depends on the current unobserved response (y_{ij}), $\gamma_1 \neq 0$. If the dropout process is CRD or RD, the *response model* and the *dropout model* can be estimated separately. But if the dropout process is ID, Θ and Γ must be estimated jointly.

It is obvious how the parameters γ_0 and γ_2 can be estimated, but how do we estimate a parameter that is a function of missing observations? It is only possible by making the assumption that the distribution of the complete (observed and unobserved) data has a specific parametric form such as a normal distribution. Figure 12.1 illustrates the assumption. Suppose that our assumption that the complete missing data are normally distributed is correct (left figure). If a selection model was fit to similar data, the model for dropout would indicate a dependence on the values of the missing scores. In contrast, if the distribution of the observed scores is normal (right figure) but the complete data is not, the model for dropout would indicate <u>no</u> dependence on the values of the missing scores. My experience is that situation described in Figure B is more typical of the observed distribution of HRQoL scores with dropout likely to be associated with poorer HRQoL. Thus, these selection models are not likely to be useful.

12.2.1 Lung Cancer Trial (Study 3)

Data from the lung cancer trial are used to illustrate this approach. Note that this is for illustrative purposes only, as there are some constraints imposed by the model and the estimation procedure that require exclusion of a portion of the data. First, we will have to exclude roughly 20% of the patients who have either intermittent missing data or are missing the initial assessment. Second we will have to assume that the interval between the third and fourth measurements are equivalent to the intervals between the first, second and third with respect to the dropout model. In practice, we would not use a model that excludes such a large portion of the data, nor would we assume equal spacing of the assessments.

Dropout as a Function of Time and Treatment (CRD)

In the following example, we used the `pmcid` function from the Oswald user-contributed `S-Plus` library. The first step is to explore models describing the dropout process under the CRD assumption. $\mathcal{X}_i$ can include any patient characteristic, but the following example will focus on time and treatment assignment. In model 1 (CRD1), we assume that the probability of dropout is the same for the second, third and fourth assessment ($\mathcal{X}_{i1} = 1$).

$$logit[P_j|\mathcal{X}_i] = \gamma_{01} \tag{12.6}$$

$$Pr(T_i^D = t_j) = \frac{e^{\gamma_{01}}}{1 + e^{\gamma_{01}}}, j = 2, 3, 4 \tag{12.7}$$

The estimated parameters for the model are displayed in Table 12.3. The estimated probability of dropout (Table 12.1) at each follow-up visit is

$$\hat{P}_j = e^{-0.806}/(1 + e^{-0.806}) = 0.31.$$

This implies that 31% of the remaining subjects drop out at each of the follow-up visits. The probability of completing the HRQoL assessment at the final visit is the product of the probability of remaining in the study at each followup. Thus, the model predicts that 69% of the subjects will have an assessment at 6 weeks $[(1 - \hat{P}_2) = .69]$, 48% at 12 weeks $[(1 - \hat{P}_2)(1 - \hat{P}_3) = .48]$ and 33% at 26 weeks $[(1 - \hat{P}_2)(1 - \hat{P}_3) * (1 - \hat{P}_4) = .33]$. The estimated probability of dropout and of remaining in the study are compared to the observed probabilities in Tables 12.1 and 12.2.

In model 2 (CRD2), we allow the probability to differ across the two treatments by adding an indicator for the Experimental group ($\mathcal{X}_{i2} = 0$ if Control, $\mathcal{X}_{i2} = 1$ if Experimental).

$$logit[P_j, \mathcal{X}_i] = \gamma_{01} + \gamma_{02}\mathcal{X}_{i2} \tag{12.8}$$

The estimated probability of dropout is higher among the subjects not assigned to the Experimental therapy ($\hat{P}_k = .35$) than among those assigned to the Experimental therapy ($\hat{P}_k = .29$).

TABLE 12.1 Study 3: Probability of dropout at the jth assessment if observed at j-1 $(Pr[R_{ij} = 0|R_{ij-1} = 1])$

Group	Weeks	Obs	CRD1	CRD2	CRD3	CRD4
Control	6	.37	.31	.35	.28	.37
	12	.27	.31	.35	.28	.27
	26	.45	.31	.35	.40	.45
Experimental	6	.24	.31	.29	.28	.24
	12	.28	.31	.29	.28	.28
	26	.38	.31	.29	.40	.38

TABLE 12.2 Study 3: Probability of a subject remaining on study at the jth assessment $(Pr[R_{ij} = 1])$

Group	Weeks	j	Obs	CRD1	CRD2	CRD3	CRD4
Control	6	2	.63	.69	.65	.72	.63
	12	3	.41	.48	.42	.52	.46
	26	4	.25	.33	.27	.31	.25
Experimental	6	2	.76	.69	.71	.72	.76
	12	3	.54	.48	.51	.52	.54
	26	4	.34	.33	.36	.31	.34

In model 3 (CRD3), the probability is the same across the two treatments but differs by time ($\mathcal{X}_{i1} = 1$ if t_2, $\mathcal{X}_{i2} = 1$ if t_3, $\mathcal{X}_{i3} = 1$ if t_4, 0 otherwise).

$$logit[P_j, \mathcal{X}_i] = \gamma_{01}\mathcal{X}_{i1} + \gamma_{02}\mathcal{X}_{i2} + \gamma_{03}\mathcal{X}_{i3} \tag{12.9}$$

The predicted dropout rate at 6 weeks ($\hat{P}_k = .28$) is very similar to 12 weeks ($\hat{P}_k = .28$) and increases at 26 weeks ($\hat{P}_k = .40$). This model fit the observed data better than the model where we assume a constant dropout rate (Table 12.3).

Finally, in model 4 (CRD4), we allow the probability to differ across the two treatments by adding indicators for the Experimental group at each time. ($\mathcal{X}_{i4} = \mathcal{X}_{i5} = \mathcal{X}_{i6} = 0$ if Control, $\mathcal{X}_{i2} = \mathcal{X}_{i5} = \mathcal{X}_{i6} = 1$ if Experimental).

$$logit[P_j, \mathcal{X}_i] = \gamma_{01}\mathcal{X}_{i1} + \gamma_{02}\mathcal{X}_{i2} + \gamma_{03}\mathcal{X}_{i3}$$
$$+\gamma_{04}\mathcal{X}_{i4} + \gamma_{05}\mathcal{X}_{i5} + \gamma_{06}\mathcal{X}_{i6} \tag{12.10}$$

This model fit the observed data better than the previous models (Table 12.3). Note that none of the parameter estimates in the model for the HRQoL outcome measure ($\beta_1 \cdots \beta_4$)have changed. This is to be expected as the longitudinal and the models are distinct (estimated separately) under the CRD assumptions.

Dropout as a Function of Previously Observed Outcomes (RD)

Building on the best CRD model, we fit the corresponding RD model by allowing dropout to depend on the value of the previous observation (Y_{ij-1}).

TABLE 12.3 Study 3: Logistic selection models assuming completely random dropout (CRD).

Parameter		CRD1	CRD2	CRD3	CRD4
$\hat{\beta}_1$	Intercept	63.9	63.9	63.9	63.9
$\hat{\beta}_2$	Group	1.69	1.69	1.69	1.69
$\hat{\beta}_3$	Time	-0.266	-0.266	-0.266	-0.266
$\hat{\beta}_4$	Group:Time	0.073	0.073	0.073	0.073
$\hat{\gamma}_0$	Intcpt (Time 2)	-0.806	-0.597	-0.933	-0.549
	(Time 3)			-0.954	-1.005
	(Time 4)			-0.399	-0.198
	Group (Time 2)		-0.307		-0.592
	(Time 3)				0.071
	(Time 4)				-0.285
-2logL		16179.39	16174.77	16166.90	16158.19
Comparison			CRD1	CRD1	CRD3
LR Statistic			$\chi_1^2 = 4.62$	$\chi_2^2 = 13.53$	$\chi_3^2 = 8.69$
p-value			0.032	0.0012	0.034

Note that this model assumes that this relationship is the same for each follow-up assessment and the previous measurement. Thus, the relationship between dropout at 6 weeks and the baseline value of the FACT-Lung TOI is assumed to be the same as between dropout at 26 weeks and the 12-week value of the FACT-Lung TOI.

$$logit[P_j, \mathcal{X}_i] = \gamma_{01}\mathcal{X}_{i1} + \gamma_{02}\mathcal{X}_{i2} + \gamma_{03}\mathcal{X}_{i3}$$
$$+ \gamma_{04}\mathcal{X}_{i4} + \gamma_{05}\mathcal{X}_{i5} + \gamma_{06}\mathcal{X}_{i6} + \gamma_2 Y_{ij-1} \qquad (12.11)$$

This RD model fits the data much better than the CRD model, with strong evidence to reject the CRD assumption (Table 12.4). As expected, there is still no change in the mean and variance parameters for the longitudinal HRQoL data. The RD model predicts that the probability of dropout will decrease with increasing FACT-Lung TOI scores during the previous assessment. Thus, in the patient assigned to the treatment that did not include Experimental, the predicted probability of dropout at 6 weeks is 44%, 35% and 27% for subjects with baseline scores of 55, 65 and 75 respectively.

$$\hat{P}_2 = \frac{e^{\hat{\gamma}_{01} + \hat{\gamma}_2 Y_{ij-1}}}{1 + e^{\hat{\gamma}_{01} + \hat{\gamma}_2 Y_{ij-1}}} = \frac{e^{1.872 - 0.0385*55}}{1 + e^{1.872 - 0.0385*55}} = .44, \mathcal{X}_{i4} = 0, Y_{i1} = 55$$

$$\hat{P}_2 = \frac{e^{\hat{\gamma}_{01} + \hat{\gamma}_2 Y_{ij-1}}}{1 + e^{\hat{\gamma}_{01} + \hat{\gamma}_2 Y_{ij-1}}} = \frac{e^{1.872 - 0.0385*65}}{1 + e^{1.872 - 0.0385*65}} = .35, \mathcal{X}_{i4} = 0, Y_{i1} = 65$$

$$\hat{P}_2 = \frac{e^{\hat{\gamma}_{01} + \hat{\gamma}_2 Y_{ij-1}}}{1 + e^{\hat{\gamma}_{01} + \hat{\gamma}_2 Y_{ij-1}}} = \frac{e^{1.872 - 0.0385*75}}{1 + e^{1.872 - 0.0385*75}} = .27, \mathcal{X}_{i4} = 0, Y_{i1} = 75$$

It is also possible to let dropout depend on the observed scores lagging back two observations. However, to do this in the current study we would have had to restrict the data to subjects with the first two observations; less than half of the subjects would remain. So, in this study, we are limited to a single lag.[*]

TABLE 12.4 Study 3: Logistic selection models contrasting completely random dropout (CRD), random dropout (RD) and informative dropout (ID).

Parameters		CRD4	RD4	ID4
$\hat{\beta}_1$	Intercept	63.9	63.9	63.9
$\hat{\beta}_2$	Group	1.69	1.69	1.70
$\hat{\beta}_3$	Time	-0.266	-0.266	-0.254
$\hat{\beta}_4$	Group:Time	0.073	0.073	0.068
$\hat{\gamma}_0$	Time2	-0.549	1.872	1.810
	Time3	-1.005	1.377	1.317
	Time4	-0.198	2.286	2.228
	Time2*Group	-0.592	-0.574	-0.577
	Time3*Group	0.071	0.134	0.002
	Time4*Group	-0.285	-0.274	-0.281
$\hat{\gamma}_1$	y_{it}			0.0022
$\hat{\gamma}_2$	y_{it-1}		-0.0386	-0.0397
-2logL		16158.19	16078.13	16078.11
Comparison			CRD4	RD3
LR Statistic			$\chi_1^2 = 80.1$	$\chi_1^2 = 0.018$
p-value			<0.001	0.89

Dropout as a Function of the Current Measure of the Outcome (ID)

Finally, we examine the ID model by adding the term that allows dropout to depend on the current observed and unobserved FACT-Lung TOI measure (Y_{ij}).

$$logit[P_j, \mathcal{X}_i)] = \gamma_{01}\mathcal{X}_{i1} + \gamma_{02}\mathcal{X}_{i2} + \gamma_{03}\mathcal{X}_{i3} + \gamma_{04}\mathcal{X}_{i4}$$
$$+\gamma_{05}\mathcal{X}_{i5} + \gamma_{06}\mathcal{X}_{i6} + \gamma_1 Y_{ij} + \gamma_2 Y_{ij-1} \qquad (12.12)$$

The ID4 model was not significantly different from the RD4 model. This is at first rather surprising as there was evidence of non-ignorable missing data for

---

[*]The Oswald routine will run without error messages other than the note that the algorithm failed to converge. The resulting parameters describing dropout at 6 weeks make no sense.

all other models considered in the previous chapters. This illustrates a very important point. The failure to reject a hypothesis of informative dropout (ID versus RD) is not conclusive proof that the dropout is ignorable (RD). *The assumption of random dropout (RD) is acceptable only if the ID model was the correct alternative and the parametric form of the ID process is correct.* A number of factors could explain the lack of evidence. In this example, the most likely explanation is that the assumption of a normal distribution for both the observed and unobserved data may be the problem. Another contributor may be the omission of the second random effect[†] corresponding to variation in the rates of change among individuals.

12.3   Summary

- All these models require the analyst to make strong assumptions.

- These assumptions cannot be formally tested. Defense of the assumptions must be made on a clinical basis rather than statistically.

- Lack of evidence of non-ignorable missing data for any particular model does not prove the missing data are ignorable.

- Estimates are not robust to model misspecification, thus more than one model should be considered (a sensitivity analysis).

[†]Oswald (Version 3.4) does not allow this option.

13

Multiple Endpoints

13.1 Introduction

It is well known that performing multiple hypothesis tests and basing inference on unadjusted p-values increase the overall probability of false positive results (Type I errors). Multiple hypothesis tests in trials assessing HRQoL arises from three sources: 1) multiple HRQoL measures (scales or subscales), 2) repeated post-randomization assessments and 3) multiple treatment arms. As a result, multiple testing is one of the major analytic challenges in these trials [Korn and O'Fallon, 1990]. For example, in the lung cancer trial (Study 3), there are five primary subscales in the FACT-Lung instrument (physical, functional, emotional and social/family well-being plus the disease specific concerns). There are three follow-up assessments at 6, 12 and 26 weeks and three treatment arms. If we consider the three possible pairwise comparisons of the treatment arms at each of the three follow-ups for the five primary subscales, we have 45 tests. Not only does this create concerns about type I error, but reports containing large numbers of statistical tests generally result in a confusing picture of HRQoL that is hard to interpret.

Although widely used in the analysis of HRQoL in clinical trials [Schumacher et al., 1991], univariate tests of each HRQoL domain or scale and time point can seriously inflate the type I (false positive) error rate for the overall trial such that the researcher is unable to distinguish between the true and false positive differences. Post hoc adjustment is often infeasible because, at the end of analysis, it is impossible to determine the number of tests performed.

In this and the following chapter, I will illustrate various strategies for addressing the multiple comparisons problem. I will use two examples. The first is the breast cancer trial of adjuvant therapy (Study 1), in which the seven domains of the Breast Chemotherapy Questionnaire (BCQ) were measured at three time points. For the purposes of illustration, I will assume that the aims are to identify the relative impact of the two therapeutic regimens on each of these seven components both on- and post-therapy. This example will be used to illustrate single step (Section 13.4) and sequentially rejective (Section 13.5) methods. The second example is the renal cell carcinoma trial (Study 4). For this trial, I will illustrate designs that integrate both the traditional disease response and survival endpoints with HRQoL measures using closed testing procedures that utilize gatekeeping strategies (Section 13.6).

13.1.1   Aims and Goals/Role of HRQoL

Aims and Goals of Trial

To develop a strategy to handle the multiple endpoints that are inherent in most clinical trials, the aims and goals of the trial and the intended audience must be clearly specified. The goals of the trial may range from registration of a new drug to an exploratory description of the impact of a new therapy. The intended audience may be individuals who will make a decision about whether a therapy will be used in practice or those planning new research. In a trial designed to support the registration of a new drug the risk of marketing an ineffective drug mandate tight control of Type I errors. At the other extreme, a trial in which the analysis of the HRQoL measure is truly exploratory and the results would be confirmed in subsequent studies, control of Type I errors should be relaxed and Type II errors minimized.

Role of HRQoL Assessments

The role of the HRQoL assessments in a trial should also be clearly understood as this too will impact the choice of procedures used to deal with multiple endpoints. How do the HRQoL endpoints relate to the other endpoints in the study? Is measurement of HRQoL the primary endpoint? Is it included to provide supportive evidence that an intervention has a positive effect. Or is the role to confirm that the effect of treatment does not come at the cost of additional toxicity and thus a negative impact on HRQoL. The nature of the question also influences the choice of methods. One approach may be appropriate when the question is Are there *any* differences? and another approach when the question is *Which* endpoints differ?

13.1.2   Other Critical Information

Relative Importance of Endpoints

The relative importance of the endpoints will influence the choice of methods and any logical sequence or hierarchy of the tests. In the breast cancer trial, one might decide *a priori* that all of the seven domains of the BCQ are equally important, or that two of the scales, well-being and symptoms, are of greater importance than the other five scales. In the renal cell trial, one might specify a gatekeeping strategy where only if there is a significant impact on either (or both) disease response and survival, will the HRQoL measures be tested formally. Variations include study designs with a single primary and multiple secondary endpoints (if the primary is non-significant, all other endpoints are irrelevant), multiple co-primary endpoints (significance of any of the endpoints is meaningful) and joint multiple co-primary endpoints (tests of all endpoints need to be significant).

Separate or Joint Testing of Endpoints

The possible methods of analysis will also influence the choices among the multiple comparison procedures. When the characteristics (e.g. binomial, continuous, time to event) or nature (e.g. longitudinal) of the endpoints makes joint analyses difficult, we will need to select methods that allow for separate testing of endpoints. The renal cell study is a good example as our three endpoints include a binomial variable (disease response), a time to an event (survival) and a longitudinally measured continuous measure (HRQoL). While theoretically possible, it would be very difficult to simultaneously estimate models for all three endpoints. In this setting, we would typically analyze each endpoint separately and choose one of the multiple comparison strategies that utilizes the resulting marginal p-values. In contrast, in the breast cancer trial, we have seven continuous measures at three timepoints. It would be feasible (though awkward) to construct a repeated measures model with both the seven domains and the three timepoints contributing to the 21 repeated measures, then construct a multivariate test across the seven subscales.

Communication of Results

The requirements imposed for the reporting of results may also influence the decisions. As will be discussed in more detail later in the chapter, global tests are easy to perform but all that can be reported is a "Yes/No" decision based on rejection/acceptance of hypothesis tests. At the other extreme, the Bonferroni test allows one and two-sided tests, and can produce adjusted p-values and confidence intervals, but at the cost of being the most conservative of the multiple comparisons procedures. In a trial that mandates the additional detail such as confidence intervals, the consequences of selecting a procedure which does not provide those details will be problematic. Thus, it is important to decide during the planning of the analysis whether the benefits of additional power outweigh the ability to produce more detailed reporting.

13.2 General Strategies for Multiple Endpoints

There are three typical strategies to reduce the problem of multiple comparisons: 1) a priori specification of a limited number of *confirmatory* tests, 2) the use of summary measures or statistics, and 3) multiple comparison procedures including alpha adjustments (e.g. Bonferroni) and closed multiple testing. In practice, a combination of focused hypotheses, summary measures and multiple comparison procedures is necessary.

13.2.1   Limiting the Number of Confirmatory Tests

One recommended approach to the multiple testing problem is to specify a limited number (≤ 3) of a priori endpoints in the design of the trial [Gotay et al., 1992] (Table 13.1). While theoretically improving the overall Type I error rate for the study, in practice investigators are reluctant to ignore the remaining data. Descriptive or graphical comparisons of the remaining scales and/or time points [Schumacher et al., 1991] are often proposed as alternatives. Without some measure of precision of the estimates (e.g. standard errors or confidence intervals) the results are uninterpretable. These presentations are essentially disguised statistical tests and there is a danger that they will be treated as such. Finally there is the issue of patient burden. If the patient reported outcomes are not included in the a priori endpoints there needs to be a strong argument for their inclusion.

TABLE 13.1 General strategies for addressing concerns about multiple testing in HRQoL studies.

Limit confirmatory tests

Advantage	• Does not require any adjustments or special statistical procedures.
Disadvantage	• Does not strictly control Type I error.
	• What is done with measures not included and what is the justification for their collection?

Summary measures and statistics

Advantage	• Reduce number of tests
	• Increase power to detect consistent small differences
Disadvantage	• Obscure differences in opposite directions

Multiple comparison procedures

Advantage	• Control of type I errors
Disadvantage	• Decrease power

13.2.2 Summary Measures and Statistics

Well-chosen summary measures or statistics often have greater power to detect patterns of consistent HRQoL differences across time or measures. They also facilitate interpretation, especially when used to summarize information over time. However, they have the potential to blur differences when components of the summary measure are in opposite directions or only one component contributes to the change. Additional details on their advantages and disadvantages are discussed in detail in the following chapter.

In the breast cancer trial (Study 1), we could choose to use the composite score based on all the items of the measure rather than the seven domain scores. This would be appropriate if our aim was to answer "Do the two treatments have a differential effect on overall HRQoL as measured by the BCQ?" and we would be satisfied with statements such as "There was an overall negative impact on HRQoL during therapy as measured by the BCQ in the experimental regimen." This would be especially true if we expected the effects to be in a similar direction across all the domains. But if we were interested in the impact of therapy on the various domains or were concerned that the effects might be in opposite directions, we should not select the composite score. Because the two follow-up timepoints, during therapy and post therapy, are so distinct we would not consider a composite score across time.

In the renal cell carcinoma trial (Study 4), we have six domains and six planned assessments. The same arguments apply to the different domains in this study. A composite score such as the FACT-BRM TOI, combining the physcial, functional and treatment specific domains (see Section 1.6.3), reduces the number of comparisons, is more sensitive to differences that are in the same direction over the four subscales, but obscures effects in different directions. In contrast to the breast cancer trial, summary measures across time may be useful because treatment will continue until either disease progression or unacceptable toxicity occurs. A summary measure across time such as the area under the QOL versus time curve (AUC) could facilitate interpretation, improve power if differences are in the same direction and minimize the multiple comparisons.

13.2.3 Multiple Testing Procedures

The remainder of this chapter will describe selected procedures that can be used to control the type I error rate for K multiple tests. It would be impossible to cover all possibilities in a single chapter, so I have selected several that illustrate the concepts and are potentially applicable to trials in which HRQoL is of interest. Although the selected procedures can generally be applied to any set of hypotheses, the discussion here is presented for a typical situation of two treatment groups with K distinct measures of HRQoL. These measures can be across time, domains or both. Some special cases that are not as common among HRQoL studies, such as dose finding studies with three or more ordered treatment arms, will not be addressed. For more complete discussion of multiple comparisons procedures, the reader is advised to consult books and review articles devoted solely to this topic.

13.3   Background Concepts and Definitions

Before proceeding further a number of definitions are needed. $H_{0(1)}, \ldots, H_{0(K)}$ denotes the K null hypotheses that are to be tested and $T_{(1)}, \ldots, T_{(K)}$ denotes the corresponding K test statistics. $p_{(k)}$ denotes the (unadjusted or marginal) probability of observing the test statistic, $T_{(k)}$, or a more extreme value if the null hypothesis, $H_{0(k)}$, is true.

When describing the multiple comparison procedures, it is often useful to order the p-values from smallest to largest: $p_{[1]} \leq \cdots \leq p_{[K]}$ and then to reorder the corresponding hypotheses, $H_{0[1]}, \ldots, H_{0[K]}$, and test statistics $T_{[1]}, \ldots, T_{[K]}$. Note that square brackets are used to indicate the ordered values.

13.3.1   Univariate versus Multivariate Test Statistics

In this chapter, I am going to use the term *univariate* test statistic to refer a test statistic, $T_{[k]}$, associated with a single hypothesis (e.g. $\theta = 0$). This test statistic can be based on either univariate or multivariate data. In some cases this is a test statistic derived from a longitudinal (multivariate) analysis. For example, a set of five univariate test statistics (t-statistics) could be generated from tests of differences in the slopes from the longitudinal analyses of the five distinct subscales in the lung cancer trial. There is no restriction on whether the K univariate statistics are generated from K separate models or from a joint multivariate model.

In contrast, a *multivariate* test statistic corresponds to the joint test of K (or a subset of K) hypotheses (e.g. $\theta_1 = \theta_2 \ldots \cdots = \theta_K = 0$). An example is an F-test of treatment differences that includes all K subscales. The critical difference is that the multivariate test statistic is a function of the correlation among the subscales (or other components) of the K hypotheses and the univariate tests statistics are not.

There are a number of practical advantages to multiple comparison procedures based on univariate test statistics (marginal p-values). In the context of HRQoL studies, these include: 1) Any of the analytic methods described in the previous chapters that generate a p-value associated with a test of a hypothesis can be used. 2) The procedures can be adapted to one-sided tests. 3) The univariate analyses do not require that all K endpoints are measured on all subjects (although all issues of non-random missing data are still applicable). This might occur if a subset of the K endpoints were not measured because a translation was not available for some of the HRQoL measures. 4) Non-parametric methods as well as parametric methods can be used.

13.3.2 Global Tests

A *global test* generates a single statistic that tests a set (family) of hypotheses and results in the acceptance or rejection of that set of hypotheses.

$$H_0 : H_{0(1)}, \ldots, H_{0(K)} \tag{13.1}$$

As will be illustrated later in this chapter, a global test can be based on either a set of univariate tests (e.g. the Bonferroni global test) or be constructed as a multivariate test statistic. It is important to note that a global test allows one to reject or accept the family of hypotheses, but does not allow inferences to be made about individual hypotheses.

In the renal cancer study, the global test might compare a selected HRQoL measure at 2, 8, 17 and 23 weeks. Based on the global test, we can conclude that the outcome differs between the two treatment groups for at least one of the time points, but we can not say when they differ. Thus, when the global test of H_0 has been rejected, the question remains Which of the individual hypotheses can be rejected?

13.3.3 Error Rates

The *comparisonwise error rate* (CER) is the probability of rejecting a hypothesis test for a single endpoint when the null hypothesis is true. The *familywise error rate* (FWE) is generally defined as the probability of rejecting a null hypothesis for a set (family) of hypotheses when some or all of null hypotheses in the family are true. Thus the FWE depends on which null hypotheses are true. It also depends on the distribution of the data and the correlation among the endpoints. Statisticians often differentiate between weak and strong control of the FWE. *Strong control* refers to control of the error rate for each component; basically it controls the error for the statements such as "The difference is in the physical functioning component of HRQoL." In contrast, *weak control* refers to control of the error rate for the global test of the family of hypotheses, thus controlling the error rate for statements such as "There is a difference in at least one of the domains."

The *false discovery rate* (FDR) is useful when examining very large numbers of hypotheses such as are typically seen in genetic studies or assessments of toxicity. It is defined as the expected number of incorrectly rejected hypotheses among all rejected hypotheses. When all the null hypotheses are true it is equal to the FWE, but otherwise it does not strictly control the FWE.

13.4   Single Step Procedures

13.4.1   Global Tests Based on Multivariate Test Statistics

An example of multivariate statistics used to construct global tests are the F-statistics for joint tests of multiple hypotheses (see Chapters 3 and 4). For purposes of illustration, consider the 7 subscales of the BCQ measured in the adjuvant breast cancer trial (Study 1). If our intent is to control the type I error for testing treatment effects separately for change from baseline to either the on- or post-therapy assessments, we could perform two multivariate analyses of variance (Table 13.2). Using the change from baseline as the outcome, the global test contrasting the two treatment arms was highly significant during therapy ($F_{7,169} = 4.83, p < 0.0001$), but not post therapy ($F_{7,159} = 1.03, p = 0.41$). At this point there have been no adjustments in the p-values, thus if we consider tests significant when $p < 0.05$, we are only controlling the Type I error rate for each of the time points, but not for both simultaneously. If we had decided to split the Type I error rate across the two time points, $\alpha = 0.025$, we could claim that the FWE was less than 5%.

While the global test allows us to make a decision about the multiple endpoints, we are rarely satisfied with only being able to say that there is a difference for at least one endpoint. The question always follows Which of the 7 domains of the BCQ are affected by the intervention? This question motivates all of the subsequent methods.

TABLE 13.2 Study 1: Treatment differences in the change from baseline to the on-therapy and post-therapy assessments for the 7 domains of the BCQ in the adjuvant breast cancer trial. Marginal p-values (two-sided tests) are reported for individual endpoints.

	During-Pre-therapy			Post - Pre-therapy		
Multivariate Global Test	$F_{7,169}=$	4.83,	$p < 0.0001$	$F_{7,159}=$	1.03,	$p = 0.41$
Univariate	DF	t	p-value	DF	t	p-value
Hair Loss (H)	174	-0.66	0.51	167	1.14	0.26
Well-being (W)	175	0.72	0.47	167	-0.50	0.62
Symptoms (S)	175	3.44	0.0007	167	0.94	0.35
Trouble (T)	175	-0.74	0.46	166	-1.20	0.23
Fatigue (F)	175	4.66	<0.0001	167	1.60	0.11
Emotional (E)	175	-0.65	0.51	167	-0.15	0.88
Nausea (N)	174	1.58	0.12	167	1.46	0.15

13.4.2   Equally Weighted Univariate Statistics

In general, multiple comparison procedures using a set of K marginal p-values are much easier to implement and report than those using multivariate test statistics. The single step procedure that equally weights each of the K endpoints is the well known Bonferroni correction. The global Bonferroni test is based on the smallest p-value, $p_{[1]}$. The global null hypothesis is rejected when

$$p_{[1]} \leq \alpha/K. \tag{13.2}$$

In the breast cancer trial, we would reject the global null hypothesis for a test of the seven domains during therapy as at least one of the unadjusted (marginal) p-values is less than $0.05/7$, but we would not for the post therapy assessments (Table 13.2). With this global test we have weak control of the FWE, but can only say that there is a difference in at least one of the seven domains during therapy.

To be able to make definitive statements about specific domains, we need to establish strong control of the FWE. For individual endpoints the procedure is to accept as statistically significant only those tests with p-values that are less than α/K. Adjusted p-values are calculated by multiplying the raw (marginal) p-values (p_k) by K; values greater than 1 are reported as 1.

$$\tilde{p}_k^B = min(1, p_k * K) \tag{13.3}$$

The Bonferroni adjusted p-values for the on-therapy comparisons are illustrated in Table 13.3. Computation of confidence intervals is also straight forward, with the usual α replaced by α/K. For example, if the unadjusted 95% confidence interval is:

$$\hat{\theta} \pm t_{(1-\alpha/2)} \sqrt{Var[\hat{\theta}]} \tag{13.4}$$

then the adjusted confidence interval would be:

$$\hat{\theta} \pm t_{(1-\alpha/2K)} \sqrt{Var[\hat{\theta}]} \tag{13.5}$$

The Bonferroni procedure results in strong control of the FWE, but is well known to be quite conservative. If the K test statistics are uncorrelated (the tests are independent) and the null hypotheses are all true, then the probability of rejecting at least one of the K hypotheses is approximately[*] αK when α is small. However, when the tests are correlated, the procedure over corrects. Another limitation is that the Bonferroni procedure focuses on the detection of large differences in one or more endpoints and is insensitive to a pattern of smaller differences that are all in the same direction. Options that address this problem will be presented later in this chapter.

---

[*]$Pr[min(\text{p-value}) \leq \alpha] = 1 - (1 - \alpha)^K \approx \alpha K$

TABLE 13.3 Study 1: Unadjusted and adjusted p-values for contrasts between the treatment arms for the during-therapy measures of the 7 domains of the BCQ. Each domain is indicated by its first letter (e.g. F=Fatigue)

BCQ domain		F	S	N	T	W	H	E
Method	k=	1	2	3	4	5	6	7
Unadjusted	$p_{[k]}$	0.0001	0.0007	0.12	0.46	0.47	0.51	0.52
Bonferroni	$\tilde{p}_{[k]}^{B}$	0.0007	0.0049	0.84	1.0	1.0	1.0	1.0
Weighted*	$\tilde{p}_{[k]}^{Bw}$	0.0010	0.0028	1.0	1.0	1.0	1.0	1.0
Holm	$\tilde{p}_{[k]}^{H}$	0.0007	0.0042	0.60	1.0	1.0	1.0	1.0
Weighted*	$\tilde{p}_{[k]}^{Hw}$	0.0010	0.0025	1.0	1.0	1.0	1.0	1.0
Hochberg	$\tilde{p}_{[k]}^{\mathcal{H}}$	0.0007	0.0042	0.52	0.52	0.52	0.52	0.52
FDR	$\tilde{p}_{[k]}^{FDR}$	0.0001	0.0025	0.28	0.52	0.52	0.52	0.52
* Weights=(1, 2.5, 1, 1, 2.5, 1, 1)								

13.4.3 Importance Weighting/ Spending α

In some settings, a subset of the HRQoL domains is of particular interest. There may be reasons that only some of the domains would be expected to change as a result of the interventions. In these trials, we may wish to spend more of α on those prespecifed endpoints. This strategy is also referred to as *importance weighting*. Instead of allocation (or spending α equally among the endpoints), we may choose to spend more of the total α on selected endpoints. If the total α_T equals 0.05, we might spend $\alpha = .0125$ on two prespecifed endpoints (well-being and symptoms) and $\alpha = .005$ on the remaining five endpoints. Note that the sum is 0.05. To determine weights, first assign the endpoint with the smallest portion of α_T a weight of 1, then the remaining endpoints weights that reflect the relative values of α_T spent on that endpoint. This would be equivalent to giving the two selected endpoints a weight of 2.5 and the remaining five a weight of 1. The sum of the weights ($\sum w_k$) is 10. The adjusted p-value for the kth endpoint is

$$\tilde{p}_k^{Bw} = min(1, p_k * (\sum_{k=1}^{K} w_k)/w_k). \tag{13.6}$$

Thus, for the two pre-selected endpoints, $\tilde{p}_k^{Bw} = p_k * 10/2.5 = p_k * 4$ and for the remaining endpoints $\tilde{p}_k^{Bw} = p_k * 10/1 = p_k * 10$. Adjusted p-values greater than 1 are set to 1. In the breast cancer example (Table 13.3), the marginal p-values for the well-being and symptom scales are multiplied by 4 and the remaining five scales by 10.

A few notes of caution are appropriate. First, the weights must be pre-specified prior to any analyses of the data. Second, while this procedure increases the power to detect differences in those endpoints given greater weights, it decreases the power for the remaining endpoints. Finally, importance weighting should not be confused with a pre-specified ordering of tests (see Section 13.6).

13.5 Sequentially Rejective Methods

13.5.1 Equal Weighting of Endpoints

Step-Down Procedure

A less conservative alternative to the classical Bonferroni adjustments was proposed by Holm [1979]. The marginal p-values are ordered from smallest to largest. The hypothesis associated with the smallest p-value is tested in exactly the same manner as in the Bonferroni procedure. If that hypothesis is rejected, then the remaining K-1 hypotheses are considered, using $\alpha/(K-1)$ to determine the critical values of the test statistic (or to adjust the p-values) for the hypothesis associated with the second smallest p-value. As long as the hypotheses are rejected, the procedure continues using smaller subsets of the endpoints. The entire procedure is as follows: the smallest p-value, $p_{[1]}$, is compared to α/K. If $p_{[1]} \leq \alpha/K$, we reject the corresponding hypothesis and continue, comparing $p_{[2]}$ to $\alpha/(K-1)$. The procedure is continued, comparing $p_{[k]}$ to $\alpha/(K-k+1)$. At the point any null hypothesis can not be rejected, the procedure stops and all remaining null hypotheses are accepted.

To maintain the same ordering as observed for the raw p-values, the adjusted p-values are calculated as follows:

$$\tilde{p}_{[1]}^{H} = min(1, p_{[1]} * K) \tag{13.7}$$
$$\tilde{p}_{[2]}^{H} = min(1, max(\tilde{p}_{[1]}^{H}, p_{[2]} * (K-1)))$$
$$\vdots$$
$$\tilde{p}_{[K]}^{H} = min(1, max(\tilde{p}_{[K-1]}^{H}, p_{[K]}))$$

When more than one of the null hypotheses are false, this procedure substantially increases the power. For example, it is much easier to reject the hypothesis associated with the second smallest p-value with this procedure than with the single step procedure. The cost is that we can not construct confidence intervals that directly correspond to the procedure.

Step-Up Procedure

Hochberg proposed an alternative to Holm's step-down procedure that is slightly more powerful, though it relies on an assumption of independence of the test statistics. The adjusted p-values for the step-up procedure are defined in the reverse order.

$$\tilde{p}^{\mathcal{H}}_{[K]} = p_{[K]} \tag{13.8}$$
$$\tilde{p}^{\mathcal{H}}_{[i]} = min(\tilde{p}^{\mathcal{H}}_{[i+1]}, p_{[i]} * (K - i + 1)), \quad i = K - 1, \cdots, 1$$

The procedure is illustrated for the seven domains of the BCQ (Table 13.3). The largest p-value, $p_{[7]} = 0.80$, remains unchanged, setting $\tilde{p}^{\mathcal{H}}_{[7]}$ to 0.80. The second largest is multiplied by 2 and compared to the largest; the minimum of the two values is 0.80. The procedure continues and in the last step $p_{[1]}$ is multiplied by 7 and compared to $\tilde{p}^{\mathcal{H}}_{[2]}$.

False Discovery Rate

A sequential procedure can also be applied using the FDR. The adjusted p-values are defined as follows:

$$\tilde{p}^{FDR}_{[K]} = p_{[K]} \tag{13.9}$$
$$\tilde{p}^{FDR}_{[i]} = min(\tilde{p}^{FDR}_{[i+1]}, \tilde{p}_{[i]} * \frac{K}{i}), \quad i = K - 1, \cdots, 1$$

The procedure is illustrated for the seven domains of the BCQ (Table 13.3). The largest p-value, $p_{[7]} = 0.80$, remains unchanged, setting $\tilde{p}^{FDR}_{[7]}$ to 0.80. The second largest is multiplied in this procedure by 7/6 and compared to the largest; the minimum of the two values is 0.80. The procedure continues and in the last step $p_{[1]}$ is multiplied by 7/1 and compared to $\tilde{p}^{FDR}_{[2]}$.

13.5.2   Implementation in SAS

The SAS procedure MULTTEST will calculate the adjusted p-values using a dataset (work.pvalues) that contains the unadjusted p-values. The variable containing the unadjusted p-values must be named Raw_P. The procedure to generate the Bonferroni, Holm, Hochberg and FDR adjusted values is:

```
proc multtest inpvalues=work.pvalues bon holm hoc fdr;
   run;
```

13.5.3   Implementation in SPSS

SPSS built-in options are limited to the Bonferroni and Sidak adjustments. In MIXED these are further limited to the EMMEANS subcomand and can be implemented by adding ADJ(BONFERRONI) or ADJ(SIDAK). The Sidak adjustment replaces α/k with a slightly more accurate criteria $1 - (1 - \alpha)^{1/k}$. For example, when $k = 5$ the criterion is 0.0100 for the Bonferroni adjustment and 0.0102 for the Sidak adjustment.

13.5.4   Implementation in R

The R function `p.adjust` will calculate the adjusted p-values. If we have created a vector of p-values called `pval`, the following statements will generate the same four adjustments:

```
> pvals=c(0.0001,0.0002,0.081,0.27,0.60,0.75,0.80)
> p.adjust(pvals,method="bonferroni")
> p.adjust(pvals,method="holm")
> p.adjust(pvals,method="hochberg")
> p.adjust(pvals,method="fdr")
```

13.5.5   Importance Weighting

The sequential rejection procedure can also be applied when the endpoints are given different weights. The modification is as follows: the smallest p-value, $p_{[1]}$, is compared to $\alpha/(\sum_{k=1}^{K} w_{[k]})/w_{[k]}$. If that hypothesis is rejected, then next smallest p-value, $p_{[2]}$, is compared to $\alpha/(\sum_{k=2}^{K} w_{[k]})/w_{[k]}$. The procedure continues until one of the hypotheses is not rejected, at which point all subsequent hypotheses are accepted. In the previous example, because the smallest p-value (fatigue) was not one of the two selected endpoints, the critical value would correspond to $\alpha/10/1 = \alpha/10$. The second smallest p-value was one of the selected endpoints; the critical value is $\alpha/9/2.5 = \alpha/3.6$. This is also rejected. Finally, the comparison of $p_{[3]}$ to $\alpha/6.5/1$ is not rejected and all subsequent hypotheses are accepted.

Again, to maintain the same ordering as observed for the raw p-values, the adjusted p-values are calculated as follows:

$$\tilde{p}_{[1]}^{Hw} = min(1, p_{[1]} * (\sum_{k=1}^{K} w_{[k]})/w_{[1]}) \tag{13.10}$$

$$\tilde{p}_{[2]}^{Hw} = min(1, max(\tilde{p}_{[1]}, p_{[2]} * (\sum_{k=2}^{K} w_{[k]})/w_{[2]}))$$

$$\vdots$$

$$\tilde{p}_{[K]}^{Hw} = min(1, max(\tilde{p}_{[K-1]}, p_{[K]}))$$

13.6   Closed Testing and Gatekeeper Procedures

The closed-testing procedure proposed by Marcus et al. [1976] provides a theoretical basis for controlling the experimentwise Type I error in a wide variety of settings. While the notation initially appears complicated, most

TABLE 13.4 Decision matrix for a closed testing procedure based on a Bonferroni correction with three hypothesis tests.

Intersection hypothesis	Rule for p-value	Implied hypotheses H_A	H_B	H_C
H_{ABC}	$p_{ABC} = 3 * min(p_A, p_B, p_C)$	p_{ABC}	p_{ABC}	p_{ABC}
H_{AB}	$p_{AB} = 2 * min(p_A, p_B)$	p_{AB}	p_{AB}	0
H_{AC}	$p_{AC} = 2 * min(p_A, p_C)$	p_{AC}	0	p_{AC}
H_{BC}	$p_{BC} = 2 * min(p_B, p_C)$	0	p_{BC}	p_{BC}
H_A	$p_A = p_A$	p_A	0	0
H_B	$p_B = p_B$	0	p_B	0
H_C	$p_C = p_C$	0	0	p_C

applications simplify and the wide range of applications justifies the initial effort to understand the procedure. To illustrate the notation, assume that we have three endpoints. The corresponding marginal hypotheses are H_A, H_B, and H_C. The intersection of the hypotheses associated with the first two endpoints is designated as H_{AB} and the intersection of all three hypotheses as H_{ABC}. There are $2^K - 1$ possible combinations. In the closed-testing procedure, the adjusted p-value for each hypothesis is the maximum p-value of the set (family) of hypotheses implied by the marginal hypothesis. For example, H_A would imply all combinations that contained A: H_A, H_{AB}, H_{AC}, and H_{ABC}. The adjusted p-value would be the maximum of the p-values associated with these four combinations. The simplification occurs when it is sufficient to report that the test of a specific hypothesis has been accepted (not significant at α); if any of the set of hypotheses is accepted, testing the remaining hypotheses is unnecessary.

13.6.1 Closed Testing Based on a Bonferroni Correction

First, recall the global test described in the single step procedures. The rule was to reject if the smallest p-value, $p_{[1]} \leq \alpha/K$ where K is the number of hypotheses being tested. Alternatively, the adjusted p-value for this global test is $\tilde{p} = p_{[i]} * K$. In the closed testing procedure, we first examine all K hypotheses simultaneously, H_{ABC}. The p-value for the global test of H_{ABC} is $3 * min(p_{[1]}, p_{[2]}, p_{[3]}) = 3P_{[1]}$. If we reject H_{ABC}, we then examine all of K-1 (two-way) combinations of hypotheses, H_{AB}, H_{AC}, and H_{BC}. The p-values for these combinations are adjusted using K-1. The procedure continues in a similar manner with smaller subsets. After all of the combinations are tested, the adjusted p-value is the maximum p-value of all the implied hypotheses. This closed testing procedure with a Bonferroni correction is identical to the Holm stepwise procedure (see Section 13.5.1).

Dmitrienko et al. [2003] present a formal way of displaying the procedure. The *decision matrix* (Table 13.4) contains a row for each of the $2^K - 1$ intersections. The second column designates the Bonferroni adjusted p-value for the respective intersection hypothesis. The next three columns indicate which of the intersection hypotheses belong to the set of implied hypotheses. The adjusted p-values for H_A, H_B, and H_C are the maximum of the values in each column. If the unadjusted p-values were $p_A = 0.08$, $p_B = 0.02$, and $p_C = 0.03$, then $p_{ABC} = 3*min(0.08, 0.02, 0.03) = 0.06$, $p_{AB} = 2*min(0.08, 0.02) = 0.04$, $p_{AC} = 2*min(0.08, 0.03) = 0.06$, $p_{BC} = 2*min(0.02, 0.03) = 0.04$. The adjusted p-values would be the maximum value in the columns that indicate the implied hypotheses: $\tilde{p}_A = max(p_{ABC}, p_{AB}, p_{AC}, p_A) = 0.08$, $\tilde{p}_B = max(p_{ABC}, p_{AB}, p_{BC}, p_B) = 0.06$, and $\tilde{p}_C = max(p_{ABC}, p_{AC}, p_{BC}, p_C) = 0.06$.

13.6.2 Sequential Families

In some settings, there is a prespecifed sequence of testing families of hypotheses. In Section 13.1.2, I mentioned trial designs with a single primary and multiple secondary endpoints (if the primary is non-significant, all other endpoints are irrelevant), multiple co-primary endpoints (significance of any of the endpoints is meaningful) and joint co-primary endpoints (tests of all endpoints need to be significant). In all of these designs, the two families of hypotheses are tested sequentially with the first family acting as a gatekeeper for the second family. Ideally the gatekeeping strategy is based on a mechanistic model in which the first family consists of measures of a proximal effect of the intervention on outcomes and the second family consists of more distal outcomes. For example, reflecting back to the conceptual model proposed by Wilson and Cleary [1995] (Figure 1.1), the first family could consist of biological and physiological factors and the second would consist of measures of symptom status. Alternatively, the first family could consist of symptom status and the second family of measures of the perceived impact of those symptoms.

Typically, HRQoL endpoints are poorly integrated into clinical trials. However, a gatekeeping procedure with sequential families provides one strategy for better integration. As an illustration, consider the renal cell carcinoma trial with hypotheses A, B, and C testing treatment differences in disease response, survival and HRQoL. Let's assume hypothetically, that the unadjusted (marginal) p-values are $p_A = 0.08$, $p_B = 0.02$, and $p_C = 0.03$.

Design 1: Single Primary Endpoint

In the first design, assume that disease response (H_A) was designated as the primary endpoint and both survival (H_B) and HRQoL (H_C) as the secondary endpoint. The first family consists of H_A and the second family of H_B and H_C. In this design, if the null hypothesis for the primary endpoint (A) is not rejected, all of the secondary null hypotheses must be accepted. This translates to the decision matrix displayed in Table 13.5. Thus for our hypothetical

TABLE 13.5 Decision matrix for a Bonferroni gatekeeping procedure for Design 1 with a single primary (A) and two secondary endpoints (B and C).

Intersection hypothesis	p-value	Implied hypotheses H_A	H_B	H_C
H_{ABC}	$p_{ABC} = p_A$	p_{ABC}	p_{ABC}	p_{ABC}
H_{AB}	$p_{AB} = p_A$	p_{AB}	p_{AB}	0
H_{AC}	$p_{AC} = p_A$	p_{AC}	0	p_{AC}
H_{BC}	$p_{BC} = 2 * min(p_B, p_C)$	0	p_{BC}	p_{BC}
H_A	$p_A = p_A$	p_A	0	0
H_B	$p_B = p_B$	0	p_B	0
H_C	$p_C = p_C$	0	0	p_C

example, disease response is the single primary endpoint. If we apply this design using the unadjusted p-values from the previous example, $p_{ABC} = p_{AB} = p_{AC} = p_A = 0.08$, $p_{BC} = 2 * min(.02, .03) = 0.04$. The adjusted p-values are $\tilde{p}_A = max(p_{ABC}, p_{AB}, p_{AC}, p_A) = 0.08$, $\tilde{p}_B = max(p_{ABC}, p_{AB}, p_{BC}, p_B) = 0.08$, and $\tilde{p}_C = max(p_{ABC}, p_{AC}, p_{BC}, p_C) = 0.08$. Thus, none of the three hypotheses are rejected and the (adjusted) results are negative for all three endpoints. If our trial design had designated survival as the primary endpoint, both the hypotheses for survival and HRQoL would have been rejected.

Design 2: Co-Primary Endpoints

In the second design, disease control and survival are the co-primary endpoints and HRQoL the secondary endpoint. If either hypothesis in the first family (H_A or H_B) is rejected, then the second family of hypotheses will be considered. This translates to the decision matrix displayed in Table 13.6. The hypotheses in the first family are tested as if the Holm procedure was applied to two endpoints. The adjusted p-values are $\tilde{p}_A = 0.08$ and $\tilde{p}_B = 0.04$. The adjusted p-value for the second family can not be smaller than the smallest in the first family because the gatekeeping procedure requires that H_C can not be rejected unless one of the hypotheses in the first family is rejected. Thus $\tilde{p}_B = 0.04$. With design 2, we would reject the null hypotheses associated with one of the primary endpoints, survival, and for the secondary endpoint, HRQoL.

Design 3: Joint Co-Primary Endpoints

In the final design, disease control and survival are joint co-primary endpoints. This design differs from the previous as it requires both H_A and H_B to be rejected before considering the second family of hypotheses. This translates to the decision matrix displayed in Table 13.7. The adjusted p-values for the first family of hypotheses is identical to those in Design 2. The difference

TABLE 13.6 Decision matrix for a Bonferroni gatekeeping procedure for Design 2 with two co-primary (A and B) and one secondary endpoint (C).

Intersection hypothesis	p-value	Implied hypotheses H_A	H_B	H_C
H_{ABC}	$p_{ABC} = 2 * min(p_A, p_B)$	p_{ABC}	p_{ABC}	p_{ABC}
H_{AB}	$p_{AB} = 2 * min(p_A, p_B)$	p_{AB}	p_{AB}	0
H_{AC}	$p_{AC} = min(p_A, p_C)$	p_{AC}	0	p_{AC}
H_{BC}	$p_{BC} = min(p_B, p_C)$	0	p_{BC}	p_{BC}
H_A	$p_A = p_A$	p_A	0	0
H_B	$p_B = p_B$	0	p_B	0
H_C	$p_C = p_C$	0	0	p_C

TABLE 13.7 Decision matrix for a Bonferroni gatekeeping procedure for Design 3 with two joint primary (A and B) and one secondary endpoint (C).

Intersection hypothesis	p-value	Implied hypotheses H_A	H_B	H_C
H_{ABC}	$p_{ABC} = 2 * min(p_A, p_B)$	p_{ABC}	p_{ABC}	p_{ABC}
H_{AB}	$p_{AB} = 2 * min(p_A, p_B)$	p_{AB}	p_{AB}	0
H_{AC}	$p_{AC} = p_A$	p_{AC}	0	p_{AC}
H_{BC}	$p_{BC} = p_B$	0	p_{BC}	p_{BC}
H_A	$p_A = p_A$	p_A	0	0
H_B	$p_B = p_B$	0	p_B	0
H_C	$p_C = p_C$	0	0	p_C

occurs in the calculation of p_{AC} and p_{BC}. Because the gatekeeping procedure requires that H_C can not be rejected unless both of the hypotheses in the first family are rejected, the adjusted p-value can not be smaller than the largest in the first family thus $\tilde{p}_C = 0.08$. Thus in design 3, only the survival hypothesis is rejected.

13.6.3 Shortcuts for Closed Testing Procedures

Hommel et al. [2007] proposed shortcuts for closed testing procedures for settings with large numbers of tests. A trial with six endpoints would produce $2^6 - 1 = 63$ intersection hypotheses. The idea is to develop rules for a stepwise procedure in which the endpoint driving the rejection of the hypothesis is dropped from the subsequent comparisons. They illustrate the procedure with a scenario that includes a composite HRQoL measure with testing of the separate domains following rejection of the intersection hypothesis driven by the composite QOL measure. Consider an example with three co-primary endpoints: disease response (E_1), survival (E_2), and HRQOL (Q).

The composite score (e.g. FACT-BRM TOI, see Section 1.6.3) has four domains (D_1, D_2, D_3, D_4) that are secondary endpoints and will be tested only if the hypothesis involving the composite score is rejected. One potential set of rules for the weights of the intersection hypotheses proposed by Hommel et al. is as follows:

- Whenever E_1 or E_2 are part of the intersection hypothesis, assign the weight of $\frac{1}{3}$ to that endpoint.

- When E_1 or E_2 are not part of an intersection, their weights are assigned to Q or are allocated equally to each of the QOL domains in the intersection hypothesis.

Thus the three co-primary endpoints initially have equal importance. The testing of Q has a greater gatekeeping role for the domain scores and if either E_1 or E_2 is rejected, Q would be allocated more weight facilitating the testing of the domain scores.

To illustrate the procedure assume that the unadjusted p-values are: $p_{E_1} = 0.082$, $p_{E_2} = 0.007$, $p_Q = 0.012$, $p_{D_1} = 0.070$, $p_{D_2} = 0.012$, $p_{D_3} = 0.0038$, and $p_{D_4} = 0.007$. In the first step, we test the intersection hypothesis for the three primary endpoints (Table 13.8) and note that E_1 is the minimum weighted p-value and thus the identified endpoint. Following the rules, the weight associated with this endpoint is transferred to Q. The composite QOL score, Q, is the identified endpoint in the second step; its weight is transferred to the four domains. The testing continues with D_3, D_4, D_2 and D_1 and finally E_1 emerging as the identified endpoints. Note that the local p-values for D_3 and E_1 are less than the proceeding adjusted p-values; to preserve the ordering of the adjusted p-value it is set to the proceeding value.

TABLE 13.8 Results from a shortcut gatekeeping procedure. Weights are ordered as E_1, E_2, Q, D_1, D_2, D_3, D_4.

Weights for current step	Rule for local p-value	Identified endpoint	Adjusted p-value
$\frac{1}{3}, \frac{1}{3}, \frac{1}{3}, 0, 0, 0, 0$	$min(\frac{3}{1}p_{E_1}, \frac{3}{1}p_{E_2}, \frac{3}{1}p_Q) = 0.021$	E_2	0.021
$\frac{1}{3}, \ , \frac{2}{3}, 0, 0, 0, 0$	$min(\frac{3}{1}p_{E_1}, \frac{3}{2}p_Q) = 0.024$	Q	0.024
$\frac{1}{3}, \ , \ , \frac{1}{6}, \frac{1}{6}, \frac{1}{6}, \frac{1}{6}$	$min(\frac{3}{1}p_{E_1}, \frac{6}{1}p_{D_1}, \cdots, \frac{6}{1}p_{D_4}) = 0.023$	D_3	0.024
$\frac{1}{3}, \ , \ , \frac{2}{9}, \frac{2}{9}, \ , \frac{2}{9}$	$min(\frac{3}{1}p_{E_1}, \frac{9}{2}p_{D_1}, \frac{9}{2}p_{D_2}, \frac{9}{2}p_{D_4}) = 0.032$	D_4	0.032
$\frac{1}{3}, \ , \ , \frac{1}{3}, \frac{1}{3}, \ $	$min(\frac{3}{1}p_{E_1}, \frac{3}{1}p_{D_1}, \frac{3}{1}p_{D_2}) = 0.036$	D_2	0.036
$\frac{1}{3}, \ , \ , \frac{2}{3}, \ , \ $	$min(\frac{3}{1}p_{E_1}, \frac{3}{2}p_{D_1}) = 0.105$	D_1	0.105
$\frac{1}{1}, \ , \ , \ , \ , \ $	$p_{E_1} = 0.082$	E_1	0.105

TABLE 13.9 Study 1: Decision matrix for a closed testing procedure based on a multivariate test. Tests of treatment differences in the pre- to during therapy change of the 7 domains of the BCQ. Each domain is indicated by the first letter (e.g. H=Hair Loss).

Intersection hypothesis	Implied hypotheses						
	H_H	H_W	H_S	H_T	H_F	H_E	H_N
$H_{HWSTFEN}$	<0.01	<0.01	<0.01	<0.01	<0.01	<0.01	<0.01
H_{WSTFEN}		<0.01	<0.01	<0.01	<0.01	<0.01	<0.01
H_{HSTFEN}	<0.01		<0.01	<0.01	<0.01	<0.01	<0.01
H_{HWSFEN}	<0.01	<0.01	<0.01		<0.01	<0.01	<0.01
H_{HWSTFN}	<0.01	<0.01	<0.01	<0.01	<0.01		<0.01
H_{HWSTFE}	<0.01	<0.01	<0.01	<0.01	<0.01	<0.01	
$\vdots$							
H_H	0.51						
H_W		0.47					
H_S			<0.01				
H_T				0.46			
H_F					<0.01		
H_E						0.52	
H_N							0.12
Max of column	≥0.51	≥0.47	<0.01	≥0.46	<0.01	≥0.52	≥0.12

13.6.4 A Closed Testing Procedure Based on a Multivariate Test

The closed testing procedure can also be based on multivariate tests. This strategy is limited to settings where a set of hypotheses can be jointly tested. This is virtually impossible when different analysis methods (Cox regression, logistic regression, linear regression) are used for the respective endpoints (survival, disease response, QOL). It is possible in settings where hypotheses for all the outcomes can be tested in the same model, although programming these analyses is a bit of a burden. Consider the test of differences in the 7 subscales between the two treatment arms of the breast cancer trial. One approach is to test all possible $2^7 - 1$ or 127 combinations and use a decision matrix strategy to compute the adjusted p-values as previously described (Table 13.9). As the number of endpoints increases this becomes a bit cumbersome. The procedure can be slightly simplified if one does not need the adjusted p-value for the null hypotheses that are not rejected. In this example, because H_H, H_W, H_T, H_F, and H_N are not rejected, it is not necessary to test the combinations that only include those hypotheses. But if we omit those tests, we can only state that the adjusted p-value for that hypothesis is above a certain value (Table 13.9).

13.6.5   Summary and Composite Measures

As will be discussed in more detail in the next chapter, multivariate tests such as Hotelling's T statistic are not as sensitive to consistent differences over all the endpoints as tests of composite measures. Noting that investigators are rarely satisfied with knowing there is a significant difference, Lechmaher et al. [1991] apply closed multiple test procedures to simple and weighted sums of the individual measures such as those described by O'Brien [1984]. It would be straightforward to apply closed testing procedure using the procedures described in this section to any of the summary or composite measures described in the next chapter.

13.7   Summary

- Multiple endpoints and testing creates a major analytic problem in clinical trials with HRQoL assessments.

- Three strategies are generally necessary:

    - Limiting the number of endpoints

    - Summary measures and statistics (see Chapter 14)

    - Multiple comparison procedures

- Multiple comparison procedures are most useful for measures of the multiple domains of HRQoL, especially when there is a concern about obscuring effects of components that move in opposite directions with the use of summary measures.

- A multiple comparison procedure based on K univariate tests is likely to be easier to report than one based on multivariate tests.

- Gatekeeping strategies utilizing closed testing procedures are useful tools for integrating HRQoL measures into the analytic strategy for the entire trial.

14

Composite Endpoints and Summary Measures

14.1 Introduction

In most clinical trials, investigators assess HRQoL longitudinally over the period of treatment and, in some trials, subsequent to treatment. Each assessment involves multiple scales that measure the general and disease-specific domains of HRQoL. For example in the lung cancer trial, there are three treatment arms, four assessments and five subscales of the FACT-Lung. As a result, addressing the problem of multiple comparisons is one of the analytic challenges in these trials [Korn and O'Fallon, 1990]. Not only are there concerns about Type I errors, but large numbers of statistical tests generally result in a confusing picture of HRQoL that is difficult to interpret [DeKlerk, 1986]. As mentioned in the previous chapter, composite endpoints and summary measures are one of three strategies that in combination will reduce Type I errors, attempt to conserve power and improve interpretation. In this chapter, the computations of composite endpoints and summary measures are presented with details concerning how their derivation is affected by missing data.

14.1.1 Composite Endpoints versus Summary Measures

The terms *composite endpoints* and *summary measures* are often interchanged, but are used differently here. The following definitions are used in this chapter: A *composite endpoint* reduces the multiple measures on each individual to a single number. The procedure is first to summarize the data within an individual subject by calculating a single value (composite endpoint) for each individual and then to perform an analysis of the composite endpoint(s). For example, we might estimate the rate of change experienced by each individual using ordinary least squares (OLS) and then apply a two-sample t-test to compare the estimates in two treatment groups. Other examples of composite endpoints include the average of the within subject post-treatment values [DeKlerk, 1986, Matthews et al., 1990, Frison and Pocock, 1992], last value minus baseline [Frison and Pocock, 1992], average rate of change over time (or slope) [Matthews et al., 1990], maximum value [DeKlerk, 1986, Pocock et al.,

1987a, Matthews et al., 1990], area under the curve [Matthews et al., 1990, Cox et al., 1992] and time to reach a peak or a pre-specified value [Pocock et al., 1987a, Matthews et al., 1990].

In contrast, a *summary measure or statistic* reduces the measurements on a group of individuals to a single value. Data are initially analyzed using multivariate techniques for longitudinal models and summary measures are constructed from the estimates of the parameters. For example, the mean rate of change (or slope) for each treatment group is estimated using a mixed-effects model and the differences in the slopes between the two treatment groups tested. Other examples include the average of the group means during the post-treatment period and area under the mean HRQoL versus time curve.

Missing data are dealt with differently in the construction of these measures and statistics [Fairclough, 1997]. For composite endpoints (Sections 14.3 and 14.5), we must develop a procedure to handle missing data at the subject level possibly by using interpolation and extrapolation or by imputing missing observations. For summary measures (Section 14.4), missing data handled by the selection of the analytic model as described in Chapters 9-12.

TABLE 14.1 Comparison of composite endpoints and summary measure for combining information across time.

Method	Composite endpoints ($S_i = \sum_{j=1}^{J} w_j f(Y_{ij})$)
Strategy	1. Summarize data within ith patient (over J repeated evaluations) 2. Univariate analysis of S_i
Advantage	Easy to describe and interpret
Disadvantage	Often difficult to develop strategy for handling every missing value on an individual basis. Some measures are biased depending on pattern and reasons for missing data.
Method	Summary measure ($S_h = \sum_{j=1}^{J} w_j g(\beta_{hj})$)
Strategy	1. Fit multivariate model, estimating means (or parameters) for repeated measures or mixed-effects model. 2. Compute summary statistic (generally linear combination of parameters) 3. Test hypothesis ($H_0 : S_h = S_{h\prime}$ or $S_h - S_{h\prime} = 0$)
Advantage	Strategies for handling missing data are model based
Disadvantage	Harder to describe procedure

14.1.2   Strengths and Weaknesses

Interpretation

There are several motivations for the use of composite endpoints and summary measures in the analysis of a longitudinal study of HRQoL [Fairclough, 1997]. The primary advantage of composite endpoints is that they may facilitate interpretation. This is particularly true when information is summarized across time. Not only are the number of comparisons reduced, but measures such as the rate of change and the area under the curve are familiar concepts in clinical medicine.

This advantage is balanced by two concerns. The first is that differences in different directions or in one but not all domains of HRQoL or transient differences at specific points in time may be obscured. The second is that when a composite endpoint is observed to be different across treatment groups, that readers are lead to or make the conclusion that all of the components contribute equally to that difference, when in many cases only one component contributes to the difference. Freemantle et al. [2003] discuss this problem. While their review focused on composites that incorporated mortality, their concerns are still relevant. Several of their recommendations concerning the transparency of results are incorporated in this chapter.

Overall, investigations that are confirmatory, designed to test the question of differences in overall HRQoL, may benefit from the use of composite endpoints. This is especially useful in studies where early toxicity in one treatment group may be balanced by later improvements in disease control. In contrast, trials that have more exploratory objectives of identifying which aspects of HRQoL are impacted by the disease or a particular therapy will not benefit from the use of composite endpoints or summary measures across multiple domains.

Increased Power

Composite endpoints and summary measures have greater power to detect small but consistent differences that may occur over extended periods of time or multiple domains of HRQoL, in contrast to a multivariate test (Hotelling's T). To illustrate, consider the two hypothetical examples displayed in Figure 14.1. In the first example (Figure 14.1 left), the measure of HRQoL is consistently better in one treatment during all four post-baseline assessments. The multivariate test of differences at the four followups is non-significant ($F_{4,100} = 1.12, p = 0.35$) however the hypothesis based on the mean of the four follow-ups is rejected ($t_{100} = -2.11, p = 0.037$). In the second example (Figure 14.1 right), the second treatment has a negative impact (toxicity) 1 month post diagnosis, but this difference almost disappears by the third month and begins to reverse by the ninth month. The results are reversed; multivariate test of differences at the four followups rejected ($F_{4,100} = 4.3, p = 0.003$) however the hypothesis based on the mean of the four follow-ups is not rejected ($t_{100} = -0.76, p = 0.45$). Although the differences between the groups in both examples are of clinical interest, in most clinical trials one would wish to have test procedures that are more sensitive to (or have greater power to detect) the consistent differences displayed in Figure 14.1 (left).

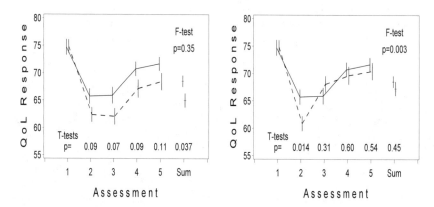

FIGURE 14.1 Hypothetical studies with consistent differences in HRQoL over time (left) or a large difference at a single point in time (right). Summary measure is the mean of the post-baseline assessments. Means are joined by horizontal line. Vertical lines indicate 1 standard error. F-test indicates multivariate test of group differences at assessments 2, 3, 4 and 5. t-tests indicate test of group difference at each assessment or for the summary measure.

14.2 Choosing a Composite Endpoint or Summary Measure

The selection of a composite or summary measure as the endpoint in a clinical trial depends on the objective of the investigation. The composite endpoint should have a clear clinical relevance and ideally should be determined prior to data collection [Matthews et al., 1990, Curren et al., 2000]. Posing the research question simply as How do the groups differ? is too vague to indicate the correct measure. The process of identifying the appropriate composite endpoint often requires the investigators to decide what specific questions the HRQoL data are expected to answer. Curren et al. [2000] describe a hypothetical trial where the objective is to reduce toxicity and maintain acceptable HRQoL. In this setting one might choose to study the worst (minimum) HRQoL score that occurred for each individual.

The selection also depends on the expected pattern of change across time and patterns of missing data. Consider several possible patterns of change in HRQoL across time (Figure 14.2). One profile is a steady rate of change over time reflecting either a constant decline in HRQoL (Figure 14.2-A) or a constant improvement (Figure 14.2-B). The first pattern is typical of patients with progressive disease where standard therapy is palliative rather than curative. This is the pattern observed in the two lung cancer trials (Studies 3 and 5). This pattern of change suggests that the rate of change or slope is a possible choice of a composite endpoint. A measure defined as the change from baseline to the last measure might initially seem relevant, but may not be desirable if patients who fail earlier and thus drop out from the study earlier have smaller changes than those patients with longer follow-up.

An alternative profile is an initial rapid change with a subsequent plateau after the maximum therapeutic benefit is realized (Figure 14.2-D). This might occur for therapies where the dose needs to be increased slowly over time or where there is a lag between the time therapy is initiated and the time maximal benefit is achieved (Studies 2 and 6). This profile illustrates the importance of identifying the clinically relevant question a priori. If the objective is to identify the therapy that produces the most rapid improvement in HRQoL, the time to reach a peak or pre-specified value is good choice. If, in contrast, the ultimate level of benefit is more important than the time to achieve the benefit, then a measure such as the post-treatment mean or mean change relative to baseline is desirable.

A third pattern of change could occur with a therapy that has transient benefits or toxicity (Figures 14.2-E and F). For example, individuals may experience transient benefits and then return to their baseline levels after the effect of the therapy has ceased. Alternatively, a therapy for cancer may significantly reduce HRQoL during therapy but ultimately result in a better HRQoL following therapy than the patient was experiencing at the time of diagnosis [Levine et al., 1988, Fetting et al., 1998] (Studies 1 and 4). For these more complex patterns of change over time, a measure such as the area under the curve might be considered as a summary of both early and continued effects of the therapy.

14.3 Summarizing across HRQoL Domains or Subscales

Almost all measures of HRQoL or health status include multiple domains or subscales. Many of these include composites of these domains. Well known examples are the Physical Component Scale (PCS) and the Mental Component Scale (MCS) of the Medical Outcome Study SF-36. Composite measures are useful when the objective is to obtain increased power to detect <u>consistent</u>

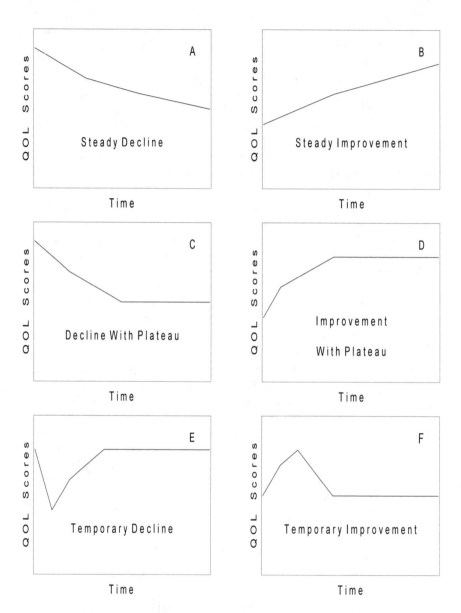

FIGURE 14.2 Patterns of change in HRQoL over time. (Reproduced from Figure 13.1, Quality of Life Assessment in Clinical Trials: Methods and Practice [Fairclough, 1998], with permission.)

differences across scales. The impact on interpretation is mixed. Reducing the number of comparisons simplifies interpretation, but we may be unclear about how the components contribute to the composite measure.

The primary focus of this section is to emphasize that each of the composites utilizes weights that place different emphasis on each of the domains or subscales. Some options for weighting include

1. weights proportional to the number of questions for each domain,

2. equal weights for each domain,

3. factor analytic weights,

4. weights derived from patient preference measures and

5. statistically derived weights (e.g. correlation among domains).

14.3.1 Weighting Proportional to the Number of Questions

Many HRQoL instruments compute an overall score where domains are weighted in proportion to the number of questions asked about each domain. In the FACT-Lung and FACT-BRM instruments, there are a number of composite endpoints. For both, a total score is computed by summing all subscales (Table 14.2). Another composite endpoint, the Trial Outcome Index is also constructed by summing the physical well-being, functional well-being and lung-cancer specific items to create the FACT-Lung TOI and by summing the physical well-being, functional well-being and the BRM specific items to create the FACT-BRM TOI. There is an implicit weighting of the subscales that is dependent on the number of items. For example, because there were only five questions assessing emotional well-being, this domain receives less weight than the other domains of physical, functional and social well-being (Table 14.2). Similarly, because there are 13 BRM specific questions and 7 lung cancer specific questions, the physical and functional well-being subscales have less weight in the FACT-BRM TOI than they do in the FACT-Lung TOI.

14.3.2 Factor Analytic Weights

The Physical Component Scale (PCS) and the Mental Component Scale (MCS) of the Medical Outcome Study SF-36 are examples of summary scores where weights are derived from factor analysis. These widely used scores present an excellent example of summary scores that need to be carefully examined when interpreting the results of a trial. The weights used to construct the summary scores were derived from both orthogonal [Ware et al., 1994] and oblique [Farivar et al., 2007] factor rotations. Orthogonal rotations identify factor weights that minimize the correlation between the PCS and MCS; oblique rotations allow the composite measures to be correlated. Note that in

TABLE 14.2 Composite measures from the FACT-Lung and FACT-BRM Version 2 instruments. Weights based on number of items used in constructing the total scores and the Trial Outcome Index (TOI).

Subscale	Items	Total Score Lung	Total Score BRM	TOI Lung	TOI BRM
Physical well-being	7	.200	.171	.333	.259
Social/Family well-being	7	.200	.171		
Relationship with doctor	2[†]	.057	.049		
Emotional well-being	5[‡]	.143	.122		
Functional well-being	7	.200	.171	.333	.259
Lung cancer subscale	7	.200		.333	
BRM Physical subscale	7		.171		.259
BRM Mental subscale	6		.146		.222

[†] Dropped from Version 4　　　　[‡] Six items in Versions 3 and 4

TABLE 14.3 Factor analytic weights for the Physical Component Scale (PCS) and the Mental Component Scale (MCS) of the Medical Outcome Study SF-36 using orthogonal rotations (UC) [Ware et al., 1994] and oblique rotations (C) [Farivar et al., 2007].

Component		PF	RP	BP	GH	V	SF	RE	MH
Physical	UC	0.42	0.35	0.32	0.25	0.03	-0.01	-0.19	-0.22
	C	0.20	0.31	0.23	0.20	0.13	0.11	0.03	-0.03
Mental	UC	-0.23	-0.12	- 0.10	-0.02	0.24	0.27	0.43	0.49
	C	-0.02	0.03	0.04	0.10	0.29	0.14	0.20	0.35

PF=Physical function, RP=Role-Physical, BP=Bodily Pain, GH=General Health, V=Vitality, SF=Social Function, RE=Role-Emotional, MH=Mental Health

the orthogonal scoring algorithms, physical function, role physical and bodily pain subscales make a modest negative contribution to the MCS and the mental health and role-emotional subscales make a modest negative contribution to the PCS score (Table 14.3). These negative contributions can produce surprising results. Simon et al. [1998] describe this in a study of antidepressant treatment where there were modest positive effects over time on the physical function, role-physical, bodily pain and general health, but a negative score (non-significant) was observed for the PCS because of the very strong positive effects in the remaining scales. The negative contribution of these remaining subscales overwhelmed the smaller contributions of the first four subscales. The point of this illustration is that investigators should be aware of the weights that are used and examine the individual components descriptively to fully understand the composite measures.

14.3.3 Patient Weights

Weights derived based on patient preferences are currently uncommon, but have a conceptual lure. For example, it is possible that most patients on adjuvant breast cancer therapy do not consider that physical well-being during a limited treatment period and disease-free survival have equal weight. They are willing to undergo adjuvant therapy with its associated morbidity including severe fatigue, hair loss and weight gain even after there is no detectable disease to maximize the chance that their disease will never recur. If weights that reflect patient preferences or values are available, they are likely to be more relevant than statistically derived weights.

A series of experimental questions are included in the FACT instruments (Versions 1-3) asking the patient to indicate how much the items in each subscale affect the patient's quality of life. For example, following the seven questions asking the patient to comment on energy, pain, nausea, side effects, ability to meet needs of family, feeling ill and spending time in bed, the following question appears:

> Looking at the above 7 questions, how much would you say your PHYSICAL WELL-BEING affects your quality of life?
>
> 0 1 2 3 4 5 6 7 8 9 10
> Not at all   Very much so

Similar questions appear for the other subscales. Responses to these questions could be used to weight the responses to each of the subscales.

Interestingly, these experimental questions have become optional in Version 4 and are not recommended for use in clinical trials. The developer cites two basic reasons [Cella, 2001]. First, using weighted scores and unweighted scores produce essentially the same results in all analyses examined. Second was the concern that the respondents were not answering the question as intended. Although some appeared to answer as a true weight, others seemed to answer the question as a summary of their response to the items and as many as 15-25% did not seem to understand at all and left the questions blank or responded in rather unusual ways. Other considerations may be a) a more complicated scoring system that would preclude hand scoring of the scale, 2) requirements for additional validation studies and 3) non-equivalence of scales from study to study.

14.3.4 Statistically Derived Weights: Inverse Correlation

Composite Endpoints

In a procedure proposed by O'Brien [1984], the weights are proportional to the inverse of the correlation of the K domains. The result is that the more strongly correlated domains are down-weighted. Two subscales that measure very similar aspects of HRQoL will contribute less to the overall score than two subscales that measure very different aspects of HRQoL. For example, consider results from the lung cancer trial (Study 3). Table 14.4 displays the correlations among the subscales. The physical well-being scores have the strongest correlation with the other subscales ($\hat{\rho} = 0.45 - 0.77$) and thus that scale has the smallest weight (Table 14.5). In contrast, the social well-being scores have the weakest correlation with other scales and the largest weight. The procedure is first to compute standardized scores (z_{ik}) for each of the K

TABLE 14.4 Study 2: Correlations among the AUC composite endpoints in the lung cancer trial.

	Phys	Func	Emot	Socl	LCS
Physical well-being	1.00	0.77	0.64	0.45	0.65
Functional well-being	0.77	1.00	0.56	0.36	0.68
Emotional well-being	0.64	0.56	1.00	0.41	0.49
Social well-being	0.45	0.36	0.41	1.00	0.36
Lung cancer subscale (LCS)	0.65	0.68	0.49	0.36	1.00

domains or subscales. Then compute a weighted sum of these standardized scores using the column sum of the inverse of the correlation (Table 14.5). $\hat{S}_i = J'\hat{R}^{-1}\hat{\mathbf{z}}_i$, where $\mathbf{z}_i = (z_{i1}, \ldots, z_{iK})'$, $J = (1, \ldots, 1)'$ and R is the estimated common correlation matrix of the observations ($\hat{\Sigma}$).

TABLE 14.5 Study 2: Inverse correlation (R^{-1}) and weights ($J'R^{-1}$) of the AUC composite endpoints in the lung cancer trial.

	Phys	Func	Emot	Socl	LCS
Physical well-being	3.21	-1.57	-0.76	-0.40	-0.51
Functional well-being	-1.57	2.91	-2.25	0.08	-0.86
Emotional well-being	-0.76	-0.25	1.79	-0.25	-0.12
Social well-being	-0.40	0.08	-0.25	1.30	-0.13
Lung cancer subscale (LCS)	-0.51	-0.86	-0.12	-0.13	2.02
Sum ($J'R^{-1}$)	-0.02	0.31	0.40	0.59	0.40

Composite endpoints with weights based on the inverse correlation are the most powerful [O'Brien, 1984, Pocock et al., 1987a] and do not require specification prior to analysis because the weights are determined by the data. The disadvantages are that they vary from study to study [Cox et al., 1992] and they may not reflect the importance that patients place on different domains.

Summary Measures

The weighted average of the individual values proposed by O'Brien [1984] also extends to the construction of a summary measure with the use of a weighted average of asymptotically normal test statistics such as the two-sample t-statistic.

$$t_{hk} = \frac{\hat{\theta}_{hk}}{\hat{\sigma}_{(\hat{\theta})hk}}, \quad t_h = (t_{h1}, \ldots, t_{hK})', \tag{14.1}$$

$$\hat{S}_h = J' R^{-1} t_h, \quad J = (1, \ldots, 1)' \tag{14.2}$$

R is the estimated common correlation matrix of the raw data $(\hat{\Sigma})$ or the pooled correlation matrix of the estimated means $(\hat{\mu}_{jk})$. An alternate way to express the summary statistic is

$$\hat{S}_h = \sum_{k=1}^{K} w_k g(\hat{\beta}_{kj}) \tag{14.3}$$

where $g(\hat{\beta}_{kj}) = \hat{\mu}_{kj}/\hat{\sigma}_{(\hat{\mu}_{kj})}$ and $(w_1, \ldots, w_K) = J'R^{-1}$. Because $\hat{S}_h$ is a linear combination of asymptotically normal parameter estimates, the asymptotic variance of the composite endpoint is

$$Var(\hat{S}_h) = W' Cov[g(\hat{\beta}_{hk})]W. \tag{14.4}$$

For two treatment groups, we can test the hypotheses $S_1 = S_2$ or $\theta = S_1 - S_2 = 0$ using a t-test with $N - 4$ degrees of freedom

$$t_{N-4} = (\hat{S}_1 - \hat{S}_2) \left[Var(\hat{S}_1 - \hat{S}_2) \right]^{-1/2} = \hat{\theta} \left[Var(\hat{\theta}) \right]^{-1/2} \tag{14.5}$$

for small samples [Pocock et al., 1987a]. More generally, for large samples we can test the hypothesis $S_1 = S_2 \cdots = S_k$ using a Wald χ^2 statistic:

$$\chi^2_{k-1} = \hat{\phi}' \left[Var(\hat{\phi}) \right]^{-1} \hat{\phi}, \quad \hat{\phi} = (\hat{S}_2 - \hat{S}_1, \ldots, \hat{S}_n - \hat{S}_1)'. \tag{14.6}$$

14.4 Summary Measures across Time

Summary measures are constructed by combining group measures over time. Examples of these group measures are the parameter estimates from growth curve models or means from repeated measures models. Summary measures across time include the change between two prespecifed time points, mean post baseline, and area under the curve (AUC). In practice the use of summary measures is often preferable when it may be much easier to develop a model-based method for handling missing data than to develop strategies for imputing each individual missing value required to compute the composite measures.

14.4.1　Notation

The general procedure for the construction of summary measure is to obtain parameter estimates for the hth group $(\hat{\beta}_{hj})$ and then reduce the set of J estimates to a single summary statistic:

$$\hat{S}_h = \sum_{j=1}^{J} w_j g(\hat{\beta}_{hj}). \tag{14.7}$$

In a repeated measures design, $g(\hat{\beta}_{hj})$ is generally a vector of the estimates of the means over time $(\hat{\mu}_{hj})$ adjusted for important covariates [Fairclough, 1997]. In a growth curve model, $g(\hat{\beta}_{hj})$ contains the parameter estimates of the polynomial or piecewise regression model. $g(\hat{\beta}_{hj})$ may also be a direct estimate of a summary statistic such as the slope or a test statistic such as the ratio of the estimate to its standard error (t_{hj}).

If the data are complete, one can use any multivariate analysis method to estimate β_{hj}. When data are missing, one must use an analytic method that is appropriate for the missing data mechanism as described in Chapters 3, 4, 6 and 9-12.

TABLE 14.6 Examples of summary measures over time calculated as a linear function of parameter estimates: $\hat{S}_h = \sum_{j=1}^{p} w_j g(\hat{\beta}_{hj})$.

Description	$g(\hat{\beta}_{hj})$	Weights (w_j)
Mean of r follow-up observations	$\hat{\mu}_{hj}$	$0, \ldots, \frac{1}{r}, \ldots, \frac{1}{r}$
Mean of follow-up - first observation	$\hat{\mu}_{hj}$	$-1, \ldots, \frac{1}{r}, \ldots, \frac{1}{r}$
Average Rate of Change $\hat{\beta}_{h2}$ (slope)		1
Area Under the Curve	$\hat{\mu}_{hj}$	$\frac{t_2-t_1}{2}, \ldots, \frac{t_{j+1}-t_{j-1}}{2}, \ldots, \frac{t_J-t_{J-1}}{2}$

14.4.2　Simple Linear Functions

First let us consider the migraine prevention trial (Study 2) and assume that the primary endpoint for this trial is the change from baseline to the average of the post-baseline assessments. The choice was based on the expected trajectory (Figure 14.2-D). Next let us consider the lung cancer trial (Study 3) and assume that the primary endpoint for this trial was the change from baseline to 26 weeks (or the fourth assessment). The choice was based on the expected trajectory (Figure 14.2-A). For both examples, let us presume that we have selected an analysis that appropriately handles the missing data or is being used as part of a sensitivity analysis.

Repeated Measures Models

To illustrate the construction of a summary measure of statistic in a repeated measures let us assume that we have fit a reference cell model with the reference cell defined as the baseline assessment (Table 14.7). (See Sections 3.3.4-3.3.6 for examples in SAS, SPSS, and R). The summary measures are simple linear combinations of the parameter estimates. (See Sections 3.5.1-3.5.3). The change from baseline to the last assessment given this parameterization is estimated as:

$$\text{Control:} \quad \hat{S}_0 = \underbrace{(\hat{\beta}_0 + \hat{\beta}_3)}_{Time4} - \underbrace{\hat{\beta}_0}_{Time1}$$

$$\text{Expermntl:} \quad \hat{S}_1 = \underbrace{(\hat{\beta}_0 + \hat{\beta}_3 + \hat{\beta}_6)}_{Time4} - \underbrace{\hat{\beta}_0}_{Time1}$$

$$\text{Difference:} \ \hat{S}_1 - \hat{S}_0 = \underbrace{\hat{\beta}_6}_{Time4} - \underbrace{0}_{Time1}$$

The average change from baseline to the mean follow-up is:

$$\text{Control:} \ \hat{S}_0 = (\underbrace{(\hat{\beta}_0 + \hat{\beta}_1)}_{Time2} + \underbrace{(\hat{\beta}_0 + \hat{\beta}_2)}_{Time3} + \underbrace{(\hat{\beta}_0 + \hat{\beta}_3)}_{Time4})/3 - \underbrace{\hat{\beta}_0}_{Time1}$$

$$= \hat{\beta}_1/3 + \hat{\beta}_2/3 + \hat{\beta}_3/3$$

$$\text{Expermntl:} \ \hat{S}_1 = (\underbrace{(\hat{\beta}_0 + \hat{\beta}_1 + \hat{\beta}_4)}_{Time2} + \underbrace{(\hat{\beta}_0 + \hat{\beta}_2 + \hat{\beta}_5)}_{Time3} + \underbrace{(\hat{\beta}_0 + \hat{\beta}_3 + \hat{\beta}_6)}_{Time4})/3 - \underbrace{\hat{\beta}_0}_{Time1}$$

$$= \hat{\beta}_1/3 + \hat{\beta}_2/3 + \hat{\beta}_3/3 + \hat{\beta}_4/3 + \hat{\beta}_5/3 + \hat{\beta}_6/3$$

$$\text{Difference:} \ \hat{S}_1 - \hat{S}_0 = (\underbrace{\hat{\beta}_4}_{Time2} + \underbrace{\hat{\beta}_5}_{Time3} + \underbrace{\hat{\beta}_6}_{Time4})/3 - \underbrace{0}_{Time1}$$

$$= \hat{\beta}_4/3 + \hat{\beta}_5/3 + \hat{\beta}_6/3$$

These examples are simple and it is possible to figure out the summary measures in one's head. But to insure that it is done correctly when models get more complicated, I recommend that you create tables of the form displayed in Table 14.7 and double check the order in which the parameters are listed to insure that the summary measure is correctly computed. When additional covariates are added, they should also be included. Centering the covariates (See Section 5.23) simplifies these computations as they drop out of the contrasts.

TABLE 14.7 Models with a common baseline for studies 2 and 3.

Repeated measures reference cell model

Treatment	Time 1	Time 2	Time 3	Time 4
Control	β_0	$\beta_0 + \beta_1$	$\beta_0 + \beta_2$	$\beta_0 + \beta_3$
Experimntl	β_0	$\beta_0 + \beta_1 + \beta_4$	$\beta_0 + \beta_2 + \beta_5$	$\beta_0 + \beta_3 + \beta_6$
Difference	0	β_4	β_5	β_6

Growth-curve model with single change in slope

Treatment	Week 0	Week 6	Week 12	Week 26
Control	β_0	$\beta_0 + 6\beta_1$	$\beta_0 + 12\beta_1 + 6\beta_2$	$\beta_0 + 26\beta_1 + 20\beta_2$
Experimntl	β_0	$\beta_0 + 6\beta_3$	$\beta_0 + 12\beta_3 + 6\beta_4$	$\beta_0 + 26\beta_3 + 20\beta_4$
Difference	0	$6(\beta_3 - \beta_1)$	$12(\beta_3 - \beta_1)$	$26(\beta_3 - \beta_1)$
			$+6(\beta_4 - \beta_2)$	$+20(\beta_4 - \beta_2)$

Mixed-Effects Growth Curve Models

A similar procedure is used for models fit with a mixed-effect growth curve. If a piecewise linear model had been used in Study 3, the expected values at the planned assessment times (0, 6, 12 and 26 weeks) are displayed in Table 14.7. The change from baseline to the last assessment given this parameterization is estimated as:

$$\text{Control:} \quad \hat{S}_0 = \underbrace{(\hat{\beta}_0 + 26\hat{\beta}_1 + 20\hat{\beta}_2)}_{Week26} - \underbrace{\hat{\beta}_0}_{Week0}$$

$$\text{Expermntl:} \quad \hat{S}_1 = \underbrace{(\hat{\beta}_0 + 26\hat{\beta}_3 + 20\hat{\beta}_4)}_{Week26} - \underbrace{\hat{\beta}_0}_{Week0}$$

$$\text{Difference:} \quad \hat{S}_1 - \hat{S}_0 = \underbrace{26(\hat{\beta}_3 - \hat{\beta}_1) + 20(\hat{\beta}_4 - \hat{\beta}_2)}_{Week26} - \underbrace{0}_{Week0}$$

The average change from baseline to the mean follow-up is:

$$\text{Control:} \quad \hat{S}_0 = \underbrace{((\hat{\beta}_0 + 6\hat{\beta}_1)}_{Week6} + \underbrace{(\hat{\beta}_0 + 12\hat{\beta}_1 + 6\hat{\beta}_2)}_{Week12}$$
$$+ \underbrace{(\hat{\beta}_0 + 26\hat{\beta}_1 + 20\hat{\beta}_2))/3}_{Week26} - \underbrace{\hat{\beta}_0}_{Week0}$$
$$= (6 + 12 + 26)\hat{\beta}_1/3 + (6 + 20)\hat{\beta}_2/3$$

$$\text{Expermntl:} \quad \hat{S}_1 = \underbrace{((\hat{\beta}_0 + 6\hat{\beta}_3)}_{Week6} + \underbrace{(\hat{\beta}_0 + 12\hat{\beta}_3 + 6\hat{\beta}_4)}_{Week12}$$
$$+ \underbrace{(\hat{\beta}_0 + 26\hat{\beta}_3 + 20\hat{\beta}_4))/3}_{Week26} - \underbrace{\hat{\beta}_0}_{Week0}$$

$$= (6 + 12 + 26)\hat{\beta}_3/3 + (6 + 20)\hat{\beta}_4/3$$

$$\text{Difference: } \hat{S}_1 - \hat{S}_0 = 44(\hat{\beta}_3 - \hat{\beta}_1)/3 + 26(\hat{\beta}_4 - \hat{\beta}_2)/3$$

See Chapter 4 for details of implementation of estimation and hypothesis testing in SAS, SPSS and R.

14.4.3 Area Under the Curve (AUC)

Another measure summarizing HRQoL over time is the area under the curve (AUC) of the HRQoL scores (Y_{hj}) plotted against time (t) [Cox et al., 1992, Matthews et al., 1990]. The area under the curve is applicable in virtually every setting. It is particularly useful when the expected trajectories are complicated (Figure 14.2-E and F), such as the renal cell carcinoma trial (Study 4). The classical application for the AUC occurs in pharmacokinetics, where the cumulative dose of a drug available is of interest. When the HRQoL measure is scored as a utility measure (with a range of 0 to 1), the AUC can be interpreted as quality-adjusted time. When we are looking at other measures, interpretation of the AUC will be facilitated when we scale time so that the period of interest is 1 unit of time: the AUC for each treatment group can be interpreted as the *average score* over the period of interest and the difference as the *average difference* between the curves.

Repeated Measures

When the model has been structured as a repeated measures analysis, the AUC can be estimated for each of the H groups by using a trapezoidal approximation (Figure 14.3). The area of each trapezoid is equal to the product of the height at the midpoint ($(Y_{hj} + Y_{h(j-1)})/2$) and the width of the base ($t_j - t_{j-1}$). The total area is calculated by adding areas of a series of trapezoids:

$$AUC_h(t_J) = \hat{S}_h = \sum_{j=2}^{J} (t_j - t_{j-1}) \frac{\hat{\mu}_{hj} + \hat{\mu}_{h(j-1)}}{2} \tag{14.8}$$

The equation can be rewritten as a weighted function of the means :

$$AUC_h(t_J) = \hat{S}_h = \frac{t_2 - t_1}{2} \hat{\mu}_{h1} + \sum_{j=2}^{J-1} \frac{t_{j+1} - t_{j-1}}{2} \hat{\mu}_{hj} + \frac{t_J - t_{J-1}}{2} \hat{\mu}_{hJ} \tag{14.9}$$

Because these summary measures are a linear function (contrast) of parameters of the form $\hat{\theta} = C\hat{\beta}$, estimation and testing hypotheses are straightforward and use the same principles as presented in Chapters 3 and 4.

For example, in the lung cancer trial, the planned times of the assessments were 0, 6, 12 and 26 weeks. The AUC over 26 weeks for the hth group is:

$$AUC_h(26) = \frac{t_2 - t_1}{2} \hat{\mu}_{h1} + \frac{t_3 - t_1}{2} \hat{\mu}_{h2} + \frac{t_4 - t_2}{2} \hat{\mu}_{h3} + \frac{t_4 - t_3}{2} \hat{\mu}_{h4}$$

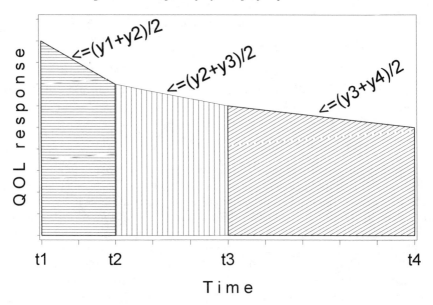

FIGURE 14.3 Calculation of the AUC using a trapezoidal approximation.

$$= \frac{6-0}{2}\hat{\mu}_{h1} + \frac{12-0}{2}\hat{\mu}_{h2} + \frac{26-6}{2}\hat{\mu}_{h3} + \frac{26-12}{2}\hat{\mu}_{h4}$$

Dividing this quantity by t_J or scaling time so that $t_J = 1$ allows us to interpret the summary measure as the average score over the period of interest.

14.4.3.1 Mixed-Effect Growth Curve Models

When the model has been structured as a growth curve model, the AUC is computed by integration from 0 to T. If a polynomial model has been used to describe the change in HRQoL over time:

$$AUC_h(T) = \int_{t=0}^{T} \sum_{j=0}^{J} \hat{\beta}_{hj} t^j \, \partial t = \sum_{j=0}^{J} \frac{t^{j+1}}{j+1}\hat{\beta}_{hj}\Bigg|_{t=0}^{T} = \sum_{j=0}^{J} \frac{T^{j+1}}{j+1}\hat{\beta}_{hj} \quad (14.10)$$

where $\hat{\beta}_{h0}$ is the estimate of the intercept for the hth group, $\hat{\beta}_{h1}$ is the linear coefficient for the hth group, etc.

For example, in the renal cell carcinoma study if we assumed a cubic model, the AUC is:

$$AUC_h(T) = \sum_{j=0}^{J=3} \frac{T^{j+1}}{j+1}\hat{\beta}_{hj}$$

$$= \frac{T^1}{1}\hat{\beta}_{h0} + \frac{T^2}{2}\hat{\beta}_{h1} + \frac{T^3}{3}\hat{\beta}_{h2}$$

If we were interested in the AUC during the initial period of therapy, defined as the first 8 weeks, the AUC is:

$$AUC_h = \underbrace{\frac{8^1}{1}}_{8} \hat{\beta}_{h0} + \underbrace{\frac{8^2}{2}}_{32} \hat{\beta}_{h1} + \underbrace{\frac{8^3}{3}}_{170.67} \hat{\beta}_{h2}$$

Estimates for longer periods of time, such as 26 and 52 weeks, are generated using the same procedure. In this study, the results would appear as follows where T is rescaled to be equal to 1. The estimates are now on the same scale as the original measure and have the alternative interpretation of the average score over the period from 0 to T.

For a piecewise regression model, one could estimate the means at each *knot* and then use a trapezoidal approximation. Integration provides a more direct method:

$$AUC_h(T) = \hat{S}_h = \int_{t=0}^{T} \sum_{j=0}^{J} \hat{\beta}_{hj} t^{[j]} \partial t$$

$$= \hat{\beta}_0 t \Big|_{t=0}^{T} + \sum_{j=1}^{J} \hat{\beta}_{hj} \frac{t^2}{2} \Big|_{t=T^{[j]}}^{T}$$

$$= \hat{\beta}_{h0} T + \sum_{j=1}^{J} \hat{\beta}_{hj} \frac{max(T - T^{[j]}, 0)^2}{2} \tag{14.11}$$

where $\hat{\beta}_{h0}$ is the estimate of the intercept for the hth group, $\hat{\beta}_{h1}$ is the initial slope and $\hat{\beta}_{hj}, j > 2$ is the change in slope at each of the knots, $T^{[l]}$. $t^{[0]} = 1$, $t^{[1]} = t$ and $t^{[j]} = max(t - T^{[j]})$.

In the renal cell carcinoma study, the piecewise regression model has two knots, one at 2 weeks and one at 8 weeks. Thus, the estimated AUC (rescaled to T=1) is

$$AUC_h(T) = (\hat{\beta}_{h0} T + \hat{\beta}_{h1} \frac{T^2}{2} + \hat{\beta}_{h2} \frac{max(T - 2, 0)^2}{2} + \hat{\beta}_{h3} \frac{max(T - 8, 0)^2}{2}) / T$$

If we were interested in the early period defined as the first 8 weeks, then

$$AUC_h(8) = (\hat{\beta}_{h0} 8 + \hat{\beta}_{h1} \underbrace{\frac{8^2}{2}}_{=32} + \hat{\beta}_{h2} \underbrace{\frac{max(8 - 2, 0)^2}{2}}_{=18} + \hat{\beta}_{h3} \underbrace{\frac{max(8 - 8, 0)^2}{2}}_{=0}) / 8.$$

14.5 Composite Endpoints across Time

The approach for constructing composite endpoints is to reduce the repeated measures from each individual to a single value. This approach is popular because simple univariate tests (e.g. t-tests) can be used for the analysis. For example, one might compute the slope of the scores observed for each subject and test the hypothesis that the slopes differed among the experimental groups. When the period of observation varies widely among subjects or data collection stops for some reason related to the outcome, this construction of composite endpoints is challenging. Easy fixes without careful thought only hide the problem. Many of the procedures for constructing composite endpoints assume data are missing completely at random (MCAR) [Omar et al., 1999] and are inappropriate in studies of HRQoL.

14.5.1   Notation

The construction of a composite endpoint that reduces the set of J measurements (Y_{ij}) on the ith individual to a single value (S_i), can be described as a weighted sum of the measurements (Y_{ij}) or a function of the measurements $(f(Y_{ij}))$. The general form is

$$S_i = \sum_{j=1}^{J} w_j \, f(Y_{ij}) \tag{14.12}$$

TABLE 14.8 Examples of composite endpoints constructed within individual across time: $S_i = \sum_{j=1}^{n} w_j f(Y_{ij})$.

Description	$f(Y_{ij})$	Weights (w_j)
Average Rate of Change	$Y_{ij} - \bar{Y}_i$	$(t_i - \bar{t})/(\sum t_i - \bar{t})^2$
Mean of r follow-up observations	Y_{ij}	$0, \ldots, \frac{1}{r}, \ldots, \frac{1}{r}$
Mean of r follow-up - baseline	Y_{ij}	$-1, \ldots, \frac{1}{r}, \ldots, \frac{1}{r}$
Area Under the Curve	Y_{ij}	$\frac{t_2 - t_1}{2}, \ldots, \frac{t_{j+1} - t_{j-1}}{2}, \ldots, \frac{t_n - t_{n-1}}{2}$
Average of Ranks	$\text{Rank}(Y_{ij})$	$1/n, \ldots, 1/n$
Minimum value	$\text{Min}(Y_i)$	1

Table 14.8 illustrates how this applies to a number of examples. Although in some cases, such as the average rate of change (slope), there are easier ways of constructing the composite endpoints, the table illustrates the common structure of all composite endpoints [Fairclough, 1997].

14.5.2 Missing Data

The calculation of composite endpoints is straightforward in the absence of missing and mistimed observations. It becomes much more challenging when there are missing data or the length of follow-up differs by individual. Strategies for handling missing data often need to be developed on a case by case basis. All of the following approaches make assumptions that may or may not be reasonable in specific settings and it is advisable to examine the sensitivity of the conclusions to the various assumptions (Table 14.9).

For example, if intermediate observations are missing, one could interpolate between observations. This approach assumes that these intermediate missing values are random and that the previous and following measures are taken under similar conditions. Interpolation is reasonable when the expected pattern of change over time is roughly linear (Figure 14.2-A, B) or constant. Interpolation would not make sense in the design used for the adjuvant breast cancer study (Study 1) for missing assessments during therapy. Interpolation between the pre- and post-therapy assessments would obviously overestimate the HRQoL of subjects during therapy. Nor would interpolation during the early phase of the renal cell carcinoma study (Study 4) make sense given the rapid drop in HRQoL followed by recovery.

Dropout and other causes of differences in the length of follow-up among individuals is another challenge. For a patient who dropped out, the last measurement could be imputed by 1) carrying the last value forward, 2) extrapolating from the last two observations or 3) implementing one of the imputation techniques described in Chapters 6 and 7. The most popular approach is to carry the value of the last observation forward (LVCF). Unfortunately, LVCF is often implemented without careful thought. This is a reasonable strategy if the expected pattern of change within individuals is either a steady improvement (Figure 14.2-B) or improvement with a plateau (Figure 14.2-D). But with other patterns of change (Figure 14.2-A,C,E), this strategy could bias the results in favor of interventions with early dropout.

Assigning zero is a valid approach for HRQoL scores that are explicitly anchored at zero for the health state of death. These are generally scores measured using multi-attribute, time trade off (TTO) or standard gamble (SG) techniques to produce *utility* measures (see Chapter 15). However, the majority of HRQoL instruments are developed to maximize discrimination among patients. In these instruments a value of zero would correspond to the worst possible outcome on every question. Even as the patients approach death, this is unlikely for most scales. Assigning zero also has some statistical implications. If the proportion of deaths is substantial, the observations may mimic a binomial distribution and the results roughly approximate a Kaplan-Meier analysis of survival.

TABLE 14.9 Possible strategies for handling missing data in the calculation of composite endpoints.

Problem	Solution	Assumptions / Limitations
Intermittent missing values	Interpolation	Change approximately linear over time period; Obs at t_{ij-1} and t_{ij+1} measured under similar conditions as t_{ij}
Mistimed last observation $(t_{iJ} \neq T)$	Estimate Y_{iT}	$Y_{iT} = \frac{(T-t_{iJ-1})Y_{iJ}+(T-t_{iJ})Y_{iJ-1}}{t_{iJ}-t_{iJ-1}}$
Incomplete follow-up	Extrapolation or LVCF	Potential bias favoring early dropout
Death	Minimum value	Potential bias favoring early death
	Zero	Mimics survival analysis; Questionable interpretation except for utilities

14.5.3   Average Rate of Change (Slopes)

When the changes over time are approximately linear, the average rate of change (or slope) may provide an excellent summary of the effect of an intervention. When there is virtually no dropout during the study or the dropout occurs only during the later part of the study, it is feasible to fit a simple regression model to the available data on each individual. This is often referred to as the ordinary least squares slope (OLS slope). $\hat{\beta}_{i2}$ is the estimated slope from a simple linear regression,

$$\hat{\beta}_i^{OLS} = \sum_{}^{J} \frac{(X_{ij} - \bar{X}_i)(Y_{ij} - \bar{Y}_i)}{(X_{ij} - \bar{X}_i)^2} = (X_i'X_i)^{-1}X_i'Y_i \qquad (14.13)$$

Lung Cancer Trial

At first glance, estimating individual slopes might be an approach for the lung cancer trial. But as a friend of mine often quotes, "The devil is in the details". Recall that a fourth of the subjects had only a single HRQoL assessment and would contribute nothing to the analysis. Further, less than half of the subjects had three or more observations, so that a substantial proportion of the subjects is likely to have unstable estimates of their slopes. Finally, there is a suspicion that the data are MNAR. As a practical design issue, it is advisable to plan frequent assessments during the early phase of a trial if one is intending to use this approach and dropout is likely.

Impact of Missing Data

Obviously, slopes for each individual can be estimated if all subjects have two or more observations. However, the estimates of the slope will have a large associated error when the available observations span a short period of time relative to the entire length of the study. The wide variation in slopes estimated with OLS is displayed in Figure 14.4. If there is a substantial proportion of subjects with only one or two observations, it may be necessary to use either imputed values for later missing values or the empirical Bayes (EB) estimates from a mixed-effects model. Because this second estimate also uses information from other individuals, it is more stable especially with highly unbalanced longitudinal studies where some individuals have only a few observations. The EB slopes display shrinkage toward the average slope as the estimator is a weighted average of the observed data and the overall average slope [Laird and Ware, 1982] (See Section 5.6). For individuals with only a few observations, the EB slope is very close to the overall average. This is illustrated by the narrow distribution of estimates displayed in Figure 14.4. Note that both approaches assume the data are missing at random (MAR). The distribution of the slopes derived using LVCF illustrates the tendency of these values to center around zero. This is by definition for those who drop out after the first observation. Finally, the distribution of slopes is displayed from the multiply imputed data. Values are more widely distributed than for either the EB or LVCF strategies. Clearly, the distribution of the composite endpoints can be sensitive to the method used to handle the missing data.

14.5.4 Area Under the Curve (AUC)

The AUC for the ith individual can be estimated using a trapezoidal approximation from the observed scores (Figure 14.3). The area of each trapezoid is equal to the product of the height at the midpoint $((Y_{ij} + Y_{i(j-1)})/2)$ and the width of the base $(t_j - t_{j-1})$. The total area is calculated by adding areas of a series of trapezoids

$$S_i = AUC_i = \sum_{j=2}^{J} (t_j - t_{j-1}) \frac{Y_{ij} + Y_{i(j-1)}}{2} \tag{14.14}$$

With a little algebraic manipulation, this calculation can also be expressed as a weighted function of the HRQoL scores where the weights are determined by the spacing of the assessments over time:

$$AUC_i = \frac{t_2 - t_1}{2} Y_{i1} + \sum_{j=2}^{J-1} \frac{t_{j+1} - t_{j-1}}{2} Y_{ij} + \frac{t_J - t_{J-1}}{2} Y_{iJ} \tag{14.15}$$

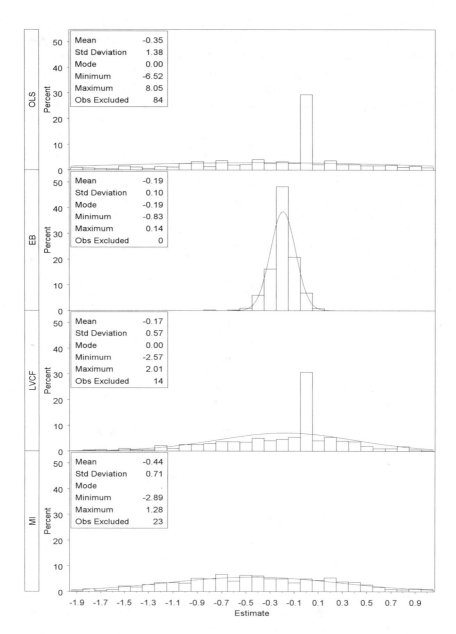

FIGURE 14.4 Study 3: Distribution of composite endpoints using different methods of estimating the slope. Ordinarily Least Squares (OLS), Empirical Bayes (EB), Last Value Carried Forward (LVCF), Multiple Imputation (MI).

Impact of Missing Data

There are a number of options for constructing a measure of the AUC in the presence of missing data (Table 14.9). All have some limitations. The best choice will depend on the objectives and the reasons for missing assessments or dropout.

Fayers and Machin [Fayers and Machin, 2000] describe one alternative, the average AUC, which may be useful in some settings where the length of follow-up varies among subjects. This composite endpoint is calculated by dividing the total AUC by the total time of observation. $S_i = AUC_i/T_i$ where T_i is the total time of observation for the ith individual. If the research question concerns the average HRQoL of patients during a limited period such as the duration of a specific therapy, this may be a reasonable approach. However, if early termination due to toxicity or lack of efficacy results in similar or higher summary scores, then the results are biased. This is illustrated in Figure 14.5, where the average areas are the same for the two curves, but the scores decline more rapidly in the subject who terminated the study early. As always, the choice between these two approaches depends primarily on the research question.

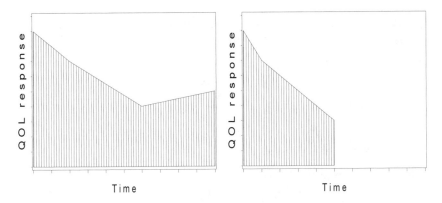

FIGURE 14.5 Contrast of two subjects with different lengths of follow-up. Both subjects have the same AUC when adjusted by each individual's length of follow-up.

The issue of selecting a strategy for computing the AUC also occurs when patients die during the study. One strategy is to extrapolate the curve to zero at the time of death. Other proposed strategies include assigning values of 1) the minimum HRQoL score for that individual or 2) the minimum HRQoL score for all individuals [Hollen et al., 1997]. One strategy will not work for all studies. Whichever strategy is chosen, it needs to be justified and the sensitivity of the results to the assumptions examined.

One might be inclined to present the AUC values calculated to the time of censoring, as one would present survival data. This approach would appear to have the advantages of displaying more information about the distribution of the AUC values and accommodating administrative censoring. Unfortunately, administrative censoring is informative on the AUC scale [Gelber et al., 1998, Glasziou et al., 1990, Korn, 1993] and the usual Kaplan-Meier estimates are biased. Specifically, if the missing data are due to staggered entry and incomplete follow-up is identical for two groups, the group with poorer HRQoL will have lower values of the AUC and are censored earlier on the AUC scale. Knowing when a subject is censored on the AUC scale gives us some information about the AUC score and thus the censoring is informative. Korn [Korn, 1993] suggests an improved procedure to reduce the bias of the estimator by assuming that the probability of censoring in short intervals is independent of the HRQoL measures prior to that time. Although this assumption is probably not true, if the HRQoL is measured frequently and the relationship between HRQoL and censoring is weak, the violation may be small enough that the bias in the estimator will also be small.

A practical problem with the use of the AUC or the mean of post-baseline measures as a composite endpoint occurs when the baseline HRQoL scores differ among groups. If one group contains more individuals who score their HRQoL consistently higher than other individuals, small (possibly statistically non-significant) differences are magnified over time in the composite endpoint. One possible solution is to calculate the AUC relative to the baseline score.

$$AUC_i^* = AUC_i - Y_{i1}(t_J - t_1) \tag{14.16}$$

$$= \left[\frac{t_2 - t_1}{2} - (t_J - t_1) \right] Y_{i1} + \sum_{j=2}^{J-1} \frac{t_{j+1} - t_{j-1}}{2} Y_{ij} + \frac{t_J - t_{J-1}}{2} Y_{iJ}$$

14.5.5 Average of Ranks

Another method proposed for combining information across repeated measures uses ranks [O'Brien, 1984]. The measurements on all subjects are ranked at each time point and then the average of the ranks across the n time points is computed for each individual. In the notation of equation 14.12 and Table 14.8, $f(Y_{ij})$ is the rank of Y_{ij} among all values of the jth measure and S_i is the average of the ranks for the ith individual ($w_j = 1/n$). When the data are complete, this procedure is straightforward.

Impact of Missing Data

If the reasons for missing data were known and one could make reasonable assumptions about the ranking of HRQoL in patients at each time point, one could possibly adapt this approach to a study with missing data. For example, it would not be unreasonable to assume that the HRQoL of patients who died or left the study due to excessive toxicity was worse than the HRQoL of those patients who remained on therapy. They would then be assigned the lowest possible rank for measurements scheduled after death or during the time of excessive toxicity. Other strategies that might be considered were discussed in Chapter 6 (see Table 6.7).

14.5.6 Analysis of Composite Endpoints

Univariate Analysis of Composite Endpoints

After constructing the composite endpoints, statistical tests (e.g. two-sample t-test, Wilcoxon Rank Sum test) are used to compare treatment groups. In most cases these tests assume that the observations are independent and identically distributed (i.i.d). The assumption of homogeneity of variance of the composite endpoints is often violated when the duration of follow-up is vastly different among subjects. For example, slopes estimated for individuals who drop out of the study early will have greater variation than slopes for those who complete the study. One solution is to weight the slopes using their standard errors, giving greater weight to those individuals with the longest follow-up. Unfortunately, unless dropout is MCAR, this will bias the analysis. The alternative procedure is to ignore the possible heterogeneity giving equal weight to all subjects. This later approach is generally more appropriate in studies of HRQoL where the MCAR assumption is rarely appropriate.

14.5.6.1 Stratified Analysis of Composite Endpoints

Dawson and Lagakos [1991, 1993], Dawson [1994] proposed a strategy for handling monotone dropout. First, we identify strata (g) defined by the dropout pattern. Composite endpoints are then calculated for each individual within the strata using just the observed data. This avoids the need to extrapolate past the point of dropout. Then a standardized test statistic, Z_g, for the two-arm comparison is calculated for each stratum. They use the non-parametric van der Waerden scores in their applications. These stratum specific test statistics are then combined into an overall test statistic: $Z = \sum w_g Z_g / \sqrt{\sum w_g^2}$. Dawson uses $w_g = \sqrt{j_g n_{g1} n_{g2} / (n_{g1} + n_{g2})}$ as a general set of weights [Dawson, 1994] and $w_g = \sqrt{\sum (x_{gj} - \bar{x}_g)^2 n_{g1} n_{g2} / (n_{g1} + n_{g2})}$ when the composite endpoints are slopes [Dawson and Lagakos, 1993].[*] Note that these weights will tend to increase the contribution of strata with longer follow-up.

When the data are missing completely at random, this approach will increase the power, since the across-strata variation is removed [Dawson and Lagakos, 1993, Dawson, 1994]. However, it is unclear how it will perform

---

[*]n_{gh} is the number of subjects in the gth stratum and the hth treatment arm. j_g is the number of observations used to compute the composite endpoint in the gth group. x_{gj} denotes the times when subjects in the gth group contribute observations.

TABLE 14.10 Hypothetical example illustrating
problem with stratified analysis of composite
endpoints when dropout rates differ across groups.

Strata (g)	Treatment	Subjects (n_{gh})	$\hat{S}_{h(g)}$	Z_g
1	A	10	-5	0
	B	40	-5	
2	A	40	20	0
	B	10	20	

when dropout is non-ignorable and the pattern of dropout differs by treatment group [Curren et al., 2000]. For example, there may not be any treatment difference in the summary statistic conditional on dropout: All $Z_g \approx 0 \rightarrow Z \approx 0$. But if the dropout patterns differ and the composite endpoints differ across the strata, then there are real differences that are not detected. To illustrate, consider a hypothetical example (Table 14.10) where there was extensive early dropout in one arm of the study. Higher scores indicate an improvement in HRQoL. Among those who drop out early $(g=1)$, the average composite endpoint score is -5 indicating a decline in HRQoL regardless of treatment arm in these subjects. Similarly, among those who remain on the study $(g=2)$, the composite endpoints average 20 in both groups. If we test for differences within each stratum we observe none, so the standardized test statistics are both approximately 0 $(Z_g \approx 0)$. However, it is clear that in arm A there were more individuals who remained on the study and experienced a greater benefit than on arm B. This example is highly exaggerated, but it illustrates the problem. One could imagine a similar, but less dramatic, scenario on a placebo controlled trial where there was early dropout among individuals who did not perceive any benefit from the intervention.

14.6   Summary

- Composite endpoints and summary measures

  1. facilitate interpretation by reducing the number of comparisons,
  2. increase the power to detect consistent differences over time or over HRQoL domains and
  3. may obscure differences in different directions.

- Selection of a composite or summary measure should depend on the research question, expected pattern of change over time and missing data patterns.

- Investigators should be aware of the weights used to construct composite and summary measures.

- Descriptive analyses of each of the components of a composite or summary measure should be generated to facilitate interpretation.

  Does one component drive the results or are there consistent differences across all the components?

  Are lack of differences due to components moving in different directions?

- In the presence of substantial missing data, construction of summary measures using models that are appropriate for the missing data mechanism may be more feasible than composite endpoints.

15

Quality Adjusted Life-Years (QALYs) and Q-TWiST

15.1 Introduction

In this chapter, I will change the focus to outcomes that can be interpreted on a time scale. Most studies of HRQoL consider measurement from one of two perspectives, outcomes expressed in the metric of the QOL scale and outcomes expressed in the metric of time. The latter group includes outcomes such as quality adjusted survival (QAS), quality adjusted life years (QALYs), and Q-TWiST that incorporate both quantity and quality of life. In some trials, these outcomes are measured as one component of an economic analysis. This is beyond the scope of this book and I will not attempt to address the analytic issues that arise in economic analyses; the reader is advised to consult books that have this as their sole focus [Drummond, 2001]. In other trials, the interest is in balancing improvements in survival with the impact of treatment on HRQoL. Questions of this nature are particularly relevant in diseases that have relatively short expected survival and the intent of treatment is palliative such as advanced-stage cancer. Scientific investigation of the balance between treatment options in diseases that have extended survival are generally outside the context of clinical trials and typically utilize larger population based observational studies.

This chapter will briefly present two approaches that might be encountered in a clinical trial. In the first, measures of patient preferences are measured repeatedly over time (Section 15.2). In the second approach, the average time in various health states is measured and weighted using preference measures that are specific to each of the health states (Section 15.3).

15.2 QALYs

This section describes calculation of quality-adjusted-life-years in trials where patient preferences are measured repeatedly over time. Trials in which patient preferences are measured directly using standard gamble (SG) or time-trade-off (TTO) measures are difficult to implement. This is balanced by the value of obtaining the patient's own preferences for their current health state. It is more common in clinical trials to obtain *multi-attribute* measures (e.g. HUI, EQ-5D, QWB) or transform health status scales (e.g. SF-36) to utility measures [Franks et al., 2003, Feeny, 2005]. Both of these methods rely on transformations of measures of current health states using formulas derived from the relationship between health states and utilities based on preferences from the general population. There are valid arguments for both approaches. The focus of the remainder of this section is on the analysis of longitudinal data obtained from clinical trials.

The basis for all of the methods is estimation of the area under a curve (AUC) generated by plotting the utility measure versus time. There are two approaches. The first strategy estimates the average trajectory in each treatment group and then calcuates the AUC using the parameter estimates (see Chapter 14). The second strategy, which will be the focus of this section, starts with the calculation of a value for each individual, $QALY_i$, that is a function of the utility scores and time. These values will then be subsequently analyzed as univariate measures.

15.2.1   Estimation of $QALY_i$

In an ideal trial, with the primary objective of estimating QALYs, we would have complete data measured on a regular schedule until death (t_D). If the measure was based on recollection of the past month, the schedule would be monthly. Two strategies are possible as illustrated in Figure 15.1. The first assumes that the utility measured at time j is an accurate reflection the entire period prior to the assessment (Figure 15.1 left).

$$QALY_i^R = \sum_{j=2}^{J_i} u_j * t + \frac{u_{J_i}}{2} * (t_D - t_{J_i}) \qquad (15.1)$$

The second approach assumes that u_j is an accurate assessment of the patients current preferences at time j and uses a trapezoidal function to approximate the average utility during the previous period (Figure 15.1 right).

$$QALY_i^T = \sum_{j=2}^{J_i} \frac{(u_j + u_{j-1})}{2} * t + \frac{u_{J_i}}{2} * (t_D - t_{J_i}) \qquad (15.2)$$

In both approaches, the contribution of the final interval that includes death uses a trapezoidal function. The calculations are illustrated in Table 15.1.

These conditions are obviously infeasible in most trials. The schedule is more infrequent, there are missing and mistimed assessments, and all subjects are not followed to death. So how do we calculate QALYs under more realistic conditions?

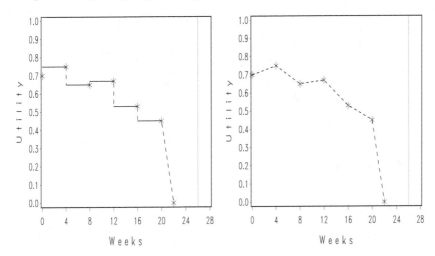

FIGURE 15.1 Illustration of two techniques to estimate $QALY_i$ when time between assessments (4 weeks) equals the period of recall using equation 15.1 (left) and 15.2 (right). Observations are indicated by $\star$. Periods using trapezoidal approximation are indicated by a dashed line.

Limited Follow-Up

Most trials are not designed to follow all subjects to death. In these trials, we need to estimate QALYs over a fixed period of time, t_C. The choice of what period of time is influenced by the length of follow-up of those subjects who have not experienced death. Computationally, the estimation of QALYs will be easiest if we use the minimum follow-up time. It requires no assumptions about surviving subjects after their last follow-up but ignores data on individuals who survive longer. Equations 15.1 and 15.2 are modified slightly for subjects who did not die during the follow-up period, where J_i is now the number assessment before the minimum follow-up time (t_C), and $u_C = u_{J_i} + (u_{J_i+1} - u_{J_i})/(t_{J_i+1} - t_{J_i}) * (t_C - t_{J_i})$ is the estimated utility at t_C (using a trapezoidal estimate for the partial follow-up time).

$$QALY_i^R = \sum_{j=2}^{J_i} u_j * t + u_C(t_C - t_{J_i}) \tag{15.3}$$

$$QALY_i^T = \sum_{j=2}^{J_i} \frac{(u_j + u_{j-1})}{2} * t + \frac{(u_{J_i} + u_C)}{2} * (t_C - t_{J_i}) \tag{15.4}$$

At the other extreme is the maximum follow-up time of all survivors. This procedure is unjustified both in terms of the precision of the estimate and tractability of estimation procedures. Choosing the median follow-up time (or some value close to it) is a reasonable compromise. This requires identifying

TABLE 15.1 Example calculations for $QALY_i$ using the two techniques (Recall Period and trapezoidal Approximation) for defining the curve when time between assessments equals period of recall. T_j is in weeks, so the last step will be to convert the sum to years.

j	T_j	U_j	Recall Period (Equation 15.1)		Trapezoidal Approximation (Equation 15.2)	
1	0	0.70				
2	4	0.75	0.75*4=	3.00	(0.75+0.70)/2*4=	2.90
3	8	0.65	0.65*4=	2.60	(0.65+0.75)/2*4=	2.80
4	12	0.67	0.67*4=	2.68	(0.67+0.65)/2*4=	2.64
5	16	0.53	0.53*4=	2.12	(0.53+0.67)/2*4=	2.40
6	20	0.45	0.45*4=	1.80	(0.45+0.53)/2*4=	1.96
7	22	0.00	0.45/2*(22-20)=	0.45	0.45/2*(22-20)=	0.45
Sum in Weeks				12.65		13.15
Sum in Years				0.242		0.252

a strategy to deal with individuals who are censored prior to the median follow-up time. A potential, though not necessarily recommended, method of extrapolation would be a form of last value carried forward.

Timing of Assessments

The timing of the assessments are likely to vary from subject to subject and will be less frequent than the period of recall (Figure 15.2). For the method relying solely on trapezoidal approximation, the equations are are only slightly modified. In equation 15.6, t is replaced by the observed difference between the assessments $t_j - t_{j-1}$ as illustrated in Table 15.2. Modifying equation 15.3 to obtain equation 15.5 is slightly more complicated. When the time between assessments is less than the period of recall (t), the length of the interval is $t_j - t_{j-1}$. When the time between assessments is greater than the period of recall, the value of the utility is extended back for the recall period and a trapezoidal approximation is used for the period of time that precedes the period of recall. This is illustrated in Figure 15.2 (left).

$$QALY_i^R = \sum_{j=2}^{J_i} [u_j * min(t, t_j - t_{j-1}) \tag{15.5}$$
$$+ \frac{(u_j + u_{j-1})}{2} * max(0, (t_j - t) - t_{j-1}]$$
$$+ u_C * (t_C - (t_{J_i} - t))$$
$$+ \frac{(u_j + u_{j-1})}{2} * max(0, min(t_C, (t_{J_i} - t)) - t_{j-1})$$

$$QALY_i^T = \sum_{j=2}^{J_i} \frac{(u_j + u_{j-1})}{2} * (t_j - t_{j-1}) \tag{15.6}$$
$$+ \frac{(u_{J_i} + u_C)}{2} * (t_C - t_{J_i})$$

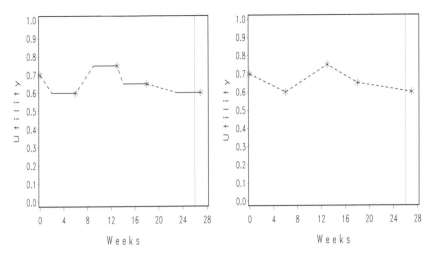

FIGURE 15.2 Illustration of two techniques to estimate $QALY_i$ when time between assessments is greater than the period of recall (4 weeks) using equation 15.5 (left) and 15.6 (right). Observations are indicated by $\star$. Vertical line indicates t_C.

If death occurs prior to t_C, then the last two terms of equation 15.5 and the last term of equation 15.6 are replaced by $\frac{u_{J_i}}{2} * (t_D - t_{J_i})$ as was done in equations 15.1 and 15.2.

Missing Assessments

When the time between assessments is extended due to missing assessments, the above approach extrapolates between the observed data. This is appropriate when the changes over time occur at a constant rate. If missing assessments occur because of abrupt changes in health states, this approach may result in bias estimates.

15.2.2   Analysis of $QALY_i$

Analysis of the individual measures, $QALY_i$, will involve univariate methods (e.g. t-tests, Wilcoxon Rank Sum test, simple linear regression) that are appropriate for the distribution of the $QALY_i$ values and sample size. When there is censoring due to limited follow-up, one tempting strategy is to analyze the $QALY_i$ values as if they were times to an events, censoring those who have not died. When I first approached this problem, I considered this option but fortunately learned that it violates the assumption of non-informative censoring before I publicly proposed it. In this situation, censoring is informative as the contribution to the $QALY_i$ value that is observed before censoring is correlated with the value that would be observed after censoring. This problem

TABLE 15.2 Example calculations for $QALY_i$ using the two techniques (Recall Period and Trapezoidal Approximation) for defining the curve when time between assessments <u>does not</u> equal the period of recall. Period of assessment is limited to 26 weeks.

			Recall Period (Equation 15.5)		Trapezoid (Equation 15.6)	
j	T_j	U_j				
1	0	0.70				
2	6	0.60	.60*4+(.60+.70)/2*2=	3.00	(.60+.70)/2*(6-0)=	2.90
3	13	0.75	.75*4+(.75+.60)/2*3=	2.60	(.75+.60)/2*(13-6)=	2.80
4	18	0.65	.65*4+(.65+.75)/2*1=	2.68	(.65+.75)/2*(18-13)=	2.64
5	27	0.60	.60*3+(.61+.65)/2*5=	2.12	$(.61^*+.65)/2*(26-18)=$	2.40
Sum in Weeks				17.59		17.78
Sum in Years				0.337		0.341

*Week 26 trapezoidal approx.: $u_C = 0.65 + (0.60 - 0.65)/(27 - 18) * (26 - 18) = 0.61$

is one of the issues that the developers of the Q-TWiST methodology cite as a motivation to develop that method [Glasziou et al., 1990].

15.3   Q-TWiST

A second method to integrate quality and quantity of life is Q-TWiST. A fundamental requirement for this approach is that we can define distinct health-states. In the original application of this method [Glasziou et al., 1990] in breast cancer patients, four health states were defined:

TOX   the period during which the patients were receiving therapy and presumably experiencing toxicity;

TWiST   the period after therapy during which the patients were without symptoms of the disease or treatment;

REL   the period between relapse (recurrence of disease) and death;

DEATH   the period following death.

The second assumption is that each health state is associated with a weight or value of the health state relative to perfect health that is representative of the entire time the subject is in that health state (e.g. utility or preference measures). The assumption that the utility for each health state does not vary with time has been termed *utility independence* [Glasziou et al., 1990].

   A third assumption is that there is a natural progression from one health state to another. In the above example, it was assumed that patients would progress from TOX to TWiST to REL to DEATH. The possibility of skipping health states, but not going backwards, is allowed. Thus, a patient might progression from TOX directly to REL or DEATH, but not from TWiST back to TOX or REL back to TWiST. Obviously, exceptions could occur, and if very rare they might be ignored. The quantity Q-TWiST is a weighted score of the average time spent in each of these health sates, where the weights are based on perference scores. Additional assumptions are made in particular analyses and will be discussed in the remainder of this section.

15.3.1 Kaplan-Meier Estimates of Time in Health States

How do we estimate the average time in each of the health states? If all of the patients in the study have been followed to death, finding the average time in each health state is quite easy as the time for each is known for every patient. But when there is censoring, we need to use methods developed for survival analyses. Figure 15.3 illustrates Kaplan-Meier estimates for the time to the end of treatment (TOX), the end of the disease free survival (DFS), and the end of survival (SURV) for the patients in the breast cancer trial (Study 1) with up to 60 months of follow-up. The average time in TOX is equal to the AUC for the time to the end of treatment. The heath state TWiST is defined as the time between the end of TOX and DFS. The average time spent in TWiST is equal to the area between the two curves. Similarly, the health state REL is defined as the time between the end of DFS and SURV. The average time in REL is again the area between the curves. When follow-up is incomplete, we must estimate restricted means which estimate the average times in each health state up to a set limit, L. At first glance it might appear that 60 months (5 years) would be a good choice. However, for practical reasons related to estimation of the variance of the estimates (discussed later), it is more appropriate to pick a time where follow-up is complete for 50-75% of the subjects who are still being followed.

More formally, estimation of the mean times in each health state starts with identifying a common origin for the measurement of the transition times (T_0). Let $T_1, \cdots T_K$ denote the times at which a patient makes transitions between the health states. If a state is skipped, then $T_{k-1} = T_k$. The final health state (usually death), $K + 1$, can not be skipped or exited. The time spent in each state is

$$\Delta_k = T_k - T_{k-1}, \quad k = 1, \cdots, K \tag{15.7}$$

When there is no censoring (or the last observation is an event), most programs will provide estimates of the mean and standard error of $T_k - T_0$, but not for $T_k - T_{k-1}$. The major difficulty is obtaining the variance $T_k - T_{k-1}$. As a consequence, a bootstrap procedure is used to estimate the mean and standard errors associated with $T_1, \cdots T_K$ and their differences. (See Appendices for additonal details about bootstrap procedures.)

The procedure is as follows:

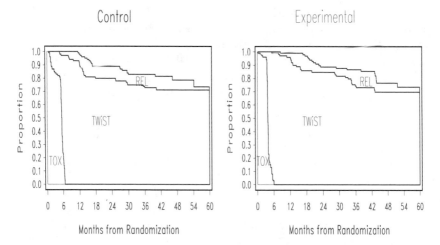

FIGURE 15.3 Study 1: Partitioned survival plots for the control and experimental groups of the breast cancer trial. Each plot shows the estimated curves for TOX, DFS and Surv. Areas between the curves correspond to time spent in the TOX, TWiST and REL health states.

1. Generate a random sample (with replacement) of patients from each of the treatment groups.

2. Estimate a "survival" curve $(\hat{S}_k(t))$ for each of the K transition times.

3. Calculate the area under the curve (AUC) from the origin to the t_c.

$$
\begin{aligned}
\hat{T}_k &= \int_{t=0}^{t_c} \hat{S}_k(t) \partial t \\
&= \sum_{j=1} \hat{S}(t_{j-1})(t_j - t_{j-1}) + \hat{S}(t_j) max(t_c - t_j, 0)
\end{aligned}
$$

where t_j are the times where an event occurs, $t_0 = 0$, t_c is the truncated follow-up time. The final term only is relevant when the last event time is greater than t_c.

4. Compute the mean time spent in each state, $\hat{\Delta}_k = \hat{T}_k - \hat{T}_{k-1}$.

5. Save results and repeat the above procedure for each bootstrap sample.

6. Compute the mean and standard error of $\hat{\Delta}_k$, $k = 1, \cdots, K$ over all the bootstrap samples. (Note that the standard error is the standard deviation of the bootstrap samples.)

As a follow-up to the previous comment about the restricted means, choosing a value for t_c where roughly 50% of subjects still alive are in active follow-up avoids bootstrap samples in which the last person is censored prior to t_c.

TABLE 15.3 Study 1: Summary of average times in months of various health states. Time is truncated at 48 months. Q-TWiST estimates assume that $U_{TOX}=0.8$ and 0.7 (s.e=0.05) for the control and experimental groups respectively and $U_{REL}=0.5$ (s.e=0.10) for both groups.

	Control		Experimental		Difference	
Outcome	Est	(s.e.)	Est	(s.e.)	Est	(s.e.)
TOX	4.78	(0.16)	3.77	(0.08)	-1.01	(0.20)
DFS	38.7	(1.57)	40.2	(1.37)	1.44	(1.03)
SURV	42.5	(1.20)	43.4	(1.02)	0.94	(1.67)
TWiST =DFS-Tox	34.0	(1.57)	36.4	(1.35)	2.45	(2.01)
REL=SURV-DFS	3.77	(0.79)	3.27	(0.65)	-0.50	(0.90)
Q-TWiST	39.7	(1.42)	40.7	(1.23)	1.00	(1.83)

Table 15.3 illustrates a typical summary of the estimation of the times in each health state for each treatment group and the differences between them. The estimates represent restricted means for 48 months (4 years) and are derived from 1000 bootstrap samples. The times in TOX and REL are shorter and TWiST are longer for the experimental arm. If the weights (U_x) were known, the Q-TWiST values would be:

$$Q - TWiST = T_{TOX} * U_{TOX} + T_{TWiST} * \underbrace{U_{TWiST}}_{=1} \qquad (15.8)$$

$$+ \; T_{REL} * U_{REL} + T_{DEATH} * \underbrace{U_{DEATH}}_{=0}$$

Typically the weight for the period of time without symptoms U_{TWiST} is fixed at a value of 1 implying no loss of QALYs and for the period after death U_{DEATH} is fixed at a value of 0. Thus, for this example, there are only two potentially unknown weights, U_{TOX} and U_{REL}.

15.3.2   Case 1: Known Estimates of U_{TOX} and U_{REL}

Suppose that we had estimates of U_{TOX} and U_{REL} that were derived from another source of data. Recognizing that both time and utilities are estimates, there are two approaches to estimate the variance of the Q-TWiST estimates: the delta method (a Taylor series approximation) or bootstrap procedure. The delta method approximates the variance of the product of two independent random variables as:

$$Var(xz) = x^2 Var(z) + z^2 Var(x).$$

This could be applied to equation 15.9. Alternatively, as we are already using a bootstrap procedure to obtain variance estimates for the average times in

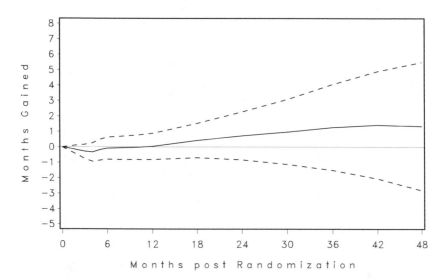

FIGURE 15.4 Study 2: Q-TWiST gain function. Assumes that $U_{TOX}=0.8$ and 0.7 (s.e=0.05) for the control and experimental groups respectively and $U_{REL}=0.5$ (s.e=0.10) for both groups.

each health state, adding this to the bootstrap procedure requires very little effort. In this illustration, we assume that our estimates are $U_{TOX}=0.8$ and 0.7 (s.e=0.05) for the control and experimental groups respectively and $U_{REL}=0.5$ (s.e=0.10). In addition to obtaining a random sample of the subjects, we would also sample values of the utilities. For example, the values of U_{TOX} would be sampled from a normal distribution with mean 0.8 and standard deviation of 0.05. Estimates of Q-TWiST obtained in this manner over a four year time span are displayed in Table 15.3. An alternative presentation of the results examines the differences in the Q-TWiST scores as a function of time (Figure 15.4).

15.3.3   Case 2: Two Unknown Weights That Are Equal across Treatments

When there are two unknown weights that can reasonably be assumed to be equal across the intervention arms, the developers of the Q-TWiST approach used a *threshold plot* to present the results. This plot uses the two unknown utility weights as the axes. It has four regions: two associated with values of Q-TWiST that favor the first treatment arm (one where the difference is statistically significant) and two that favor the second treatment arm. The central dividing line is defined by values of U_{TOX} and U_{REL} for which the

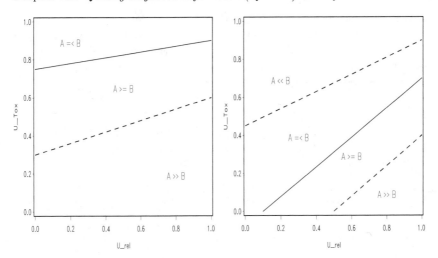

FIGURE 15.5 Threshold plots for two hypothetical trials. The region in which the differences between the two treatments are not statistically significant are indicated by $A >= B$ and $A <= B$. The region where treatment A is superior is indicated by $A >> B$.

value of Q-TWiST is equal for the two treatment arms. In our example it would be the line where

$$\Delta \text{Q-TWIST} = \Delta T_{TOX} U_{TOX} + \Delta T_{TWiST} + \Delta T_{REL} U_{REL} = 0 \quad (15.9)$$

Each of the regions defined by equation 15.9 is then divided unto the region where the differences are non-significant or significant at some prespecified level, generally $\alpha = 0.05$. The region of non-significance would correspond to the regions

$$z_{-\alpha/2} \leq \Delta \text{Q-TWIST}/s.e.(\text{Q-TWIST}) \leq z_{1-\alpha/2} \quad (15.10)$$

Solving equation 15.9 for U_{TOX} as a function of U_{REL} and substituting the estimates of the times in each health state from the breast cancer trial, the central line would be:

$$U_{TOX} = -(\Delta T_{TWiST} + \Delta T_{REL} * U_{REL})/\Delta T_{TOX}$$
$$= -(2.45 - 0.50 * U_{REL})/ - 1.01 = 0.49 * U_{REL} + 2.42$$

In the breast cancer trial, there are no possible values of U_{TOX} and U_{REL} that satisfy equation 15.9 when the follow-up time is 48 weeks. So to illustrate the principal of threshold plots, Figure 15.5 is based on made up data. The basic idea is that an individual would express their preferences with respect to the toxicity associated with treatment (U_{TOX}) and relapse (U_{REL}). In the

TABLE 15.4 Study 1: Differences between treatments of average times in months of various health states by presence of concurrent chronic disease and 4 or more positive nodes. Time is truncated at 48 months. See text for weights used to generate Q-TWiST estimates.

| | No chronic disease | | | | Chronic disease | | | |
| | 0-4 nodes | | 4+ nodes | | 0-4 nodes | | 4+ nodes | |
Outcome	Est	(s.e.)	Est	(s.e.)	Est	(s.e.)	Est	(s.e.)
TOX	-1.13	(0.24)	-1.58	(0.18)	-0.96	(0.23)	-1.41	(0.22)
DFS	-2.26	(2.13)	6.53	(4.03)	-2.19	(1.52)	1.05	(3.68)
SURV	1.63	(1.57)	3.69	(4.03)	-0.94	(1.31)	-5.73	(3.61)
TWiST	1.13	(2.09)	8.11	(3.99)	-1.23	(1.54)	2.46	(3.70)
REL	3.88	(1.58)	-2.83	(1.98)	-1.25	(0.82)	-6.78	(2.24)
Q-TWiST	-0.46	(1.76)	5.07	(3.93)	-1.77	(1.39)	-2.46	(3.57)

plot on the left, only three regions are present, two in which the differences between the two treatments are not statistically significant ($\alpha = 0.05$) as indicated by $A >= B$ and $A <= B$ and the lower portion ($A >> B$) where treatment A is superior. Note that in this plot, the results are virtually insensitive to the choice of U_{REL} because the time in this health state is very similar in both treatment groups. In the plot on the right, all four regions are present and the choice between the two treatments is more sensitive to patient's preferences.

As the number of unknown utilities increases, presenting the results becomes increasingly more complicated. The results in the breast cancer trial based on the Breast Chemotherapy Questionnaire (BCQ) measures suggest that the value of U_{TOX} differ between the two treatments (see Chapter 3) and there are at least three unknown utilities. If the trial is designed with primary endpoints such as Q-TWiST, it would be advisable to develop strategies to obtain estimated values of the utilities using multi-attribute measures or health status scales (e.g. SF-36) with validated conversions to utility measures [Franks et al., 2003, Feeny, 2005].

15.3.4 Proportional Hazards Estimates of Time in Health States

Cole at al. [1993] proposed a method for incorporating patient characteristics into a Q-TWiST analysis using Cox's proportional hazards models. This approach is useful when the outcomes depend on prognostic factors. In this method, the area under the curve corresponding to the time to each transition depends on the patient characteristics (X):

$$\int_0^L S_0(t)^{exp(\beta X)} \partial t \tag{15.11}$$

In breast cancer, the number of positive nodes is a well known prognostic factor. I have also included an indicator of having a concurrent chronic disease (other than cancer) in the following illustration. The results for the four groups are displayed in Table 15.4. From the results, it appears that for women with 4+ positive nodes without concurrent chronic disease there is an advantage (though not statistically different) associated with the experimental therapy, illustrating how this approach could be useful.

15.4 Summary

- QALY and Q-TWiST measures integrate quality and quantity of life; these measures may be useful when there are tradeoffs associated with the interventions being assessed in the clinical trial.

- When measures of patient preferences are measured repeatedly over time, QALYs can be calculated in a number of ways. The major challenges occur when assessments are missing or follow-up is limited.

- The Q-TWiST approach is useful when distinct progressive health states can be defined in which patients preferences can be assumed to be constant.

16

Analysis Plans and Reporting Results

16.1 Introduction

The analysis plan is an essential part of any randomized clinical trial. Most statisticians have considerable experience with writing adequate analysis plans for studies that have one or two univariate endpoints. For example, clinical trials of treatments for cancer have a primary and one to two secondary endpoints, which are either the time-to-an-event (e.g. disease progression or death) or a binary outcome such as a complete or partial response (measured as the change in tumor size). The analysis of these univariate outcomes is straightforward.

When multiple measures are assessed repeatedly over time, the choices for analysis are much more complex. This is true whether the outcome is HRQoL or another set of longitudinal measures. For example, an analgesic trial might include longitudinal patient ratings of the average and worst pain as well as use of additional medication for uncontrolled episodes of pain. Unfortunately, HRQoL is often designated as a secondary endpoint and the development of an analysis is postponed until after the trial begins. Because the analyses are more complex and may require auxiliary information to be gathered if missing data is expected, more attention is required during protocol development to insure an analysis can be performed that will answer the research objectives.

At the point that a detailed analysis plan is written it will become very clear whether the investigators have a clear view of their research objectives. Choices for strategies of handling multiple comparisons will require clarity about the exact role of the HRQoL data. Will it be used in any decision about the intervention or will it play only an explanatory or supportive role? The choice to use a composite endpoint or summary measure or to perform tests at each follow-up will require clarity about whether the intent is to explore the patterns of differences over time or to identify a general benefit. The choice of analysis methods and strategies for handling missing data will require clarity about the population of inference. For example, are the conclusions intended for all those started on the intervention (Intent-to-Treat) or conditional on some criteria (e.g. survival, only while on therapy, etc.).

This chapter focuses on selected issues that are critical to the development of a detailed analysis plan for the HRQoL component of a clinical trial. Even when it is a policy not to include details of the analysis of secondary endpoints in the protocol, these details should be established before the protocol is finalized. Failure to do so may result in the omission of critical information from the data collection or the ability to make a definitive inference from the data.

16.2 General Analysis Plan

16.2.1 Goals of the Trial and Role of HRQoL

From my personal experience, developing the analysis plan is straightforward once the goals of the trial and role of HRQoL are clear. But clarifying these may be the most challenging step. Too often, when I ask specific questions about the role of HRQoL in the trial, the answer is "All of them." It is important to persist and identify which of the possible roles are the most important. In each of the following sections, I will present the decisions that need to be made among the strategies that have been presented in the previous chapters.

16.2.2 Primary versus Secondary Endpoints

The need for clarity about the role of the HRQoL assessments in the clinical trial becomes obvious when defining the primary and secondary endpoints. The intent of the trial could be as strong as demonstrating the efficacy of a drug solely on the basis of HRQoL for the purposes of product registration, advertising claims, or changing practice. At the other extreme, the intent may be solely exploratory with no decisions or claims to be made on the basis of the HRQoL assessments. Typically the role of HRQoL will be somewhere between the two extremes. For example, when there are no effective therapies for a life-threatening condition, a decision to declare a drug *effective* might be made solely on the basis of clinical measures. Tumor response (measurable shrinkage of a tumor) and the time to disease progression are typical measures of response for cancer treatments. On the other hand, a decision to declare a drug *beneficial* might be made on the basis of either survival or improvements in a global measure of HRQoL.

The first step is to clarify the relative roles of all the trial endpoints. If the intent is to make a decision about the efficacy or benefits of the intervention based on the dimensions of HRQoL and other primary endpoints, then HRQoL is taking on the role of a primary endpoint (regardless of the language used in the protocol). This implies a need for an explicit strategy for handling or reducing multiple comparisons (see Chapter 13). Note that an explicit strategy does not always mean the use of a formal procedure to control the experimentwise error rate simultaneously for all endpoints, but may include other options such as the use of summary measures (see Chapter 14) or controlling error rates within clusters of related endpoints [Proschan and Waclawiw, 2000].

The second step is to clarify the roles of the multiple dimensions of HRQoL. Is the intent to claim a generic HRQoL benefit or only benefits in certain dimensions? If generic, what are the criteria that will establish that inference? When the HRQoL assessments are considered supportive of primary endpoints, then HRQoL is taking the role of a secondary endpoint. Less stringent criteria are generally required for secondary endpoints, however, HRQoL and other patient reported outcomes are often held to a higher standard. It is wise to consider both control of type I and II error rates as well options to reduce the multiplicity of endpoints as a means to improve interpretability of the results.

16.2.3   Composite Endpoints or Summary Measures

Identifying composite endpoints or summary measures consistent with the objectives will reduce multiplicity of data over time. As discussed in detail in Chapter 14, the choice will be determined by the expected pattern of change over time and the period of the study where differences are clinically relevant. Well-chosen summary measures or statistics often have greater power to detect patterns of small but consistent HRQoL differences across time or measures. This is a particular advantage in smaller studies, where the power to detect meaningful differences is limited.

16.2.4   Comparison Procedures

The next step is to select a strategy for controlling the type I error rate. Details are presented in Chapter 13. As an example, consider several scenarios for drugs to treat a fatal disease. In the first scenario, there are no effective drugs. Thus, either extending the duration of survival or the quality of life during survival could be considered a benefit. If this is the first in a series of trials and the decision is only whether to continue development of the drug, then no multiple comparison procedures are mandatory. However, if the intent is to ask for approval of the drug if either survival or HRQoL is improved, then an explicit procedure is necessary. There are still numerous options. One is based on the argument that because there are no effective drugs, the analyses of survival and HRQoL should each be performed at $\alpha = 0.05$, with multiple comparison procedures for the K HRQoL measures. At worst, the experimentwise error rate is no more than 10%. In a second scenario, there exist current therapies that delay the progression of the disease but do not result in a cure. If the intent was to obtain approval if either survival or HRQoL was improved, an option is to split the alpha between survival (α_1) and HRQoL (α_2). However, if the intent is to ask for approval only if the drug shows a survival benefit and then examine HRQoL for other reasons, then a gatekeeper strategy may be warranted.

16.2.5   Who Is Included?

The design of the longitudinal assessment of any outcome measure will determine the inferences that can be made from a trial. One aspect of this is who is assessed and for how long. Ideally, all subjects are assessed at all of the planned assessments; but this ideal can rarely be achieved in practice. In addition to attrition due to the patient's decision to drop out, subjects can be excluded from the analysis as a result of the study design or implementation. Some exclusions present no threat to the scope and validity of inference that is possible at the end of the trial. For example, a very small proportion of subjects may be excluded because appropriate translations are not available. Because the exclusion is completely unrelated to both treatment assignment and to future outcomes it can be safely ignored.

Trial designs and analysis plans often create exclusions that limit the questions that can be answered. At this point, it may be helpful to differentiate between two research questions. The first type of question has the intent to compare the outcomes of subjects on each treatment arm with the goal of determining the superiority (or equivalence) of a particular treatment. The inference associated with this question relies on randomization and intent-to-treat (ITT) principles to avoid selection bias. However, designs that mandate follow-up be discontinued when treatment is discontinued may induce a selection bias in a randomized trial. Similarly, criteria that limit analysis to a subset of the subjects, such as those based on the number of assessments or a minimum dose of the intervention, may also induce a selection bias. Some exclusions, such as failure to start therapy, are easily justified in a blinded study if the exclusion is equally likely across treatment arms. Other exclusions may depend on treatment and should be very carefully justified with plans for sensitivity analysis and documentation of the impact of this exclusion on results.

In a very small number of trials, the research questions explicitly limit the analysis to a subset of subjects who are responders, treatment compliant or survivors. While these questions may be clinically relevant, causal inferences based on comparisons of the groups are no longer possible. Differences (or lack of differences) between the subjects selected from two treatment groups may be attributable to selection rather than the effects of treatment. For example, the HRQoL trajectories of survivors may be very similar among treatment groups, but the proportion of subject surviving are quite different. Analysis plans for this type of question should address the issues of selection bias and the possible presence of confounders.

16.2.6   Models for Longitudinal Data

Chapters 3 and 4 summarize the two major options for modeling longitudinal data. When the design is event-driven or there will be a limited number of assessments (2-4) occurring close to the planned time, repeated measures models are appropriate (Chapter 3). Event-driven designs are particularly common for interventions that have a fixed duration. In contrast, when interventions do not have a fixed duration and the assessments occur over extended periods of time, growth curve models are appropriate (Chapter 4). There are within each of these groups, a number of options for the primary analysis and sensitivity analyses when missing data is a concern.

Event-Driven Designs and Repeated Measures Models

The basic strategies for the analysis of event-driven designs are presented in Chapter 3. When missing data is a concern, sensitivity analyses for event driven designs include the following options. When the analyst has good auxiliary information about the subject's cause of dropout and status after dropout that is related to the HRQoL measure, multiple imputation using MCMC or a sequential procedure is a possible approach (Chapter 9). Mixture models can also be used for repeated measures models (Chapter 10, Section 4). A sensitivity analysis that includes the CCMV restriction and Brown's protective estimate is a feasible strategy (see Section 10.4.1) for the simplest design with only two assessments (pre-/post-) when missing data are limited to follow-up.

Time-Driven Designs and Mixed-Effects Growth Curve Models

The basic strategies for the analysis of trials with time-driven designs involve using growth curve models. There are several options for sensitivity analyses. The joint or shared parameter models rely on the presence of variation in the slopes that is associated with the time of dropout or another event (see Chapter 11). A mixture model with parametric restrictions is possible when subgroups (strata) can be defined for which missing data are ignorable (see Chapter 10).

16.2.7   Missing Data

Missing HRQoL assessments are generally not random. This may introduce bias that can not be controlled with statistical methods [Fayers and Machin, 2000] or through imputation [Revicki et al., 2001]. As indicated by the number of chapters in this book, handling missing data is a challenge and requires careful planning. Appropriate strategies will depend on the objectives and the nature and extent of the missing data. No single approach is useful in all settings [Bernhard et al., 1998b].

Ignorable Missing Data

With minimal missing data or the expectation that the data will be predominately MAR or MCAR, the recommendation is to use a likelihood-based method that uses all available data (see Chapters 3-6). Depending on the design of the study, the proposal can be to use either a repeated measures model (Chapter 3) or a mixed-effects growth curve model (Chapter 4). Even when there is a concern that the data may be MNAR, these models may be proposed 1) for initial analysis to be followed by sensitivity analyses, 2) as a means for identifying feasible models for the covariance structure or 3) for generating initial estimates required for other models.

Non-Ignorable Missing Data

A strategy for checking the sensitivity of the results should be included in the analysis plan when there is any suspicion that the missing data will be related to events or outcomes that will affect HRQoL. The analyst should consider at least two candidate models for the proposed sensitivity analysis because, as we noted in Chapter 9, it is possible that a particular model may suggest ignorable missing data when other models contradict that finding.

Final Modification of Analysis Plan

Most of the analytic methods for non-ignorable missing data are dependent on the characteristics of the data. For example, neither the conditional linear model nor the joint mixed-effects/dropout model (Chapter 9) are feasible if there is no random variation in the slopes among subjects. Thus, final decisions about the analytic methods may require preliminary looks at blinded data. Initial analysis plans should consider possible options, followed by an updated plan based on preliminary analyses of blinded data.

16.3 Sample Size and Power

Although repeated measures and growth curve models are often used for the analysis of longitudinal studies, it is rare to see sample size calculations for clinical trials that correspond to these analyses. One of the most common approaches is to pick a single point in time (often the last), calculate the sample size for the expected difference in the group means and inflate that sample size for dropout. Basically, this calculation provides the sample size for a univariate analysis. In most cases, this will provide a conservative (larger than necessary) estimate of the sample size. In this section, a procedure is described for the estimation of the sample size when the analysis is based on MLE of a repeated measures or growth curve model with missing data.

FIGURE 16.1 Checklist for the statistical analysis plan.

Endpoints

✓ Definitive research objectives and specific a priori hypotheses

✓ Superiority versus equivalence

✓ Define primary and secondary endpoints; specify summary measures

Scoring of HRQoL Instruments

✓ Specify method (or reference if it contains specific instructions)

✓ State how missing responses to individual items are handled

Primary Analysis

✓ Power or Sample Size Requirements

✓ Procedures for handling multiplicity of HRQoL measurements:

    ✓ What summary measures are proposed?

    ✓ Adjustment procedures for multiple comparisons

✓ What statistical procedure is used to model the repeated measures/longitudinal data?

✓ What assumptions are made about the missing data? What are the expected rates of missing data and how does that affect the analysis?

Sensitivity Analysis

✓ What is the plan for sensitivity analyses?

✓ What models were considered and why were the particular models selected?

✓ Is the description specific enough for another analyst to implement the analysis?

Secondary Analysis

✓ If some scales are excluded from the primary analysis, what exactly will be reported for these scales?

✓ What is the justification for including these assessments if not part of the primary analysis?

✓ What exploratory analyses are planned? (Psychometric characteristics of HRQoL instrument, Relationship between clinical outcomes and HRQoL measures, Treatment effects in specific subgroups)

While this approach will provide a more accurate estimate of the required sample size, the real usefulness is that it provides a method for estimating the required sample size for any hypothesis that is based on a linear functions of the parameter estimates.

16.3.1   Simple Linear Combinations of β

Consider the case where the hypothesis of interest is a univariate test of a linear combination of the parameters,

$$H_0 : \theta = C\beta = 0 \text{ versus } H_A : \theta = \delta_\theta,$$

where C is a known $1 \times p$ vector and δ_θ is the value of θ under the alternative hypothesis. The hypothesis can be as simple as a contrast of the means at a specific time point (.g. time 4) across treatment groups, $H_0 : \mu_{B4} - \mu_{A4}$ or $H_0 : \theta = \mu_{B4} - \mu_{A4} = 0$ or as complex as the difference between the area under the curves (AUC).

If the sample size is sufficiently large, then the distribution of the test statistic $z_\theta = \hat\theta / \sqrt{\varsigma_\theta^2 / N}$ is well approximated by a univariate standard normal distribution, where $\sqrt{\varsigma_\theta^2 / N}$ is the standard error of $\hat\theta$ and ς_θ^2 is N times the variance of the estimate of θ. That is, $\varsigma_\theta^2 = N \, Var(\hat\theta)$ where N is the total sample size.

The general form of the sample size approximation for a two-sided test is:

$$N = (z_{\alpha/2} + z_\beta)^2 \frac{\varsigma_\theta^2}{\delta_\theta^2}. \tag{16.1}$$

For any hypothesis of the form $\theta = C\beta$, we can estimate the required sample size if we can determine ς_θ^2 and δ_θ^2.

Familiar Special Cases

Equation 16.1 may not be exactly familiar, but there are two well-known sample size formulas that are special cases of this general formula. In the first, a test of the equality of means from two independent samples of the same size with equal variance corresponds to $N = n_A + n_B$, $\delta_\theta = \mu_A - \mu_B$, $\varsigma_\theta^2 = N \times Var(\hat\mu_A - \hat\mu_B) = N \times 2\sigma_Y^2/n = 4\sigma_Y^2$. Thus, the total sample size is

$$N = (z_{\alpha/2} + z_\beta)^2 \frac{\varsigma_\theta^2}{\delta_\theta^2} = (z_{\alpha/2} + z_\beta)^2 \frac{4\sigma_Y^2}{(\mu_A - \mu_B)^2} \tag{16.2}$$

or the more familiar formula for the number required in each group

$$n = (z_{\alpha/2} + z_\beta)^2 2\sigma_Y^2 / (\mu_A - \mu_B)^2.$$

The second special case is the test of equality of means in a paired sample:
$N = n$, $\delta_\theta = \mu_A - \mu_B$, $\varsigma_\theta^2 = N \times Var(\mu_A - \mu_B) = N \times 2\sigma_Y^2(1 - \rho)/N =$

$2\sigma_Y^2(1 - \rho)$. Thus, the number of pairs is

$$N = (z_{\alpha/2} + z_\beta)^2 \frac{\varsigma_\theta^2}{\delta_\theta^2} = (z_{\alpha/2} + z_\beta)^2 \frac{2\sigma_Y^2(1 - \rho)}{(\mu_A - \mu_B)^2} \qquad (16.3)$$

.

16.3.2 Longitudinal Studies with Repeated Measures

The following procedure is based on asymptotic approximations of the co-variance of the estimated parameters. It is applicable to any linear model, $E[Y_i] = X_i\beta + \epsilon_i$, where the data are approximately multivariate normal $(Y_i \sim N(X_i\beta, \Sigma_i))$.

Complete Designs Inflated for Dropout

To illustrate, assume the design for the study includes two groups (A and B) with four repeated measurements of HRQoL: baseline and three follow-ups. Even if we decide to use a different parameterization for our analysis, it is easiest to perform sample size calculation using a cell mean model. Let us consider two possible hypotheses. The first is a contrast of the change from baseline to the last assessment and the second is a contrast of difference between the baseline assessment and the average of the three follow-up assessments.

$$H_{01} : (\mu_{B4} - \mu_{B1}) = (\mu_{A4} - \mu_{A1}) \qquad (16.4)$$
$$H_{02} : (\frac{\mu_{B2} + \mu_{B3} + \mu_{B4}}{3} - \mu_{B1}) = (\frac{\mu_{A2} + \mu_{A3} + \mu_{A4}}{3} - \mu_{A1}) \quad (16.5)$$

or

$$H_{01} : \theta_1 = (\mu_{B4} - \mu_{B1}) - (\mu_{A4} - \mu_{A1}) = 0$$
$$H_{02} : \theta_2 = (\frac{\mu_{B2} + \mu_{B3} + \mu_{B4}}{3} - \mu_{B1}) - (\frac{\mu_{A2} + \mu_{A3} + \mu_{A4}}{3} - \mu_{A1}) = 0$$

The first step is to identify the differences we expect under the alternative hypothesis. If we assume the differences are 0.0, 0.4, 0.5 and 0.6 times the standard deviation (σ) at 0, 6, 12 and 26 weeks respectively, then $\mu_{B1} - \mu_{A1} = 0.0\sigma$, $\mu_{B2} - \mu_{A2} = 0.4\sigma$, $\mu_{B3} - \mu_{A3} = 0.5\sigma$ and $\mu_{B4} - \mu_{A4} = 0.6\sigma$. With a bit of algebra, we find that $\delta_{\theta_1} = 0.6\sigma$ and $\delta_{\theta_2} = 0.5\sigma$.

The next step is to calculate the variance of $\hat{\theta}$. When the data are complete and asymptotically normal, two simple rules can be used. The rules are that when a, b and c are known constants, $Var(ax + by) = a^2Var(x) + 2abCov(x, y) + b^2Var(y)$ and $Var(cy) = c^2Var(y)$ or more generally in matrix notation: $Var(CY) = CVar(Y)C'$. Based on these principles, we would estimate the variance of θ_1 as follows:

$$\hat{\theta}_1 = \frac{\sum y_{iB4} - \sum y_{iB1}}{n_B} - \frac{\sum y_{iA4} - \sum y_{iA1}}{n_A}$$

$$Var(\hat{\theta}_1) = Var\left(\frac{\sum y_{iB4} - \sum y_{iB1}}{n_B} - \frac{\sum y_{iA4} - \sum y_{iA1}}{n_A}\right)$$

$$= Var\left(\frac{\sum y_{iB4} - \sum y_{iB1}}{n_B}\right) - Var\left(\frac{\sum y_{iA4} - \sum y_{iA1}}{n_A}\right)$$

$$= \frac{Var\left(\sum y_{iB4} - \sum y_{iB1}\right)}{n_B^2} + \frac{Var\left(\sum y_{iA4} - \sum y_{iA1}\right)}{n_A^2}$$

$$= \frac{n_B[Var(y_{iB4}) - 2Cov(y_{iB4}, y_{iB1}) + Var(y_{iB1})]}{n_B^2} +$$

$$\frac{n_A[Var(y_{iA4}) - 2Cov(y_{iA4}, y_{iA1}) + Var(y_{iA1})]}{n_A^2}$$

If we can make a simplifying assumption that the variance of Y is homoscedastic (constant) across time and treatment groups and recalling that $Cov(x, y) = \rho_{12}\sigma_x\sigma_y$, this simplifies to:

$$Var(\hat{\theta}_1) = \frac{n_B(\sigma_Y^2 - 2\sigma_Y^2\rho_{14} + \sigma_Y^2)}{n_B^2} + \frac{n_A(\sigma_Y^2 - 2\sigma_Y^2\rho_{14} + \sigma_Y^2)}{n_A^2}$$

$$= \sigma_Y^2\left(\frac{2(1 - \rho_{14})}{n_B} + \frac{2(1 - \rho_{14})}{n_A}\right)$$

Finally, if we substitute Np_A for n_B and Np_B for n_B where N is the total sample size and p_A and p_B are the proportions allocated to each of the treatment groups and multiply by N:

$$\sigma_{\hat{\theta}_1}^2 = NVar(\hat{\theta}_1) = \sigma_Y^2 2(1 - \rho_{14})\left(\frac{1}{p_B} + \frac{1}{p_A}\right)$$

At this point, we can use equation 16.1 to determine the number of subjects with complete data that we will need. For example, if the correlation between the first and fourth assessment is 0.5 and the allocation between treatments is 2:1, the required number for 90% power ($\alpha = 0.05$) is

$$N = (z_{\alpha/2} + z_\beta)^2 \frac{\varsigma_\theta^2}{\delta_\theta^2} \tag{16.6}$$

$$= (1.96 + 1.282)^2 \frac{\sigma_Y^2 2(1 - .5)\left(\frac{1}{2/3} + \frac{1}{1/3}\right)}{0.6^2\sigma_Y^2} = 131.4$$

Thus we would need 88 and 44 subjects with follow-up at the fourth assessment in the two groups, thus the number of subjects would need to be inflated for dropout. If there was a 30% dropout by the fourth assessment or 70% with the fourth assessment, the inflated numbers would be $88/.7 = 126$ and $44/.7 = 63$ or a total of 189 subjects.

Incomplete Designs

Clinical trials rarely have complete data and calculation of ς_θ for endpoints that summarize data across multiple assessments requires programs that can perform matrix manipulation (SAS or R) or manipulation of the procedure used to analyze the data (SAS).

It is assumed that the total number of subjects is large and $\left[\sum_i^N X_i' \hat{\Sigma}_i^{-1} X_i\right]^{-1}$ is a valid approximation of the covariance of the parameter estimates ($\hat{\beta}$). This variance can be expressed as a function of the number (n_k) of subjects in each of the unique design matrices, X_k (equation 16.7). It may also be expressed as a function of the total number of subjects, N, and the corresponding proportion (p_k) in each of the K groups (equation 16.8).

$$Var[\hat{\beta}] = \left[\sum_{i=1}^{N} X_i' \hat{\Sigma}_i^{-1} X_i\right]^{-1} = \left[\sum_{k=1}^{K} n_k X_k' \hat{\Sigma}_k^{-1} X_k\right]^{-1} \quad (16.7)$$

$$= \frac{1}{N}\left[\sum_{k=1}^{K} p_k X_k' \hat{\Sigma}_k^{-1} X_k\right]^{-1}. \quad (16.8)$$

The variance of $\hat{\theta}$ is $C\,Var(\hat{\beta})\,C'$ thus

$$\varsigma_\theta^2 = N\,Var(\hat{\theta}) = N\,C\,Var(\hat{\beta})\,C' = C\left[\sum_{k=1}^{K} p_k X_k' \hat{\Sigma}_k^{-1} X_k\right]^{-1} C'. \quad (16.9)$$

For incomplete designs, the sample size approximation can be written as:

$$N = (z_{\alpha/2} + z_\beta)^2\, C\, \underbrace{\left[\sum_{k=1}^{K} p_k X_k' \hat{\Sigma}_k^{-1} X_k\right]^{-1} C'}_{\varsigma_\theta^2} / \delta_\theta^2. \quad (16.10)$$

Let us assume that dropout is equal in the two groups and that all missing data are due to dropout. The rate of dropout is 1%, 5%, 10% and 20% at each of the four assessments (T1-T4). Thus 64% will complete all assessments. If subjects are equally allocated to both groups, the pattern of observations will appear as displayed in Table 16.1.

In our example, the design matrix (cell means model) for the subjects in group A with all four observations is:

$$X_k = \begin{bmatrix} 1 & 0 & 0 & 0 & 0 & 0 & 0 & 0 \\ 0 & 1 & 0 & 0 & 0 & 0 & 0 & 0 \\ 0 & 0 & 1 & 0 & 0 & 0 & 0 & 0 \\ 0 & 0 & 0 & 1 & 0 & 0 & 0 & 0 \end{bmatrix}, \quad p_k = .32.$$

The design matrix for the subjects in group A with only the first two observations is:

$$X_k = \begin{bmatrix} 1 & 0 & 0 & 0 & 0 & 0 & 0 & 0 \\ 0 & 1 & 0 & 0 & 0 & 0 & 0 & 0 \end{bmatrix}, \quad p_k = .05.$$

TABLE 16.1 Proportions in each pattern with equal (1:1) and unequal (2:1) allocation.

Pattern	Group	\multicolumn{4}{c}{Assessments}				%	Equal p_k	Unequal p_k
		T1	T2	T3	T4			
1	A					1%	.005	.0067
2	A	X				5%	.025	.0333
3	A	X	X			10%	.05	.0667
4	A	X	X	X		20%	.10	.1333
5	A	X	X	X	X	64%	.32	.4267
							.50	.6667
6	B					1%	.005	.0033
7	B	X				5%	.025	.0167
8	B	X	X			10%	.05	.0333
9	B	X	X	X		20%	.10	.0667
10	B	X	X	X	X	64%	.32	.2133
							.50	.3333

X indicates an observed assessment of HRQoL.

p_k is the proportion of the total sample with the indicated pattern.

The first step is to generate a data set with one subject representing each of the patterns. Each subject will be associated with a weight p_k. While the values of Y_i are not involved in the calculation of ς_θ, they can be used to calculate δ_θ using the expected values under the alternative hypothesis. Assuming that the standard deviation or Y is 1, we will use $Y_i = (0, 0, 0, 0)$ for group A and $Y_i = (0, .4, .5, .6)$ for group B. The dataset would contain a record for each observation observed in a particular pattern:

ID	Group	p_k	Time	Y		ID	Group	p_k	Time	Y
2	A	0.025	1	0.0		7	B	0.025	1	0.0
3	A	0.050	1	0.0		8	B	0.050	1	0.0
3	A	0.050	2	0.0		8	B	0.050	2	0.4
4	A	0.100	1	0.0		9	B	0.100	1	0.0
4	A	0.100	2	0.0		9	B	0.100	2	0.4
4	A	0.100	3	0.0		9	B	0.100	3	0.5
5	A	0.320	1	0.0		10	B	0.320	1	0.0
5	A	0.320	2	0.0		10	B	0.320	2	0.4
5	A	0.320	3	0.0		10	B	0.320	3	0.5
5	A	0.320	4	0.0		10	B	0.320	4	0.6

Note that in the generated dataset, all four assessments only appear for patterns 5 and 10. The fourth assessment is omitted in patterns 4 and 9, the third and fourth assessments are missing in patterns 3 and 8, all but the initial assessment is missing in patterns 2 and 7 and patterns 1 and 6 are omitted completely.

If we have good estimates of the variance of the HRQoL measure over time we can use them. But in their absence we will have to assume some covariance structure for the repeated measures. Suppose the variance is constant over time and $\rho = 0.5$. Then

$$\Sigma_i = \sigma_Y^2 \begin{bmatrix} 1 & .5 & .5 & .5 \\ .5 & 1 & .5 & .5 \\ .5 & .5 & 1 & .5 \\ .5 & .5 & .5 & 1 \end{bmatrix}.$$

If we again assume that the standard deviation of Y_i is 1, then $\sigma_Y^2 = 1$ and it drops out of the calculations.

Because the SAS Proc MIXED procedures allows us to supply a fixed estimate of Σ_i we can perform a single iteration of the ML algorithm to obtain δ_θ and ς_θ for the two endpoints defined in equations 16.4 and 16.5.

```
proc mixed data=work.work2  maxiter=1 method=ml;
  class ID Group Time;
  weight p_k;
  model Y=Group*Time/Noint Solution;
  repeated Time/Subject=ID type=UN;
  parms (1)
        (.5) (1)
        (.5) (.5) (1)
        (.5) (.5) (.5) (1)/noiter;
  estimate 'Theta 1' Group*Time 1 0 0 -1 -1 0 0 1;
  estimate 'Theta 2' Group*Time 3 -1 -1 -1 -3 1 1 1/divisor=3;
  run;
```

Note that we have fixed the variance parameters (noiter in the parms statement). The values of interest are δ_θ (the Estimate column) and ς_θ (the Standard Error column):

Label	Estimate	Standard Error
Theta 1	0.6000	2.3387
Theta 2	0.5000	1.7264

For a two-sided test with $\alpha = 0.05$ and 90% power, $z_{\alpha/2} = -1.96$ and $z_\beta = -1.282$, the total sample size (equation 16.10) for the two endpoints are

$$\theta_1 : N = (1.96 + 1.282)^2 \frac{(2.3387)^2}{(.6)^2} = 159.7$$

$$\theta_2 : N = (1.96 + 1.282)^2 \frac{(1.7264)^2}{(.5)^2} = 125.3$$

Note that in the above example, Y and Σ are scaled so the variance of Y_{ijk} is standard normal ($N(0, 1)$) and PARMS specifies the correlation of Y. It is not necessary to convert everything to a standard normal distribution; it is critical that one consistently use either the unstandardized or standardized values of Y (δ) and Σ.

Unequal Allocations of Subjects to Treatment Groups

Some clinical trial designs specify an unequal allocation of subjects to treatment arms. Because the sample size calculation is specified in terms of the total sample size (N), this requires only an adjustment of the proportions within each pattern of observations (p_k). For example, if subjects were allocated in a 2:1 ratio to treatments A and B, then the pattern would appear as displayed in the last column of Table 16.1.

16.3.3 Longitudinal Data and Growth Curve Model

Consider the same two-group design where the four assessments are assumed to occur at 0, 6, 12 and 26 weeks. The dropout rates are the same. Instead of using a repeated measures design we plan to use a piecewise linear growth curve model. The model is defined with four parameters per group: β_0 is the common intercept, β_{1A} is the slope for the first 6 weeks in treatment group A, β_{2A} is the change in the slope after 6 weeks and β_{3A} is the change in the slope after 12 weeks, etc. For a subject in group A with all four assessments,

$$X_i = \begin{bmatrix} 1 & 0 & 0 & 0 & 0 & 0 & 0 \\ 1 & 6 & 0 & 0 & 0 & 0 & 0 \\ 1 & 12 & 6 & 0 & 0 & 0 & 0 \\ 1 & 26 & 20 & 14 & 0 & 0 & 0 \end{bmatrix}.$$

Let us consider the sample size required for two additional endpoints: The first hypothesis (H_{03}) is the area under the HRQoL versus time curve (equation 16.11). The second hypothesis is the same as in the previous example: the averages of the estimates at 6, 12 and 26 weeks minus the baseline assessments (H_{04}). The final hypothesis is the change from baseline to week 26 (H_{05}).

$$H_{03}: \int_{t=0}^{26} \left(\beta_0 + \beta_{1A}t + \beta_{2A}t^{[6]} + \beta_{3A}t^{[12]} \right) \partial t = \qquad (16.11)$$

$$\int_{t=0}^{26} \left(\beta_0 + \beta_{1B}t + \beta_{2B}t^{[6]} + \beta_{3B}t^{[12]} \right) \partial t$$

$$H_{04}: \frac{\mu_{B6} + \mu_{B12} + \mu_{B26}}{3} - \mu_{B0} = \frac{\mu_{A6} + \mu_{A12} + \mu_{A26}}{3} - \mu_{A0} \quad (16.12)$$

$$H_{05}: (\mu_{B26} - \mu_{B0}) = (\mu_{A26} - \mu_{A0}) \qquad (16.13)$$

where $\mu_{A0} = \beta_0$, $\mu_{A6} = \beta_0 + 6\beta_{1A}$, $\mu_{A12} = \beta_0 + 12\beta_{1A} + 6\beta_{2A}$, and $\mu_{A26} = \beta_0 + 26\beta_{1A} + 20\beta_{2A} + 14\beta_{3A}$. By rearranging the terms and noting that the term for the common baseline (β_0) always drops out, we get:

$$H_{03}: \frac{26^2}{2}(\beta_{1A} - \beta_{1B}) + \frac{20^2}{2}(\beta_{2A} - \beta_{2B}) + \frac{14^2}{2}(\beta_{3A} - \beta_{3B}) = 0$$

$$H_{04} : \frac{44}{3}(\beta_{1A} - \beta_{1B}) + \frac{26}{3}(\beta_{2A} - \beta_{2B}) + \frac{14}{3}(\beta_{3A} - \beta_{3B}) = 0$$

$$H_{05} : 26(\beta_{1A} - \beta_{1B}) + 20(\beta_{2A} - \beta_{2B}) + 14(\beta_{3A} - \beta_{3B}) = 0$$

Again we would set up a dataset with the essence of our expected patterns of X_k and p_k:

ID	Group	p_k	Weeks	weeks6	weeks12
2	A	0.025	0	0	0
3	A	0.050	0	0	0
3	A	0.050	6	0	0
...					
10	B	0.320	0	0	0
10	B	0.320	6	0	0
10	B	0.320	12	6	0
10	B	0.320	26	20	14

The following SAS program is very similar to that used in the previous example; the major difference is the setup of the variables used to model change over time. We use the same method of defining the covariance structure, noting that the compound symmetry is identical to assuming a random intercept in a mixed-effects model. A more complex variance structure, with a random slope, could be used if there is sufficient information to estimate the parameters.

```
proc mixed data=work.work2 maxiter=1 method=ml;
  class ID Group Time;
  weight p_k;
  model Y=Group*Weeks Group*Weeks6 Group*Weeks12/Solution;
  repeated Time/Subject=ID type=UN;
  parms (1)
        (.5) (1)
        (.5) (.5) (1)
        (.5) (.5) (.5) (1)/noiter;
  estimate 'Theta 3' Group*Weeks 338 -338 Group*Weeks6 200 -200
                     Group*Weeks12 98 -98/divisor=26 E;
  estimate 'Theta 4' Group*Weeks 44 -44 Group*weeks6 26 -26
                     Group*Weeks12 14 -14/divisor=3 E;
  estimate 'Theta 5' Group*Weeks 26 -26 Group*weeks6 20 -20
                     Group*Weeks12 14 -14/divisor=3 E;

  ods output Estimates=work.Theta; * Outputs Estimates *;
data work.ssize;
  set work.theta;
  Z_alpha=probit(.05/2);
  Z_beta=probit(.10);
  N=((Z_alpha+Z_beta)*StdErr/Estimate)**2;
```

```
proc print data=ssize;
  id label; var Estimate StdErr N;
  run;
```

The results of the estimate statements are output to a dataset and the total sample size (N) is calculated in a subsequent DATA Step:

Label	Estimate	StdErr	N
Theta 3	-11.6000	32.6205	83.1
Theta 4	-0.5000	1.4036	82.8
Theta 5	-0.6000	2.1117	130.2

16.3.4   Other Considerations

Intermittent Missing Data Patterns and Time-Varying Covariates

In the previous two examples, we assumed that missing data only occurred as a result of dropout. We ignored the possibility of intermittent patterns of missing data. Another problem is that there may be considerable variation in the exact timing of the assessments. Both will have some impact on the power (and sample size estimates). If there is enough information to predict the expected patterns, it is possible to address these problems. One strategy is to consider all patterns of observed data. But in most cases this is cumbersome. An alternative approach is to obtain an estimate of ς_θ^2 by randomly generating a large (e.g. $N_S = 10000$) number of subjects with their expected pattern of observation (X_i) and corresponding variance (Σ_i). Then estimate $\varsigma_\theta^2 = N_S C \left[\sum^{N_S} X_i' \Sigma_i^{-1} X_i \right]^{-1} C'$. One can do this again using PROC MIXED (omitting the WEIGHT statement). The value of the standard error in the output labeled ESTIMATE Statement Results of PROC MIXED is $\varsigma_\theta / \sqrt{N_S}$, so it is necessary to multiply this value by $\sqrt{N_S}$ where N_S is the number of observations used to simulate the pattern of observations.

```
%let Niter=10000;
data work.work1;
  input K Group$ p_k Y1 Y2 Y3 Y4;
  do i=1 to  int(&Niter*p_k);
    ID=K*&NIter+i;
    Time=1; Weeks=0; Y=Y1; if Y ne . then output;
    Time=2; Weeks=6+int(ranuni(73)*3)/7; Y=Y2; if Y ne . then output;
    Time=3; Weeks=12+int(ranuni(33)*7)/7; Y=Y3; if Y ne . then output;
    Time=4; Weeks=26+int(ranuni(93)*10)/7; Y=Y4; if Y ne . then output;
  end;
  keep ID Group p_k Time Weeks Y;
  cards;
1 A .005   . . . .
2 A .025  0 . . .
3 A .05   0 0 . .
4 A .1    0 0 0 .
```

```
 5 A .32    0 0 0 0
 6 B .005   . . . .
 7 B .025   0 . . .
 8 B .05    0 .4 . .
 9 B .1     0 .4 .5 .
10 B .32    0 .4 .5 .6
data work.work2;
  set work.work1;
  if ranuni(333333) lt .1 then delete; * Extra 10% *;
  run;
```

If we extend the previous, adding an additional 10% missing data at each
point in time due to reasons other than dropout, we obtain estimates of 34.2,
1.47 and 2.17 for ς_θ for the three hypotheses and thus sample size estimates
of 115, 114 and 172 respectively. This represents an inflation of 10-12% in the
sample size requirements.

Multivariate Tests

Sample size approximations can also be created for multivariate tests. For
example, we might wish to test simultaneously for differences in the change
from baseline in our example.

$$H_0 : (\mu_{B2} - \mu_{B1}) - (\mu_{A2} - \mu_{A1}) = 0,$$
$$(\mu_{B3} - \mu_{B1}) - (\mu_{A3} - \mu_{A1}) = 0,$$
$$(\mu_{B4} - \mu_{B1}) - (\mu_{A4} - \mu_{A1}) = 0.$$

For large samples, one can generalize the univariate z-statistic to a multi-
variate χ^2-statistic. The null hypothesis is $H_0 : \theta = C\beta = G$, where $C_{(\nu \times p)}$
and $G_{(\nu \times 1)}$ are known. The χ^2 test statistic is $\hat{\theta}'(Var(\hat{\theta}))^{-1}\hat{\theta}$ and the power
of the test is:

$$Pr[\chi_\nu^2(\lambda) > \chi_{\nu,\alpha}^2] = 1 - \beta \tag{16.14}$$

where $\chi_{\nu,\alpha}^2$ is the critical value for a χ^2 distribution with ν degrees of freedom
(α). λ is the non-centrality parameter such that

$$\lambda = \theta'(Var(\hat{\theta}))^{-1}\theta$$
$$= N\theta' \left(C \left[\sum_{k=1}^{K} p_k X_k' \hat{\Sigma}_k^{-1} X_k \right]^{-1} C' \right)^{-1} \theta \tag{16.15}$$

when $\theta = C\beta - G$ is calculated under the alternative hypothesis.

We can again use the output from our SAS program to simplify the calculations. First, we calculate the critical value. In our example, this is
$\chi_{3,\alpha=0.05}^2 = 7.815.^*$ Second, we calculate the non-centrality parameter (λ)

---

*SAS: c_alpha=cinv(1-0.05,3);

solving equation 16.14 for λ. In our example, $\lambda = 14.17$.[†] Finally, we obtain the quantity

$$\theta' \left(C \left[\sum_{k=1}^{K} p_k X_k' \hat{\Sigma}_k^{-1} X_k \right]^{-1} C' \right)^{-1} \theta$$

by adding to the `Proc MIXED` statements.

```
CONTRAST 'Change from Baseline'
    GROUP*Weeks 6 -6,
    GROUP*Weeks 12 -12 GROUP*Weeks6 6  -6,
    GROUP*Weeks 26 -26 GROUP*Weeks6 20 -20 GROUP*Weeks12 14 -14
    /CHISQ;
```

The estimate of the total sample size is λ/CHISQ= 14.17/0.086=163.1 where CHISQ is obtained from the `Proc MIXED` output.

Small Sample Size Approximations

For previous sample size calculations, the approximations assume the sample size is sufficiently large that the asymptotic approximation of the covariance of the parameters is appropriate and the loss of degrees of freedom when using t- and F-statistics will not affect the results. When the sample sizes are small the above procedures can be used to obtain the first estimate of the sample size. The estimation procedure is repeated, using the t- or F-distributions with updated estimates of the degrees of freedom (ν), until the procedure converges.

$$N = (t_{\nu,\alpha/2} + t_{\nu,\beta})^2 \frac{s_\theta^2}{\delta_\theta^2}$$

$$= (t_{\alpha/2} + t_\beta)^2 C \left[\sum_{k=1}^{K} p_k X_k' \hat{\Sigma}_k^{-1} X_k \right]^{-1} C'/\delta_\theta^2. \tag{16.16}$$

Restricted Maximum Likelihood Estimation

Kenward and Roger [1997] provide the details for modifying the estimated covariance of $\hat{\beta}$ for Restricted Maximum Likelihood Estimation (REML) and propose an F-distribution approximation for small sample inference.

FIGURE 16.2 Checklist for reporting requirements for HRQoL trials.

Introduction

√ Rationale for assessing HRQoL in the particular disease and treatment.

√ State specific a priori (pretrial) hypotheses

Methods

√ Justification for selection of instrument(s) assessing HRQoL. (see Chapter 2) References to instrument and validation studies. Details of psychometric properties if a new instrument. Include copy of instrument in appendix if previously unpublished. Details of any modifications of the questions or formats.

√ Details of cross-cultural validation if relevant and previously unpublished.

√ Method of administration (self-report, face-to-face, etc.)

√ Planned timing of the study assessments.

√ Method of scoring, preferably by reference to a published article or scoring manual, with details of any deviations.

√ Interpretation of scores. Do higher values indicate better outcomes?

√ Methods of analysis. What analyses were specified a priori and which were exploratory?

√ Which dimension(s) or item(s) of the HRQoL instruments were selected as endpoints prior to subject accrual?

√ What summary measures and multiple comparison procedures were used? Were they specified a priori?

Results

√ Timing of assessments and length of follow-up by treatment group

√ Missing data:

  √ Proportions with missing data and relevant patterns.

  √ How were patients who dropped out of the study handled?

  √ How were patients who died handled?

√ Results for all scales specified in protocol/analysis plan (negative as well as positive results).

√ If general HRQoL benefit reported, summary of all dimensions.

√ If no changes were observed, describe evidence of responsiveness to measures in related settings and the lack of floor and ceiling effects in current study.

16.4   Reporting Results

All of the standard guidelines for reporting clinical trials apply to the reporting of HRQoL studies. There are multiple sources for these standard guidelines. One source, the CONSORT statement, has been adopted by numerous journals for manuscripts reporting on randomized controlled trials (RCTs). The statement comprises a 22-item checklist and a flow diagram. The checklist itemizes information on how the trial was designed, analyzed, and interpreted; the flow diagram displays the progress of all subjects through the trial. Detailed information can be found at `www.consort-statement.org`. The International Committee of Medical Journal Editors also has guidelines entitled "Uniform Requirements for Manuscripts Submitted to Biomedical Journals" [ICMJE , 2008] available on their web site: `www.icmje.org`.

Because all readers are not as familiar with some of the issues associated with measurement of HRQoL as they are with other clinical endpoints, some additional guidelines are worth mentioning. Based on a systematic review of 20 articles reporting HRQoL in cancer trials in 1997, Lee and Chi [2000] identify the major deficiencies that should be addressed as 1) the failure to provide a rationale of HRQoL assessment, and 2) inadequate description of methodology. In addition to the checklist included here (Figure 16.2), the reader is encouraged to read other published guidelines specific to HRQoL [Staquet et al., 1996].

16.5   Summary

- The analysis plan is driven by explicit research objectives.

- Analyses of HRQoL data are often more complex, because of their longitudinal and multidimensional nature, than the analyses of traditional univariate outcomes.

- The analysis plan should be developed prior to initiation of the study addressing issue of multiple endpoints and missing data regardless of whether HRQoL is a primary or secondary endpoint.

---

†SAS: lambda=cnonct(c_alpha,3,1-0.9);

Appendix C: Cubic Smoothing Splines

The varying coefficent model described in Section 11.3 utilizes a cubic smoothing spline. The following procedure to create B, a $r \times r - 2$ design matrix for the smoothing function was adapted from code provided on Xihong Lin's website. We start with, $\mathcal{T}^0$, a vector of the r distinct values of $\mathcal{T}_i^D$. Next create h^0 a $r - 1$ vector of the differences between the times (equation 17). Then calculate Q^0 an $r \times r - 2$ matrix with values on the diagonal and two off diagonal positions (equations 18-20) and R^0 an $r - 2 \times r - 2$ matrix with values on the diagonal and two off diagonal positions (equations 21-23). Then G is lower triangular component of the square root (Cholesky decomposition) of R (equation 24). Finally L and B are calculated (equations 25 and 26).

$$h_i^0 = \mathcal{T}_{i+1}^0 - \mathcal{T}_i^0 \quad i = 1 \cdots r - 1 \tag{17}$$

$$Q_{j,j}^0 = 1/h_j^0 \quad j = 1 \cdots r - 2 \tag{18}$$

$$Q_{j+1,j}^0 = -1/h_{j+1}^0 - 1/h_j^0 \tag{19}$$

$$Q_{j+2,j}^0 = 1/h_{j+1}^0 \tag{20}$$

$$R_{j,j}^0 = (h_j^0 + h_{j+1}^0)/3 \tag{21}$$

$$R_{j,j-1}^0 = (h_j^0)/6 \tag{22}$$

$$R_{j,j+1}^0 = (h_{j+1}^0)/6 \tag{23}$$

$$R = G\,G' \tag{24}$$

$$L = Q\,(G^{-1})' \tag{25}$$

$$B = L(L'L)^{-1} \tag{26}$$

A SAS macro to perform these calculations can be found on the website: *http://home.earthlink.net/~ dianefairclough/Welcome.html.*

Appendix P: PAWS/SPSS Notes

General Comments

The PAWS/SPSS software focuses on menu-driven analyses. However, many of the procedures described in this book go beyond the options that are available through the menus. When I am unfamiliar with a command, I typically start with the menu, cut the code out of the output window, paste it into the syntax window, and finally tailor that code to my needs.

Licenses for PAWS/SPSS vary with respect to the options available at each institution. For example, my university only subscribes to the basic version, which does not include the procedures tailored to missing data.[‡] You may find that you also do not have access to all the commands. Version 17 has come out just as I am finishing my proofs; as I hunt through the Help files I notice that there are additional functions that I was not aware of previously that may facilitate analyses not presented in this book. If you develop good examples applied to datasets in this book, I will post them on the web site.

Loading Datasets

Datasets that were used to generate the illustrations in the book are available on *http://home.earthlink.net/~ dianefairclough/Welcome.html*. They are in SPSS *.sav format. Datasets can be loaded by clicking on the dataset, using menu options within SPSS or embedding the following code into a program. To load the data for Study 1 use the following with .... replaced by the directory in which the data is saved.

```
GET  FILE='C:\....\Breast3.sav'.
```

[‡]I was able to obtain an expanded license for a limited time as an author to develop some of the code presented in this book.

Reverse Coding and Scoring Questionnaires

Both reverse coding and scoring using the half rule in the presence of missing items can be accomplished in a few lines of code. This minimizes the possibility of typographical errors. Suppose the item variables are named ITEM1, ITEM2, ..., ITEMK etc. where missing values are coded as a SPSS missing value. The first step is to reverse code questions that are negatively worded. While SPSS has a function to recode variables, reverse coding is quite straightforward (see Section 8.2). For a response that is coded from 1 to 5, the following code will reverse code ITEM2:

```
/* Recode Item 2 */
COMPUTE Item2r=6-(Item2).
EXECUTE.
```

I created a new variable, ITEM2r, to avoid problems of doubly recoding the same variable. To calculate a summated score using the half rule, either example of following code can be used:

```
/* Count missing values and if less than half, compute SUM score */
COUNT NMiss=Item1 Item2r Item3 Item4 Item5 Item6 Item7(MISSING).
IF  (NMiss le 3) SumScore=
               MEAN(Item1,Item2r,Item3,Item4,Item5,Item6,Item7)*7.
EXECUTE.


DEFINE !fvars()
   Item1, Item2r, Item3, Item4, Item5, Item6, Item7
!ENDDEFINE.
IF  (NMISS(!fvars) LE 3)  SumScore2=MEAN(!fvars)*7.
EXECUTE.
```

Both check that the number of missing responses is less than half (≤ 3), take the mean of the observed responses, and multiply by the number of items.

Centering Variables

The following code is an example of a procedure that can be used when there are an equal number of records per subject:

```
AGGREGATE
   /OUTFILE=* MODE=ADDVARIABLES
   /BREAK=
   /Var1_mean=MEAN(Var1).
COMPUTE Var1_c=Var1-Var1_mean.
EXECUTE.
```

To center variables within a subgroup, add that variable after BREAK=.

To center variables when there are an unequal number of observations, you must first convert the data to a single record per subject (CASESTOVARS), create the centered variables, and finally transpose that data back to multiple records per subject (VARSTOCASES).

```
/* Transpose data to one record  per subject */
SORT CASES BY PatID FUNO.
SPLIT FILE BY PatID.
CASESTOVARS
  /ID=PatID
  /INDEX=FUNO
  /AUTOFIX
  /GROUPBY=VARIABLE.
SPLIT FILE OFF.

/* Centering */
/* Calculate overall mean */
AGGREGATE
  /OUTFILE=* MODE ADDVARIABLES
  /BREAK=
  /Mean_Age=mean(Age_Tx).
/* Subtract overall mean */
COMPUTE Age_C=Age_Tx-Mean_age.
EXECUTE.

/* Transpose data to multiple records */
VARSTOCASES
  /INDEX=FUNO(4)
  /NULL=KEEP
  /MAKE FACT_T2 FROM FACT_T2.1 to FACT_T2.4
  /MAKE MONTHS FROM MONTHS.1 to MONTHS.4
  /DROP Mean_Age.
```

Bootstrap Procedures for Longitudinal Data

The BOOTSTRAP command in SPSS Version 18 is designed for data and procedures that use datasets with one record per case. It will inappropriately sample observations rather than cases for the longitudinal data considered in this book.

Appendix R: R Notes

General Comments

R is a powerful free open-source-code language that consists mainly of user-defined functions. As a result the capacity of the R language grows rapidly and is often at the forefront of methods development. The learning curve for a new user is steep, but once mastered provides the greatest flexibility of any language.

Accessing Additional Function Libraries

To fit models to the longitudinal data (see Chapters 3 and 4), I use two functions that are part of of the nlme package: gls and lme. So as a first step check that the nlme package is in your library, then load the nlme package:

```
library()          # lists packages in library
library("nlme")    # loads nlme
```

There are additional libraries for the joint shared parameter models described in Chapter 11:

```
R> library("MASS")
R> library("nlme")
R> library("splines")
R> library("survival")
R> library("JM")
```

Loading Datasets

Datasets that were used to generate the illustrations in the book are available on *http://home.earthlink.net/~ dianefairclough/Welcome.html*. They are in CSV format. The following code will load the dataset for Study 1 with ... replaced by the directory where the data is saved.

```
# Breast Cancer data set
  Breast = read.table("C:/.... /breast3.csv",header=TRUE,sep=",")
  str(Breast)                     # lists contents
```

Helpful Computations

To convert a continuous indicator variable of the treatment groups (`Trtment`) to a variable of the *factor* class (`TrtGrp`):

```
> Renal$TrtGrp=factor(Renal$Trtment)     # Creates a CLASS variable
```

Parameters for the changes in slope for the piecewise linear models (Chapter 4):

```
> WEEK2=Renal3$Weeks-2                 # Week2=Weeks-2
> WEEK2[Week2<0]=0                     # Negative values set to zero
> Renal3$WEEK2=WEEK2                   # Stored in renal3
```

Centering Variables

The following code creates a centered variable for `AGE_TX` assuming that all subjects have the same number of assessments. The variable `All` indicates the entire sample.

```
Lung$All=1
Lung$Age_C=Lung$AGE_TX-tapply(Lung$AGE_TX,Lung$All,mean)
```

For datasets with unequal numbers of assessments, identify a single record. For example, if each subject has a record for the first follow-up assessment add [Lung$FUNO==1] as below:

```
Lung$Age_C=Lung$AGE_TX-tapply(Lung$AGE_TX[Lung$FUNO==1],
+                             Lung$All[Lung$FUNO==1],mean)
```

Functions within Subgroups

To compute the mean (or other function) within subgroups requires more complex code. For example, if we wish to add a variable to the dataset `Lung` which is the mean of `Strata_S2` from each treatment group `Exp`:

```
Mean_S2<-tapply(Lung$Strata_S2[Lung$FUNO==1],
                Lung$Exp[Lung$FUNO==1],mean,na.rm=T)
Mean_S2<-data.frame(Mean_S2=Mean_S2,Exp=names(Mean_S2))
Lung<-merge(Lung,Mean_S2,by="Exp")
```

Setting up Models for the "Means"

In Chapters 3 and 4, different parameterizations are used to obtain equivalent models using both continuous indicator and factor variables. Consider the simple situation where we are fitting a simple model with a intercept and slope for two treatment groups. For the two treatment groups, we can either use a continuous indicator variable (`Trtment`) where 0 indicates the control group and 1 indicates the experimental group or a *factor* variable that has two levels(`TrtGrp`). The following statements generate identical models:

```
fixed=TOI2~ Trtment*Weeks
fixed=TOI2~ Trtment + Weeks + Trtment:Weeks
fixed=TOI2~ TrtGrp*Weeks
fixed=TOI2~ TrtGrp + Weeks + TrtGrp:Weeks
```

The output for the first two versions appears as:

```
Fixed: TOI2 ~ Trtment + Weeks + Trtment * Weeks
(Intercept)        Trtment        Weeks Trtment:Weeks
69.75192368    -5.14639184   -0.07676819     0.00623725
```

and for the last two versions as:

```
Fixed: TOI2 ~ TrtGrp + Weeks + TrtGrp:Weeks
  (Intercept)        TrtGroup1        Weeks TrtGroup1:Weeks
  69.75192368    -5.14639184   -0.07676819      0.00623725
```

The resulting models are equivalent, though the labeling differs. The resulting parameters have the interpretation of 1) the intercept in the control group, 2) the difference in the intercept between the experimental and control group, 3) the slope of the control group, and 4) the difference in the slope between the experimental and control group. Note that when the "*" symbol is used lower order terms are automatically generated. If we wished to generate a model in which the intercept and slopes were estimated for each treatment group, we would use the following, adding "0" or "-1" to the model suppresses the default intercept:

```
fixed=TOI2~0+ TrtGrp+TrtGrp:Weeks
```

The results are as follows:

```
Fixed: TOI2 ~ TrtGrp + TrtGrp:Weeks - 1
    TrtGrp0         TrtGrp1      TrtGrp0:Weeks     TrtGrp1:Weeks
  69.75192368    64.60553184     -0.07676819       -0.07053094
```

Functions

I have also created several functions. They can be found on the website *http://home.earthlink.net/~dianefairclough/Welcome.html*. To load the commands stored in an external file (`RFunctions.r`) into the working space of **R**, use the following after modifying the path:

```
source("C:/..../Rprgms/RFunctions.r")
```

Estimation of $\Theta = C\beta$

This function estimates linear functions of β and tests the hypothesis that $\Theta = C\beta = 0$ assuming that the sample size is large enough that a z-statistic is adequate.

The first step is to define C and add rownames as labels (later is optional), then to call the function:

```
R>  C1=c(-1, 1, 0, 0, 0, 0)    # Pre-Tx Diff
R>  C2=c(0, 0, -1, 1, 0, 0)    # During Tx Diff
R>  C3=c(0, 0, 0, 0, -1, 1)    # Post Tx Diff
R>  C=rbind(C1, C2, C3)
R>  rownames(C)=c("Pre-Tx Diff","During Tx Diff","Post Tx Diff")
```

When the model has been fit using gls, then *est* is the object named *model*$coef and *var* is the object named *model*$var. Thus the code might appear as:

```
R>  CMean=gls( ....)
R>  estCbeta(C,CMean$coef,CMean$var)
```

Similarly, when the model has been fit using lme, then *est* is the object named *model*$coef$fix and *var* is the object named *model*$varFix. Thus the code might appear as:

```
R>  LinMod=lme( ....)
R>  estCbeta(C,LinMod$coef$fix,LinMod$varFix)
```

The code for the function is:

```
estCbeta = function(C,est,var) {
    est.beta = as.matrix(est);   # Beta
    dim(est.beta)=c(length(est.beta),1)
    var.beta = var                    # var(Beta)
    est.theta = C %*% est.beta        # Theta=C*Beta
    var.theta = C %*% var.beta %*% t(C)  # Var(T)=C*Var(B)*C'
    se.theta  = sqrt(diag(var.theta))
    dim(se.theta)=c(length(se.theta),1)
    zval.theta= est.theta/se.theta
    pval.theta=(1-pnorm(abs(zval.theta)))*2
    results =cbind(est.theta,se.theta,zval.theta,pval.theta)
    colnames(results)=c("Theta","SE","z","p-val")
    rownames(results)=rownames(C)
    results
    }
```

Bootstrap Procedures for Longitudinal Data

The `bootstrap` function in R is designed for datasets with one record per case. It will inappropriately sample observations rather than cases for the longitudinal data considered in this book. If I discover or write a function appropriate to longitudinal data, I will post it on the website.

Appendix S: SAS *Notes*

Loading Datasets and Associated Formats

The **SAS** datasets available on the website have permanent formats associated with selected variables. If you place the associated format library in the same directory as the dataset, then the following statements will link the data and the formats. Separate subdirectories should be used for the different datasets.

```
libname BOOK V8 "path_to_directory_with_datasets";
options fmtsearch=(BOOK);
```

Datasets are available on *http://home.earthlink.net/~dianefairclough/Wel come.html*.

Reverse Coding and Scoring Questionnaires

Both reverse coding and scoring using the half rule for missing items can be accomplished in a few lines of code using macros rather than separate statements for every item and scale. This minimizes the possibility of typographical errors. Suppose the item variables are named ITEM1, ITEM2, ..., ITEMK etc. where missing values are coded as a SAS missing values. The first step is to reverse code questions that are negatively worded. The second step is to create a scoring macro that 1) checks whether the number of completed responses (N(of &ITEMS(*))) is greater than half the possible responses (DIM(of &ITEMS(*))), 2) calculates the summated score in the presence of missing items and 3) standardizes the summated score to have a range of 0 to 100. Arrays are then constructed with the items specific to each subscale included and the macro is invoked to calculate the subscales.

```
DATA WORK.SCORES;
  SET WORK.ITEMS;

  *** Reverse Code Selected Items Coded 0-4 ***;
  *** REV is the list of questions that are reverse coded ***;
  ARRAY REV ITEM1 ITEM7 ITEM13 ... ITEM31;
```

```
DO I=1 to DIM{REV};
  REV[I]=4-REV[I];
END;

*** Define Scoring Macro                               ***;
*** ITEM is the name of an array of items              ***;
*** MIN is the lowest possible response to a question  ***;
*** MAX is the highest possible response to a question ***;
*** SUMSCORE is the name of the summated score         ***;
*** STDSCORE is the name of the standardized (0-100) score ***;
%MACRO SCORE(ITEMS,MIN,MAX,SUMSCORE,STDSCORE);
    N_SCALE=DIM(&ITEMS);                   * # items in subscale *;
    IF N(of &ITEMS(*)) GE N_SCALE/2 THEN
        &SUMSCORE=MEAN(of &ITEMS(*))*N_SCALE;
    &STDSCORE=(&SUBSCORE-(&MIN*N_SCALE))
            *100/((&MAX-&MIN)*N_SCALE);
%MEND SCORE;

*** Array items for each subscale ***;
ARRAY PWB ITEM1 ITEM2 ITEM3 ITEM4 ITEM5 ITEM6 ITEM7;
ARRAY EWB ITEM20 ITEM21 ITEM22 ITEM23 ITEM24;

*** Compute summated scores and standardized scores ***;
%SCORE(PWB,0,4,PWB_SUM,PWB_STD);
%SCORE(EWB,0,4,EWB_SUM,EWB_STD);
```

Centering Variables

To create a new dataset (`work.centered`) with center variables within each
treatment group (`Trtment`) using a dataset (`work.patient`) that has one
record per subject:

```
PROC SQL;
  create table work.centered as
  select PatID,
    (Var1 - mean(Var1)) as Var1_C,
    (Var2 - mean(Var2)) as Var2_C,
    (Var3 - mean(Var3)) as Var3_C,
    (Var4 - mean(Var4)) as Var4_C
  from work.patient
  group by Trtment
  order by PatID;
quit;
```

`PatID` is included for merging with other datasets; `order by PatID` is optional
but avoids later sorting. To center variables across all subjects, drop `group`

by Trtment.

Bootstrap Procedure for Longitudinal Data

Bootstrapping is typically used to generate a distribution for statistics where it is difficult to derive these directly. The idea is to sample with replacement from the original data and compute the statistics using the proposed method of analysis, repeating the process a large number of times. Once this empirical distribution has been created, characteristics of the statistics can be derived. Versions of this bootstrap procedure are proposed in Chapter 10 (Mixture Models) and Section 15.3 (Q-TWiST). The example presented here implements one of the mixture models described for the lung cancer trial (Study 3) in Chapter 10.

The basic procedure assumes that there are two sets of data. The first will only contain one record per subject; in this example we have two datasets, one for each treatment group (**Frame1** and Frame2). The second set of data contains the longitudinal data (**work.Lung3**). The macro **Boot** runs the bootstrap procedure. It calls four macros that select the random sample (**%BootSelect**)[§], merge the sample with the longitudinal data (**%BootMerge**), analyze the longitudinal data (**%Analyze**) and saves the results into a dataset that will be used later (**%BootSave**). The user must write **%Analyze** as it will depend on the particular analysis; the other three are available later in this appendix.

```
%macro boot(B);
   %do i=1 %to &B;

   *** Select random sample from patient data frames ***;
   %bootselect(work.frame1,work.select1,&i*7,1000);
   %bootselect(work.frame2,work.select2,&i*19,2000);

   *** Merge random sample with longitudinal data   ***;
   %bootmerge(work.select1,work.Lung3,work.merged1,PatID);
   %bootmerge(work.select2,work.Lung3,work.merged2,PatID);

   *** SAS statements for the analysis of the longitudinal data ***;
   %analyze(indata,results);

   *** Estimates of interest are saved in work.results which has **;
   ***    one record which is then appended to work.bootsum    ***;
   %bootsave(work.results,work.bootsum);
```

[§]**Proc SurveySelect** performs the same function.

```
   %end;
%mend;
```

The procedure is as follows:

1. Sample with replacement N subjects from the first set of data, where N is the number of subjects. Generate a unique identifier for each of the N subjects in the bootstrap sample using the %BootSelect macro. If you wish to keep the number of subjects in any subgroups (e.g. treatment arms) constant, this step can be performed within each subgroup, using a different &StartID so that subjects in the different subgroups have different BootIDs. The datasets Frame1 and Frame2 contain the study identifiers for control and experimental groups respectively.

2. Merge the bootstrap sample with the longitudinal data (Lung3) using the %BootMerge macro.

3. Analyze the bootstrap sample as appropriate and save the estimates of interest (%Analyze). The BootSave macro can be used to create new-data to save the results, appending the results after the first iteration.

4. Repeat these three steps 1000 times. (This is adequate to estimate the standard error; but more repetitions may be necessary if the tails of the distribution need to be estimated more precisely.)

5. Calculate the required statistics. In this example we wish to know the standard errors, recalling that this is the standard deviation of the means.

Macro %Analyze

The following macro is specific to the analysis presented in Section 10.3.4.

```
*** Macro to Analyze the Bootstrap Sample                 ***;
%macro Analyze;
   *** Center the Dropout Indicators within Treatment Group ***;
   proc sql;
      create table work.centered1 as select BootID,
         (StrataB1 - mean(StrataB1)) as D1B,
         (StrataB2 - mean(StrataB2)) as D2B
         from work.select1 order by BootID;
      create table work.centered2 as select BootID,
         (StrataB1 - mean(StrataB1)) as D1B,
         (StrataB2 - mean(StrataB2)) as D2B
         from work.select2 order by BootID;
      quit;
   *** Merged Centered Indicators with Longitudinal Data ***;
   data work.merged;
      merge work.centered1 work.centered2 work.merged1 work.merged2;
```

```
      by BootID;
      run;

   *** Pattern Specific Estimates ***;
   proc mixed data=work.Merged noclprint order=internal;
      title2 'Strata B definition';
      class PatID Trtment;
      model FACT_T2=Trtment Trtment*Weeks Trtment*D1b Trtment*Weeks*D1b
            Trtment*D2b Trtment*Weeks*D2b/noint solution;
      random Intercept Weeks/subject=PatID type=UN;
      Estimate 'Control Week=0' Trtment 1 0;
      Estimate 'Exprmtl Week=0' Trtment 0 1;
      Estimate 'Control Week=26' Trtment 1 0 Trtment*Weeks 26 0;
      Estimate 'Exprmtl Week=26' Trtment 0 1 Trtment*Weeks 0 26;
      Estimate 'Control Change'  Trtment*Weeks 26   0;
      Estimate 'Exprmtl Change'  Trtment*Weeks 0 26;
      Estimate 'Difference Change' Trtment*Weeks  -26 26;
      ods output Estimates=work.Results; * Outputs Estimates *;
      run;
%mend;
```

Putting it together

The backbone of a typical **SAS** program is as follows:

```
*** Read in the file with the Bootstrap Macros              ***;
%include "C:\BootstrapMacros.sas"; * Change directory as needed *;

*** SAS statements that prepare the datasets                ***;
***   - work.frame1 and work.frame2 contain patient level data ***;
***     for the two treatment groups                        ***;
***   - work.lung3 contains the longitudinal data           ***;
```

Test the procedure with 3 iterations, then runs the full bootstrap procedure.

```
*options mprint mlogic; * Generates Details in Log if problems ***;
*%boot(3);             * Test with 3 iterations *;

*** Suppresses Information going to Output and Log          ***;
proc printto print="C:\Trash_Output.txt" log="C:\Trash_Log.txt";
   run;
*** Runs the bootstrap procedure for 1000 iterations        ***;
%boot(1000);
*** Restores Output and Log to default                      ***;
proc printto;
   run;
```

Finally, calculate the statistics of interest; in this example the standard errors of the estimates. This code will change with the application.

```
*** Calculation of the Standard Errors ***;
proc means data=work.bootsum nway N Mean Std maxdec=2;
  title "Summary of Bootstrap Estimates";
  class label; * Identifier of each estimate *;
  var estimate;
  run;
```

Macro %BootSelect

```
* Randomly Selects Subjects from the dataset &Indata       *;
* Creates a dataset &Outdata                               *;
* The dataset &Indata must have only one rec/ subject      *;
* Seed is usually a function of the iteration # such as &i*7 *;

%macro BootSelect(indata,outdata,seed,startID);
data &outdata;
    * Creates Random Variable from 1 to n *;
    choice=Ceil(ranuni(&seed)*n);
    set &indata point=choice nobs=n;
    BootID=&startID+_N_; * ID for future analysis *;
    if _N_>n then stop;
  run;
%mend;
```

Macro %BootMerge

```
* Merges data from &Bootdata with &Longdata       *;
* &ID is the subject ID on the original datasets  *;
* The merged dataset will have a new ID: BootID    *;

%macro BootMerge(bootdata,longdata,outdata,id);
proc sql;
  create table &outdata
    as select *
    from &bootdata as l left join &longdata as r on l.&id=r.&id
    order by BootID;
  quit;
%mend;
```

Macro %BootSave

```
*** Saves the results from &Indata into &Outdata ***;
*** &Indata will usually have one record          ***;

%macro BootSave(indata,outdata);
    %if &I=1 %then %do; * Saves results in &outdata *;
      data &outdata;
        set &indata;
      run;
```

```
    %end;
    %else %do;              * Appends results to &outdata *;
      proc append base=&outdata new=&indata force;
         run;
    %end;
%mend;
```

The code is available on *http://home.earthlink.net/~ dianefairclough/Wel come.html.*

References

Aaronson NK, Ahmedzai S, Bergman B, et al. (1993) The European Organization for Research and Treatment of Cancer QLQ-30: A quality-of-life instrument for use in international clinical trials in oncology. *Journal of the National Cancer Institute*, 85: 365-376.

Albert PS. (1999) Tutorial in biostatistics: Longitudinal data anlaysis (repeated measures) in clinical trials. *Statistics in Medicine*, 18: 1707-1732.

Bacik J, Mazumdar M, Murphy BA, Fairclough DL, Eremenco S, Mariani T, Motzer RJ, Cella D. (2004) The functional assessment of cancer therapy-BRM (FACT-BRM): A new tool for the assessment of quality of life in patients treated with biologic response modifiers. *Quality of Life Research*, 13: 137-154.

Barnard J, Meng XL. (1999) Applications of multiple imputation in medical studies: From AIDS to NHANES. *Statistical Methods in Medical Research*, 8: 17-36.

Barnard J, Rubin DB. (1999) Small-sample degrees of freedom with multiple imputation. *Biometrika*, 86: 948-955.

Baron RM, Kenny DA. (1986) The moderator-mediator variable distinction in social psychological research: Conceptual, strategic, and statistic considerations. *Journal Personality and Social Psychology*, 51: 1173-1182.

Bernhard J, Peterson HF, Coates AS, Gusset H, Isley M, Hinkle R, Gelber RD, Castiglione-Gertsch M, Hürny C. (1998) Quality of life assessment in International Breast Cancer Study Group (IBCSG) trials: Practical issues and factors associated with missing data. *Statistics in Medicine*, 17: 587-602.

Bernhard J, Cella DF, Coates AS, et al. (1998) Missing quality of life data in clinical trials: Serious problems and challenges. *Statistics in Medicine*, 17: 517-532.

Bonomi P, Kim KM, Fairclough D, Cella D, Kugler J, Rowinsky E, Jiroutek M, Johnson D. (2000) Comparison of survival and quality of life in advanced non-small-cell lung cancer patients treated with two dose levels of Paclitaxel combined with Cisplatin versus Etoposide-Cisplatin: Results of an Eastern Cooperative Group Trial. *Journal of Clinical Oncology*, 18: 623-31.

Bouchet C, Guillemin F, Paul-Dauphin A, Brianon S. (2000) Selection of quality-of-life measures for a prevention trial: A psychometric analysis. *Controlled Clinical Trials*, 21: 30-43.

Box GEP, Draper NR. (1987). *Empirical Model-Building and Response Surfaces*, p. 424, Wiley, New York.

Brazier JE, Roberts J, Deverill M. (2002) The estimation of a preference-based measure of health status from the SF-36. *Journal of Health Economics*, 21: 271-292.

Brooks R. (1996) EuroQoL: The current state of play. *Health Policy (Amsterdam)*, 37: 53-72.

Brooks MM, Jenkins LS, Schron EB, Steinberg JS, Cross JA, Paeth DS. (1998) Quality of life at baseline: Is assessment after randomization valid? *Medical Care*, 36: 1515-1519.

Brown CH. (1990) Protecting against nonrandomly missing data in longitudinal studies. *Biometrics*, 46: 143-155.

Buck SF. (1960) A method of estimation of missing values in multivariate data suitable for use with a electronic computer. *Journal Royal Statistical Society, Series B*, 22: 302-306.

Busch P, Schwendener P, Leu RE, VonDach B, Castiglione M. (1994) Life quality assessment of breast cancer patients receiving adjuvant therapy using incomplete data. *Health Economics*, 3: 203-220.

Cella DF, Skeel RT, Bonomi AE. (1993) Policies and Procedures Manual. Eastern Cooperative Oncology Group Quality of Life Subcommittee (unpublished).

Cella DF, Tulsky DS, Gray G, et al. (1993) The Functional Assessment of Cancer Therapy (FACT) scales: Development and validation of the general measure. *Journal of Clinical Oncology*, 11: 570-579.

Cella DF, Bonomi AE, Lloyd SR, Tulsky DS, Kaplan E, Bonomi P. (1995) Reliability and validity of the Functional Assessment of Cancer therapy - Lung (FACT-L) quality of life instrument. *Lung Cancer*, 12: 199-220, 1995.

Cella DF, Bonomi AE. (1995) Measuring quality of life: 1995 update. *Oncology*, 9 11(supplement) 47-60.

Cella DF. (2001) Personal communication.

Center for Drug Evaluation and Reserach, Food and Drug Administration. (1998) E9 Statistical principles for clinical trials. *Federal Register*, 63: 49584-49598.

Chi Y, Ibrahim JG. (2006) Joint models for multivariate longitudinal and multivariate survival data. *Biometrics*, 62, 432-445.

Chuang-Stein C, Tong DM. (1996) The impact of parameterization on the interpretation of the main-effect yerm in the presence of an interaction. *Drug Information Journal*, 30: 421-424.

Cleeland CS, Mendoza TR, Wang XS, Chou C, Harle MT, Morrissey M, Engstrom MC. (2000) Assessing smptoms distress in cancer patients: The MD Anderson Symptom Inventory. *Cancer*, 89: 1634-1646.

Cohen J. (1988) *Statistical Power Analysis for the Behavioral Sciences, 2nd edition*. Lawrence Erlbaum Associates, Hillsdale, New Jersey.

Cole BF, Gelber RD, Goldhirsch A. (1993) Cox regression models for quality adjusted survival analysis. *Statistics in Medicine* 12: 975-987.

Converse JM, Presser S. (1986) *Survey Questions: Handcrafting the Standardized Questionnaire. Survey Research Methods*. Sage Publications, Newbury Park, CA.

Cook NR. (1997) An imputation method for non-ignorable missing data in studies of blood pressure. *Statistics in Medicine*, 16: 2713-2728.

Cox DR, Fitzpatrick R, Fletcher AI, Gore SM, Spiegelhalter DJ, Jones DR. (1992) Quality-of-life assessment: Can we keep it simple? (with discussion). *Journal of the Royal Statistical Society A*, 155: 353-393.

Crawford SL, Tennstedt SL, McKinlay JB. (1995) A comparison of analytic methods for non-random missingness of outcome data. *Journal of Clinical Epidemiology*, 48: 209-219.

Curren D. (2000) *Analysis of Incomplete Longitudinal Quality of Life Data*. Doctoral dissertation, Linburgs Universitair Centrum.

Curren D, Aaronson N, Standaert B, Molenberghs G, Therasse P, Ramierez A, Keepmanschap M, Erder H, Piccart M. (2000) Summary measures and statistics in the analysis of quality of life data: an example from an EORTC-NCIC-SAKK locally advanced breast cancer study. *European Journal of Cancer*, 36: 834-844.

Daniels MJ, Hogan JW. (2000) Reparameterizing the pattern mixture model for sensitivity analyses under informative dropout. *Biometrics*, 5: 1241-1248.

Dawson JD, Lagakos SW. (1991) Analyzing laboratory marker changes in AIDS clinical trials. *Journal of Acquired Immune Deficiency Syndromes*, 4: 667-676.

Dawson JD, Lagakos SW. (1993) Size and power of two-sample tests of repeated measures data. *Biometrics*, 49: 1022-1032.

Dawson JD. (1994) Stratification of summary statistic tests according to missing data patterns. *Statistics in Medicine,* 13: 1853-1863.

DeGruttola V, Tu XM. (1994) Modeling progression of CD-4 lymphocyte count and its relationship to survival time. *Biometrics,* 50: 1003-1014.

DeKlerk NH. (1986) Repeated warnings re repeated measures. *Australian New Zealand Journal of Medicine,* 16: 637-638.

Dempster AP, Laird NM, Rubin DB. (1977) Maximum likelihood estimation from incomplete data via the EM algorithm (with discussion). *Journal of the Royal Statistical Society, Series B,* 39: 1-38.

Devellis RF. (1991) *Scale Development: Theory and Application.* Sage Publications, Newbury Park, CA.

Diehr P, Patrick DL, Hedrick S, Rothaman M, Grembowski D, Raghunathan TI, Beresford S. (1995) Including deaths when measuring health status over time. *Medical Care,* 33(suppl): AS164-172.

Diggle PJ, Kenward MG. (1994) Informative dropout in longitudinal data analysis (with discussion). *Applied Statistics,* 43: 49-93.

Diggle PJ, Liang KY, Zeger SL. (1994) *Analysis of Longitudinal Data.* Oxford Science Publications. Clarendon Press, Oxford.

Dmitrienko A, Offen W, Westfall PH. (2003) Gatekeeping strategies for clinical trials that do not require all primary effects to be significant. *Statistics in Medicine,* 22: 2387-2400.

Donaldson GW, Nakamura Y, Moinpour C. (2009) Mediators, moderators, and modulators of causal effects in clinical trials - Dynamically Modified Outcomes (DYNAMO) in health-related quality of life. *Quality of Life Research,* 18: 137-145.

Drummond M. (2001) Introducing ecomonic and quality of life measurements into clinical studines. *Annals of Medicine,* 33: 344-349.

Elashoff RM, Li G, Li N. (2007) An approach to joint analysis of longitudinal measurements and competing risks failure time data. *Statistics in Medicine,* 26: 2813-35.

Fairclough DL, Cella DF. (1996) A cooperative group report on quality of life research: Lessons learned. Eastern Cooperative Oncology Group (ECOG). *Journal of the National Cancer Institute,* 40: 73-75.

Fairclough DL, Cella DF. (1996) Functional Assessment of Cancer Therapy (FACT-G): Non-response to individual questions. *Quality of Life Research,* 5: 321-329.

Fairclough DL. (1997) Summary measures and statistics for comparison of quality of life in a clinical trial of cancer therapy, *Statistics in Medicine*, 16: 1197-1209.

Fairclough DL. (1998) Method of analysis for longitudinal studies of health-related quality of life, Chapter 13. *Quality of Life Assessment in Clinical Trials: Methods and Practice.* Staquet MJ, Hayes RD and Fayers PM, eds. Oxford University Press, New York.

Fairclough DL, Peterson H, Chang V. (1998) Why is missing quality of life data a problem in clincial trials of cancer therapy? *Statistics in Medicine*, 17: 667-678.

Fairclough DL, Peterson H, Bonomi P, Cella DF. (1998) Comparison of model based methods dependent of the missing data mechanism in two clinical trials of cancer therapy. *Statistics in Medicine*, 17: 781-796.

Fairclough DL, Fetting JH, Cella D, Wonson W, Moinpour C for the Eastern Cooperative Oncology Group. (1999) Quality of life and quality adjusted survival for breast cancer patients recieving adjuvant therapy. *Quality of Life Research*, 8: 723-731.

Farivar SS, Cunninghom WE, Hayes RD. (2007) Correlated physical and meantal health summary scores for the SF-36 and SF-12 Health Survey, V.1. *Health and Quality of Life Outcomes*, 5: 54-61.

Fayers PM, Hand DJ. (1997) Factor analysis, causal indicators and quality of life. *Quality of Life Research*, 6: 139-150.

Fayers PM, Machin D. (2000) *Quality of Life: Assessment, Analysis and Interpretation.* John Wiley and Sons, England.

Feeny D, Furlong W, Barr RD, et al. (1992) A comprehensive multi-attribute system for classifying the health status of survivors of childhood cancer. *Journal of Clinical Oncology*, 10: 923-928.

Feeny D. (2005) Preference-based measures: Utility and quality-adjusted life years. In *Assessing quality of life in Clinical Trials, 2nd edition.* pp 405-429. Fayers P and Hays R, eds. Oxford University Press.

Feeny D, Farris K, Côté I, Johnson JA, Tsuyuki RT, Eng K. (2005) A cohort study found the RAND-12 and Health Utilities Index Mark 3 demonstrated construct validity in high-risk primary care patients. *Journal of Clinical Epidemiology*, 58: 138-41.

Fetting J, Gray R, Abeloff M, et al. (1995) CAF vs. a 16-week multidrug regimen as adjuvant therapy for receptor-negative, node positive breast cancer: An intergroup study. *Proceedings of the Americal Society of Clinical Oncology*, 114: #83.

Fetting JJ, Gray R, Abeloff MD, Fairclough DL, et al. (1998) A 16-week multidrug regimen versus cyclophosphamide, doxorubicin and 5-flurouracil as adjuvant therapy for node-positive, receptor negative breast cancer: An intergroup study. *Journal of Clinical Oncology*, 16: 2382-91.

Fitzmaurice GM, Laird NM, Shneyer L. (2001) An alternative parameterization of the general linear mixture model for longitudinal data with non-ignorable drop-outs. *Statistics in Medicine*, 20: 1009-1021.

Fleiss JL. (1986) *The Design and Analysis of Clinical Experiments*. John Wiley and Sons, New York.

Floyd J, Fowler JR. (1988) *Survey Research Methods*. Sage Publications, Newbury Park, CA.

Follman D, Wu M. (1995) An approximate generalized linear model with random effects for informative missing data, *Biometrics*, 51: 151-168.

Frank-Stromborg M, Olsen S. (1997) *Instruments for Clinical Health Care Research, Second Edition* Jones and Bartlett Publishers, Boston.

Franks P, Lubetkin EI, Gold MR, Tancredi DJ. (2003) Mapping the SF-12 to preference-based instruments: Convergent validity in a low-income, minority population. *Medical Care*, 41: 1277-83.

Freemantle N, Calvert M, Wood J, Eastangh J, Griffin C. (2003) Composite outcomes in randomized trials: Great precision but with greater uncertainty? *Journal of the American Medical Association*, 239: 2554-59.

Friedman LM, Furberg CD, Demets D. (1985) *Fundamentals of Clinical Trials, 2nd edition*. John Wright PSG, Boston.

Frison L, Pocock SJ. (1992) Repeated measures in clinical trials: Analysis using mean summary statistics and its implications for design. *Statistics in Medicine* 11: 1685-1704.

Gelber RD, Gelman RS, Goldhirsh A. (1998) A quality of life oriented endpoint for comparing therapies. *Biometrics* 45: 781-95.

Glasziou PP, Simes RJ, Gelber RD. (1990) Quality adjusted survival analysis. *Statisitics in Medicine* 9: 1259-1276.

Glynn RJ, Laird NM, Rubin DB. (1993) Multiple imputation in mixture models for non-ignorable nonresponse with follow-ups. *Journal of the American Statistical Association*, 88: 984-993.

Goldhirsch A, Gelber RD, Simes RJ, et al. (1989) Costs and benefits of adjuvant therapy in breast cancer: A quality adjusted survival analysis. *Journal of Clinical Oncology* 7: 36-44, 1989.

Gotay CC, Korn EL, McCabe MS, Moore TD, Cheson BD. (1992) Building quality of life assessment into cancer treatment studies. *Oncology*, 6: 25-28.

Gould AL. (1980) A new approach to the analysis of clinical drug trails with withdrawals. *Biometrics*, 36: 721-727.

Guo X, Carlin BP. (2004) Separate and joint modeling of longitudinal and event time data using standard computer packages. *The American Statistician*, 16-24.

Guyatt GH, Townsend M, Merman LB, Keller JL. (1987) A comparison of Likert and visual analogue scales for measuring change in function. *Journal of Chronic Disease*, 40: 1129-1133.

Guyatt G et al. (1991) Glossary. *Controlled Clinical Trials*, 12: 274S-280S.

Heitjan DA, Landis JR. (1994) Assessing secular trends in blood pressure: A multiple imputation approach. *Journal of the American Statistical Association*, 89: 750-759.

Heyting A, Tolbomm TBM, Essers JGA. (1992) Statistical handling of dropouts in longitudinal clinical trials. *Statistics in Medicine*, 11: 2043-2061.

Hicks JE, Lampert MH, Gerber LH, Glastein E, Danoff J. (1985) Functional outcome update in patients with soft tissue sarcoma undergoing wide local excision and radiation (Abstract). *Archives of Physical Medicine and Rehabilitation*, 66: 542-543.

Hochberg Y. (1988) A sharper Bonferroni procedure for multiple significance testing. *Biometrika*, 75: 800-803.

Hogan JW, Laird NM. (1997) Mixture models for the joint distribution of repeated measuress and event times. *Statistics in Medicine*, 16: 239-257.

Hogan JW, Laird NM. (1997) Model-based approaches to analysing incomplete longitudinal and failure time data. *Statistics in Medicine*, 16: 259-272.

Hogan JW, Roy J, Korkontzelou C. (2004) Tutorial in biostatistics: Handling drop-out in longitudinal studies. *Statistics in Medicine*, 23: 1455-1497.

Hogan JW, Lin X, Herman G. (2004) Mixtures of varying coefficient models for longitudinal data with discrete or continuous non-ignorable dropout. *Biometrics*, 60: 854-864.

Hollen PJ, Gralla RJ, Cox C, Eberly SW, Kris M. (1997) A dilemma in analysis: Issues in serial measurement of quality of life in patients with advanced lung cancer. *Lung Cancer*, 18: 119-136.

Holm S. (1979) A simple sequentially rejective multiple test procedure. *Scandinavian Journal of Statistics*, 6: 65-70.

Holmbeck GN. (1997) Toward terminological, conceptual and statistical clarity in the study of mediators and moderators: Examples from the child-clinical and pediatric psychology literatures. *Journal of Consulting and Clinical Psychology*, 65: 599-610.

Holmbeck GN. (2002) Post-hoc probing of significant moderational and mediational effects in studies of pediatric populations. *Journal of Pediatric Psychology*, 27: 87-96.

Hommel G. (1983) Tests of overall hypothesis for arbitrary dependence structures. *Biometric Journal*, 25: 423-30.

Hommel G, Bretz F, Maurer W. (2007) Powerful sort-cuts for multiple testing procedures with special reference to gatekeeping strategies. *Statistics in Medicine*, 26: 4063-4073.

Hopwood P, Harvey A, Davies J, Stephens RJ, et al. (1997) Survey of the administration of quality of life questionniares in three multicentre randomised trials in cancer. *European Journal of Cancer*, 90: 49-57.

Hürny C, Bernhard J, Gelber RD, Coates A, Castiglione M, Isley M, Dreher D, Peterson H, Goldhirsch A, Senn HJ. (1992) Quality of life measures for patients receiving adjuvant therapy for breast cancer: An international trial. *European Journal of Cancer*, 28: 118-124.

Hürny C, Bernhard J, Bacchi M, et al. (1993) The Perceived Adjustment to Chronic Illness Scale (PACIS): A global indicator of coping for operable breast cancer patients in clinical trials. *Supportive Care in Cancer*, 1: 200-208.

Hürny C, Bernhard J, Coates AS, et al. (1996) Impact of adjuvant therapy on quality of life in node-positive patients with operable breast cancer. *Lancet*, 347: 1279-1284.

International Committee of Medical Journal Editors (2008) Uniform requirement for manuscripts submitted to biomedical journals. Retrieved from: www.jcmje.org

Jaros, M. (2008) *A Joint Model for Longitudinal Data and Competing Risks*. Doctoral dissertation, University of Colorado at Denver.

Jennrich R, Schluchter M. (1986) Unbalanced repeated-measures models with structured covariance matrices. *Biometrics*, 42: 805-820.

Jhingran P, Osterhaus JT, Miller DW, Lee JT, Kirchdoerfer L. (1998) Development and validation of the migraine-specific quality of life questionnaire. *Headache*, 38: 295-302.

Jones RH. (1993) *Longitudinal Data with Serial Correlation: A State-Space Approach*. Chapman and Hall, London.

Juniper EF, Guyatt GH, Jaeschke R. (1996) How to develop and validate a new health-related quality of life instrument. in *Quality of Life and Pharma-*

coeconomics in Clinical Trials, Chapter 6. Spilker B, ed. Lippincott-Raven Publishers, Philadelphia.

Kaplan RM, Bush JW. (1982) Health-related quality of life measurement for evaluation research and policy analysis. *Health Psychology*, 1: 61-80.

Kenward MG, Roger JH. (1997) Small sample inference for fixed effects from restricted maximum likelihood. *Biometrics*, 53: 983-997.

Kittleson JM, Sharples K, Emerson SS. (2005) Group sequential clinical trials for longitudinal data with analyses using summary statistics. *Statistics in Medicine*, 24: 2457-2475.

Korn EL, O'Fallon J. (1990) *Statistical Considerations, Statistics Working Group. Quality of Life Assessment in Cancer Clinical Trials*, Report on Workshop on Quality of Life Research in Cancer Clinical Trials. Division of Cancer Prevention and Control, National Cancer Institute.

Korn DL. (1993) On estimating the distribution function for quality of life in cancer clinical trials. *Biometrika*, 80: 535-42.

Kosinski M, Bayliss M, Bjorner JB, Ware JE. (2000) Improving estimates of SF-36 Health Survey scores for respondents with missing data. *Medical Outcomes Trust Monitor*, 5: 8-10.

Kraemer HC, Wilson GT, Fairburn CG, Agras WS. (2002) Mediators and moderators of treatment effects in randomized clinical trials. *Archives of General Psychiatry*, 59: 877-883.

Laird NM, Ware JH. (1982) Random-effects models for longitudinal data. *Biometrics*, 38: 963-974.

Lauter J. (1996) Exact t and F tests for analyzing studies with multiple end-points. *Biometrics*, 52: 964-970.

Lavori PW, Dawson R, Shera D. (1995) A multiple imputation strategy for clinical trials with truncation of patient data. *Statistics in Medicine*, 14: 1912-1925.

Law NJ, Taylor JMG, Sandler HM. (2002) The joint modeling of a longitudinal disease progression marker and the fairure time process in the presence of cure. *Biostatistics*, 3: 547-563.

Lechmaher W, Wassmer G, Reitmeir P. (1991) Procedures for two-sample comparisons with multiple endpoints controling the experimentwise error rate. *Biometrics*, 47: 511-522.

Lee CW, Chi KN. (2000) The standard of report of health-related quality of life in clinical cancer trials. *Journal of Clinical Epidemiology*, 53: 451-458.

Levine M, Guyatt G, Gent M, et al. (1988) Quality of life in stage II breast cancer: An instrument for clinical trials. *Journal of Clinical Oncology*, 6: 1798-1810.

Li L, Hu B, Greene T (2007) Semiparametric joint modeling of longitudinal and survival data. *Joint Statistical Meetings Proceedings, 2007*: 293-300.

Listing J, Schlitten R. (1998) Tests if dropouts are missed at random. *Biometrical Journal*, 40: 929-935.

Listing J, Schlitten R. (2003) A nonparametric test for random dropouts. *Biometrical Journal*, 45: 113-127.

Littel RC, Miliken GA, Stroup WW, Wolfinger RD. (1996) *SAS System for Mixed Models*, SAS Institute Inc., Cary, NC.

Little RJ, Rubin DB.(1987) *Statistical Analysis with Missing Data*. John Wiley and Sons, New York.

Little RJA. (1988) A test of missing completely at random for multivariate data with missing values. *Journal of the American Statistical Association*, 83: 1198-1202.

Little RJA. (1993) Pattern-mixture models for multivariate incomplete data. *Journal of the American Statistical Association*, 88: 125-134.

Little RJA.(1994) A class of pattern-mixture models for normal incomplete data. *Biometrika*, 81: 471-483.

Little RJA. (1995) Modeling the dropout mechanism in repeated-measures studies. *Journal of the American Statistical Association*, 90: 1112-1121.

Little RJA, Wang Y. (1996) Pattern-mixture models for multivariate incomplete data with covariates. *Biometrics*, 52: 98-111.

Little R, Yau L. (1996) Intent-to-treat analysis for longitudinal studies with dropouts. *Biometrics*, 52: 1324-1333.

MacKinnon DP, Warsi G, Dwyer JH. (1995) A simulation study of mediated effect measures. *Multivariate Behavarial Research*, 30: 4162.

MacKinnon DP, Fairchild AJ, and Fritz MS. (2007) Mediation analysis. *Annual Reviews Psychology*, 58: 593-614.

MacKinnon DP. (2008) *Introduction to Statistical Mediation Analysis*. Taylor & Francis Group, New York, NY.

Marcus R, Peritz E, Gabriel KR. (1976) On closed testing procedures with special reference to ordered analysis of variance. *Biometrika*, 63: 655-660.

Martin BC, Pathak DS, Sharfman MI, Adelman JU, Taylor F, Kwong WJ, Jhingran P. (2000) Validity and reliability of the migraine specific quality of life questionnaire (MSQ Version 2.1). *Headache*, 40: 204-215.

Matthews JNS, Altman DG, Campbell MJ, Royston P. (1990) Analysis of serial measurements in medical research. *British Medical Journal*, 300: 230-235.

McDowell I, Newell C. (1996) *Measuring Health: A Guide to Rating Scales and Questionnaires, 2nd edition.* Oxford University Press, New York.

McNeil BJ, Weichselbaum R, Pauker SG. (1981) Tradeoffs between quality and quantity of life in laryngeal cancer. *New England Journal of Medicine*, 305: 982-987.

Meinert CL. (1986) *Clinical Trials: Design, Conduct and Analysis.* Oxford University Press, England.

Michiels B, Molenberghs G, Lipsitz SR. (1999) Selection models and pattern-mixture models for incomplete data with covariates. *Biometrics*, 55: 978-983.

Miller GA. (1956) The magic number seven plus or minus two: some limits on our capacity for information processing. *Psychological Bulletin*, 63: 81-97.

Moinpour C, Feigl P, Metch B, et al. (1989) Quality of life endpoints in cancer clinical trails: Review and recommendations. *Journal of the National Cancer Institute*, 81: 485-495.

Mori M, Woodworth GG, Woolson RF. (1992) Application of empirical Bayes inference to estimation of rate of change in the presence of informative right censoring. *Statistics in Medicine*, 11: 621-631.

Motzer RJ, Murphy BA, Bacik J, et al. (2000) Phase III trial of Interferon Alfa-2a with or without 13-*cis*-retinoic acid for patients with advanced renal cell carcinoma. *Journal of Clinical Oncology*, 18: 2972-2980.

Murray GD, Findlay JG. (1988) Correcting for the bias caused by dropouts in hypertension trials. *Statistics in Medicine*, 7: 941-946.

Naughton MJ, Shumaker SA, Anderson RT, Czajkowski SM. (1996) Psychological aspects of health-related quality of life measurment: Tests and scales, in *Quality of Life and Pharmacoeconomics in Clinical Trials*, Chapter 15. Spilker B, ed. Lippincott-Raven Publishers, Philadelphia.

Neter J, Wasserman W. (1974) *Applied Linear Statistical Models*, pp 313-317, Richard Irwin, Homewood, Illinois.

Noll RB, Fairclough DL.(2004) Health-related quality of life: Developmental and psychometric issues (Editorial). *The Journal of Pediatrics*, 145: 8-9.

Norton NJ, Lipsitz SR. (2001) Multiple imputation in practice: Comparison of software packages for regression models with missing variables. *The American Statistician*, 55: 244-254.

O'Brien PC. (1984) Procedures for comparing samples with multiple endpoints. *Biometrics*, 40: 1079-1087.

Omar PZ, Wright EM, Turner RM, Thompon SG. (1999) Analyzing repeated measurements data: A practical comparison of methods. *Statistics in Medicine*, 18: 1587-1608.

Paik, SSS (1997) The generalized estimating approach when data are not missing completely at random. *Journal of the American Statistical Association*, 92: 1320-1329.

Pater J, Osoba D, Zee B, Lofters W, Gore M, Dempsey E, Palmer M, Chin C. (1998) Effects of altering the time of administration and the time frame of quality of life assessments in clinical trials: An example using the EORTC QLQ-C30 in a large anti-emetic trial. *Quality of Life Research*, 7: 273-778.

Patrick DL, Bush JW, Chen MM. (1973) Methods for measuring levels of well-being for a health status index. *Health Services Research*, 8: 228-245.

Patrick D, Erickson P. (1993) *Health Status and Health Policy: Allocating Resources to Health Care.* Oxford University Press, New York.

Pauler DK, McCoy S, Moinpour C. (2003) Pattern mixture models for longitudinal quality of life studies in advanced stage disease. *Statistics in Medicine*, 22: 795–809.

Piantadosi S. (1997) *Clinical Trials: A Methodological Perspective.* John Wiley and Sons, New York.

Pinheiro JC, Bates DM. (2000) *Mixed-Effects Models in S and S-PLUS.* Springer Verlag, New York, NY.

Pledger G, Hall D. (1982) Withdrawals from drug trials (letter to editor). *Biometrics*, 38: 276-278.

Pocock SJ, Geller NL, Tsiatis AA. (1987a) The analysis of multiple endpoints in clinical trials. *Biometrics*, 43: 487-498.

Pocock SJ, Hughes MD, Lee RJ.(1987b) Statistical problems in the reporting of clinical trials. *New England Journal of Medicine* 317: 426-432.

Proschan MA, Waclawiw MA. (2000) Practical guidelines for multiplicity adjustment in clinical trials. *Controlled Clinical Trials*, 21: 527-539.

Raboud JM, Singer J, Thorne A, Schechter MT, Shafran SD. (1998) Estimating the effect of treatment on quality of life in the presence of missing data due to dropout and death. *Quality of Life Research*, 7: 487-494.

Reitmeir J, Wassmer G. (1999) Resampling-based methods for the analysis of multiple endpoints in clinical trials. *Statistics in Medicine*, 18: 3455-3462.

Revicki DA, Gold K, Buckman D, Chan K, Kallich JD, Woodley M. (2001)

Imputing physical function scores missing owing to mortality: Results of a simulation comparing multiple techniques. *Medical Care*, 39: 61-71

Ribaudo HJ, Thompson SG, Allen-Mersh TG (2000) A joint analysis of quality of life and survival using a random-effect selection model. *Statistics in Medicine*, 19: 3237-3250.

Ridout MS. (1991) Testing for random dropouts in repeated measurement data. *Biometrics*, 47: 1617-1621.

Rizopoulos D, Verbeke G, Lesaffre E. (2009) Fully exponential Laplace approximation for the joint modelling of survival and longitudinal data. *Journal of the Royal Statistical Society, Series B*, 71: 637-654.

Rosenbaum PR, Rubin DB. (1984) Reducing bias in observational studies using subclassification in the propensity score. *Journal of the American Statistical Association*, 79: 516-524.

Rubin DB, Schenker N. (1986) Multiple imputation for interval estimation from simple random samples with ignorable nonresponse. *Journal of the American Statistical Association*, 81: 366-374.

Rubin DB. (1987), *Multiple Imputation for Nonresponse in Surveys*, Wiley, New York.

Rubin DB, Schenker N. (1991) Multiple imputation in health-care data bases: An overview and some applications. *Statistics in Medicine*, 10: 585-598.

Rubin DB. (1996) Multiple imputation after 18+ years. *Journal of the American Statistical Association*, 91: 473-489.

Russell IJ, Crofford LJ, Leon T, Cappelleri JC, Bushmakin AG, Whalen E, Barrett JA, Sadosky A. (2009) The effects of pregabalin on sleep disturbance symptoms among individuals with fibromyalgia syndrome. *Sleep Medicine*, 10: 604-610.

SAS Institute (1996) Chapter 18: The MIXED procedure. *SAS/STAT Software. Changes and Enhancements (through Release 6.11)*, SAS Institute, Cary, NC.

Schafer J. (1997) *Analysis of Incomplete Multivariate Data*. Chapman and Hall, London.

Schipper H, Clinich J, McMurray A, Levitt M. (1984) Measuring the quality of life of cancer patients. The Functional Living Index - Cancer: Development and validation. *Journal of Clinical Oncology*, 2: 472-482.

Schipper H. (1990) Guidelines and caveats for quality of life measurement in clinical practice and research. *Oncology*, 4: 51-57.

Schluchter MD. (1990) 5V: Unbalanced repeated measures models with structured covariance matrices, pp 1207-1244, 1322-1327 in *BMDP Statistical Software Manual, 2* W.J. Dixon, ed. University of California Press, Berkeley CA.

Schluchter MD. (1992) Methods for the analysis of informatively censored longitudinal data. *Statistics in Medicine*, 11: 1861-1870.

Schluchter DM, Green T, Beck GJ. (2001) Analysis of change in the presence of informative censoring: application to a longitudinal clinical trial of progressive renal disease. *Statistics in Medicine*, 20: 989-1007.

Schluchter MD, Konstan MW, Davis PB. (2002) Jointly modelling the relationship between survival and pulmonary function in cystic fibrosis patients. *Statistics in Medicine*, 21: 1271-1287.

Schumacher M, Olschewski M, Schulgen G. (1991) Assessment of quality of life in clinical trials. *Statistics in Medicine*, 10: 1915-1930.

Schuman H, Presser S. (1981) *Questions and Answers in Attitude Surveys: Experiments on Question Form, Wording and Context*. Academic Press, London.

Schwartz D, Flamant R, Lellouch J. (1980) *Clinical Trials*. Academic Press, London.

Searle SR. (1971) *Linear Models* pp 46-47, John Wiley and Sons, New York.

Simes RJ. (1986) An improved Bonferroni procedure for multiple tests of significance. *Biometrika*, 73: 751-754.

Simon GE, Revicki DA, Grothaus L, Vonkorff M. (1998) SF-summary scores: Are physical and mental health truly distinct? *Medical Care*, 36: 567-572.

Smith, DM. (1996) Oswald: Object-oriented software for the analysis of longitudinal data in S. http://www.maths.lancs.ac.uk/Software/Oswald.

Smith DM, Schwarz N, Roberts TR, Ubel PA. (2006) Why are you calling me? How study introductions change response patterns. *Quality of Life Research*, 15: 621-630.

Statistical Solutions (1997) *Solas for Missing Data Analysis 1.0 User Reference*. Statistical Solutions Ltd., Cork, Ireland.

Spilker B., ed. (1996) *Quality of Life and Pharmacoeconomics in Clinical Trials*. Lippincott-Raven Publishers, Philadelphia.

Spilker B. (1991) *Guide to Clinical Trials*. Lippincott Williams & Wilkins.

Staquet M, Aaronson NK, Ahmedzai S, et al. (1992) Editorial: Health-related quality of life research. *Quality of Life Research*, 1: 3.

Staquet M, Berson R, Osoba D, Machin D. (1996) Guidelines for reporting results of quality of life assessments in clinical trials. *Quality of Life Research*, 5: 496-502.

Staquet MJ, Hayes RD, Fayers PM. (1998) *Quality of life assessment in clinical trials: Methods and practice.* Oxford University Press, New York.

Streiner DL, Norman GR. (1995) *Health Measurement Scales - A Practical Guide to their Development and Use - Second Edition.* Oxford Medical Publications, Oxford University Press, New York.

Sugarbaker PH, Barofsky I, Rosenberg SA, Gianola FJ. (1982) Quality of life assessment of patients in extremity sarcoma clinical trials. *Surgery*, 91: 17-23.

Tandon PK. (1990) Applications of global statistics in analyzing quality of life data. *Statistics in Medicine* 9: 819-827.

Tang ST, McCorkle R. (2002) Appropriate time frames for data collection in quality of life research among cancer patients at the end of life. *Quality of Life Research*, 11: 145-155.

Thiebaut R, Jacqmin-Gabba H, Babiker A, Commenges D. (2005) Joint modeling of bivariate longitudinal data with informative dropout and left-censoring, with application to the evolution of CD4+cell count and HIV RNA viral load in response to treatment of HIV infection. *Statistics in Medicine*, 24: 65-82.

Torrance GW, Thomas WH, Sackett DL. (1971) A utility maximizing model for evaluation of health care programs. *Health Services Research*, 7: 118-133.

Touloumi G, Pocock SJ, Babiker AG, Daryshire JH. (1999) Estimation and comparison of rates of change in longitudinal studies with informative dropouts. *Statistics in Medicine*, 18: 1215-1233.

Troxel AB, Lipsitz SR, Harrington DP. (1994) Marginal models for the analysis of longitudinal measurements with nonignorable non-monotone missing data. *Biometrika* 94: 1096-1120.

Troxel A, Fairclough DL, Curren D, Hahn EA. (1998) Statistical analysis of quality of life data in cancer clinical trials. *Statistics in Medicine* 17: 653-666.

VanBuuren S, Boshuizen HC, Knook DL. (1999) Multiple imputation of missing blood pressure covariates in survival analysis. *Statistics in Medicine*, 18: 681-694.

Verbeke G, Molenberghs G. (ed.) (1997) *Linear Mixed Models in Practice: A SAS-Oriented Approach.* Springer, New York.

Verbeke G, Molenberghs G. (2000) *Linear Mixed Models for Longitudinal Data.* Springer, New York.

Vonesh EF, Greene T, Schluchter MD. (2006) Shared parameter models for the joint analysis of longitudinal data and event times. *Statistics in Medicine*, 25: 143-163.

von Hippel PT. (2004) Biases in SPSS 12.0 missing value analysis. *The American Statistician*, 58: 160-164.

Wang XS, Fairclough DL, Liao Z, Komaki R, Chang JY, Mobley GM, Cleeland CS. (2006) Longitudinal study of the relationship between chemoradiation therapy for non-small-cell lung cancer and patient symptoms. *Journal of Clinical Oncology*, 24: 4485-4491.

Ware JE, Borrk RH, Davies AR, Lohr KN. (1981) Choosing measures of health status for individuals in general populations. *American Journal of Public Health*, 71: 620-625.

Ware JE, Snow KK, Kosinski M, Gandek B. (1993) *SF-36 Health Survey: Manual and Interpretation Guide*. The Health Institute, New England Medical Center, Boston, MA.

Ware J, Kosinski M, Keller SD. (1994) *SF-36 Physical and Mental Component Summary Scales: A User's Manual*. The Health Institute, New England Medical Center, Boston, MA.

Weeks J. (1992) Quality-of-life assessment: Performance status upstaged? *Journal of Clinical Oncology*, 10: 1827-1829.

Wei LJ, Johnson WE. (1985) Combining dependent tests with incomplete repeated measurements. *Biometrika* 72: 359-364.

Westfall PH, Young SS. (1989) p-value adjustment for multiple testing in multivariate bionomial models. *Journal of the American Statistical Association*, 84: 780-786.

Wiklund I, Dimenas E, Wahl M. (1990) Factor of importance when evaluating quality of life in clinical trials. *Controlled Clinical Trials*, 11: 169-179.

Wilson IB, Cleary PD. (1995) Linking clinical variables with health-related quality of life - a conceptual model of patient outcomes. *Journal of the Americal Medical Association*, 273: 59-65.

World Health Organization (1948) Constitution of the World Health Organization. *Basic Documents*, WHO, Geneva.

World Health Organization (1958) The First Ten Years of the World Health Organization, WHO, Geneva.

Wu MC, Bailey KR. (1988) Analyzing changes in the presence of informative right censoring caused by death and withdrawal. *Statistics in Medicine*, 7: 337-346.

Wu MC, Bailey KR. (1989) Estimation and comparison of changes in the presence of informative right censoring: Conditional linear model. *Biometrics*, 45: 939-955.

Wu MC, Carroll RJ. (1988) Estimation and comparison of changes in the presence of informative right censoring by modeling the censoring process. *Biometrics*, 44: 175-188.

Wulfsohn M, Tsiatis A. (1997) A joint model for survival and longitudinal data measured with error. *Biometrics*, 53: 330-339.

Yabroff KR, Linas BP, Schulman K. (1996) Evaluation of quality of life for diverse patient populations. *Breast Cancer Research and Treatment*, 40: 87-104.

Yao Q, Wei LJ, Hogan JW. (1998) Analysis of incomplete repeated measurements with dependent censoring times. *Biometrika*, 85: 139-149.

Young T, Maher J. (1999) Collecting quality of life data in EORTC clinical trials - what happens in practice? *Psycho-oncology*, 8: 260-263.

Yu M, Law NJ, Taylor JMG, Sandler HM. (2004) Joint longitudinal-survival-cure models and their applications to prostate cancer. *Statistica Sinica*, 14: 835-862.

Zeger SL, Liang K-Y. (1992) An overview of methods for the analysis of longitudinal data. *Statistics in Medicine*, 11: 1825-1839.

Zhang J., Quan H, Ng J, Stepanavage ME. (1997) Some statistical methods for multiple endpoints in clinical trials. *Controlled Clinical Trials*, 18: 204-221.

Zwinderman AH. (1990) The measurement of change of quality of life in clinical trials. *Statistics in Medicine*, 9: 931-42.

Index